THE KEY TO LOCKJAW

THE KEY TO LOCKJAW

An Autobiography

W. E. van Heyningen

COLIN SMYTHE
Gerrards Cross, 1987

First published in 1987 by Colin Smythe Limited,
Gerrards Cross, Buckinghamshire

British Library Cataloguing in Publication Data

van Heyningen, W. E.
The key to lockjaw : an autobiography.
1. van Heyningen, W. E. 2. Medical
Research — Great Britain — Biography
I. Title
610'.92'4 R489.V/

ISBN 0-86140-251-9

Produced in Great Britain
Copy prepared by Action Typesetting Ltd., Gloucester
and printed and bound by Billing & Sons Ltd., Worcester

CONTENTS

ILLUSTRATIONS

PREFACE

An autobiography is proof of conceit; therefore I apologise for mine. My excuse is an up-to-date version of that used by a little man in a pre-war *Punch*. He had just published a best-seller, and when a reporter asked him how he had started it, he replied 'Well, I had just bought a bottle of ink'. I had just bought a word-processor, and I am most grateful to Mr L. G. Fouweather, Mr G. B. Lescott and Mr R. I. Saxton of the Oxford University Computing Service for all the kind and patient help they gave me in coming to terms with it.

In parts of this autobiography I have tried to describe other people's scientific research, or some of my own efforts at it. It is an attempt at writing about science in a way that is comprehensible to a layman. Please be so kind as to try and read it; and do not think it is necessary to understand the scientific words. Most of them are nouns, the names of various things that you do not need to understand; but most of the verbs that state what these things do, or what is done to them, are non-scientific words.

ACKNOWLEDGEMENTS

C.P. Snow's letters are used by permission of the Hon. Philip Snow, © 1986 Philip Snow, and the extracts from *The Corridors of Power,* by courtesy of Macmillan Publishers, London and Basingstoke. The passage from *The River* by Pare Lorentz is reprinted by permission of Stackpole Books.

1
SOUTH AFRICA

My first names are William Edward, after my mother's father, William Edward Higgs. I was called Willie by my family and friends when I was a boy, and am still called so by my surviving relations in South Africa, but everybody else calls me Kits. There was an unreliable legend in the family that held that when my father's father came to South Africa from Holland in 1858 he had the imposing name of Petrus Arnoldus Conradus Kits van Heyningen van Hoei Schildhouder, and that he dropped the Kits and van Hoei Schildhouder components before or soon after arrival. But the name Kits lived on in the family, with my elder brother (and only surviving sibling) being christened George Philipus Kits, and always being called Kits. When I went to the University of Stellenbosch in the Cape in 1929 my contemporaries took to calling me Kits, presumably because I must have bragged about my grandfather's legendary name; and I have recently learned that the same thing happened to my younger brother. The name has stayed with me ever since, and I like it, because in Afrikaans a *kits* is an instant. (And driving down the Mile End Road in London many years ago, before I was aware of the new DIY cult, I was startled by an exhortation over a shop — DO IT YOURSELF KITS, it said; too true, I thought.) But I would not have kept the name if I had not shaken the dust of Africa from my feet in 1934. At least one of my friends in Cambridge, Marjory Stephenson (the first woman, together with Kathleen Lonsdale, and apart from Queen Victoria, to be elected Fellow of the Royal Society), used to think, although I believe she otherwise thought well enough of me, that I was a psychological case, stealing my brother's name. There was a public discussion of my first names in Paris in 1974, when I gave the Louis Rapkine Memorial Lecture at the Pasteur Institute. I was introduced by an old and distinguished friend, André Lwoff, who had won the Nobel Prize for Medicine or Physiology in 1965. He said (in part):

Si vous le permettez, je rapellerai un souvenir personel. C'est à

Cambridge, en 1936, que van Heyningen et moi avons fait connaissance. Lui à l'Institut de Biochimie chez Sir Frederick Gowland Hopkins, cependant je passais quelques mois au Molteno Institute chez David Keilin. A ce moment déjà, dans le monde scientifique, le futur Professor Willam Edward van Heyningen était connu sous le nom de Kits. Cela semblait parfaitement naturel; mais lorsque j'ai appris que je devais présenter le conférencier j'ai commencé à me poser des questions sur la signification de ce nom. J'ai commencé par consulter un ami anglais qui m'a répondu que Kits était le diminutif de William. Cela m'a semblé étrange. J'ai alors consulté un autre ami anglais qui m'a affirmé que Kits était le diminutif d'Edward. Cela m'a paru bizarre. Des recherches personelles étaient manifestement nécessaires qui furent longues et difficiles, mai qui, finalement, connurent le succès. Je découvris qu'à la fin du 18ème siècle, l'un des arrière grand-pères de l'un des grand-pères du Professor van Heyningen avait épousé une demoiselle Wilhelmina Gerardina Kits. C'était une person impérieuse qui exigea que son époux et ses déscendants portent le nom Kits. Voila fixé un point d'histoire.

[If you will allow me, I will relate a personal recollection. It was in Cambridge in 1936 that van Heyningen and I got to know each other. He was at the Institute of Biochemistry with Sir Frederick Gowland Hopkins, while I was spending some months at the Molteno Institute with David Keilin. At that time already in the scientific world, the future Professor William Edward van Heyningen was known as Kits. That seemed perfectly natural; but when I learned that I was to present the lecturer, I started asking myself questions as to the meaning of that name. I started by consulting an English friend who replied that Kits was the diminutive of William. That seemed strange. So I consulted another English friend, who affirmed that Kits was the diminutive of Edward. That seemed bizarre. Personal research was manifestly necessary. It was long and difficult, but it was finally crowned with success. I discovered that at the end of the 18th century, one of the great-grandfathers of one of the grandfathers of Professor van Heyningen had married a Miss Wilhelmina Gerardina Kits. She was an imperious person who demanded that her husband and their descendants should bear the name of Kits. Thus was settled a point of history.]

That statement about Wilhelmina Gerardina Kits is a slightly garbled version of what I had told Lwoff the day before the lecture. In the 1950s we lived in Keble Road in Oxford, where we had a succession of *au pair* girls who came from the Continent to look after the children while Ruth and I went to work in our respective laboratories in the University. One of these was Antje Kloeke, who came from Leiden under the wing of her aunt, Dr Jacoba van Lessen, a distinguished lexicographer. Soon after her return to Holland, Dr van Lessen sent me a cutting from the *Nieuwe Amsterdamsche Courant* announcing that a Miss Adrienne

Jacqueline Marie Kits van Heyningen had gained her medical doctorate with distinction in the University of Amsterdam. I got her address from the Registrar of the University and wrote to her to arrange a meeting in Amsterdam, where I happened to be going in a few weeks. She was, like me, and Ruthie, a biochemist, newly married to a pleasant young lawyer called van Beusekom. She was proud of the Kits connection, and told me I should be too. From a study of the *Nederland's Patriciaat*, and other works in the Centraal Bureau voor Genealogie in The Hague, I have been able to trace my van Heyningen, Kits and van Hoei Schildhouder ancestors. The *Patriciaat* may sound grand, but a good Dutch dictionary will tell you it means '. . . the collective patricians, the aristocracy; both literally and figuratively . . . .' I'm sure that the figurative interpretation applies in our case, and that suits me. My enquiries into my ancestry are reported in the appendix.

Two thirds of the Nineteenth Century

My mother's people arrived in Cape Town before my father's, either in 1820 or in 1837; and my father's people arrived in 1858. Between those arrivals great changes had taken place in South Africa. The reason for these changes was the Great Trek of the Dutch *Voortrekkers* from the Cape Colony that had come under British Rule in 1814. Before 1836 all the white settlers in South Africa, Dutch, English and French Huguenots, were in the Cape Colony; but many of the Dutch (and Huguenot) farmers, always seeking more grazing land for their sheep and cattle, and wanting to get away from the meddlesome British, moved away from the vicinity of the Cape and trekked eastwards towards the Great Fish River. These migrating farmers came to be known as *Trek Boere* (diphthong rhymes with 'moo'), or Boers (diphthong rhymes with 'moor') in English . A *boer* is a farmer, and Afrikaans people are known as Boers to this day, even if most of them now are townsmen. But the British followed the Boers eastwards, imposing their rule, their language, and their recent renunciation of slavery on them; and they brought more of their own kind in from England. On this new eastern frontier the Whites were having trouble with the Blacks, mainly Xosas, who were also moving towards the Great Fish River, but from the opposite direction, the North-east. The British Government in London, needing more British Whites to defend the frontier, started the 1820 Settlers scheme. I quote now from the Standard *Encyclopaedia of Southern Africa* [32]:

'While carefully refraining from mentioning the exact locality of the intended settlement, widely distributed notices informed the public in Britain that approved persons of adequate means, to be known as 'heads' or 'directors', would each be allowed to collect an organised unit or 'party' of a number of families or adult individuals wishing to emigrate to the Cape; that the Government would grant free passage in specified ships; that on arrival rations, seed and implements would be provided at cost until the first harvest could be reaped; that tents would be loaned for a limited period; and that at the end of three years title deeds to the lands of the party's 'location' would be issued on the basis of 100 acres to each family or adult then in occupation for an annual quitrent payable only after 10 years from the initial occupation of the 'location' by the party. There were 90,000 applications for settlerships, but 4000 were deemed sufficient for the Government's frontier defence scheme, and so only about 4000 men, women and children sailed from England at the end of 1819 in 21 ships, and debarkation on the shores of Algoa Bay started on 10 April 1820. In the beginning the immigrants suffered much adversity from floods, drought, and Xosa harrassment, but by 1825 things started getting better for them.'

The *Trek Boere*, or a large number of them, decided to get completely away from the British and move northwards; and so the *Voortrekkers* set out on their Great Trek in 1836, inspired by Piet Retief, and led by Louis Trichard and Janse van Rensburg. They crossed a great river, which they called the Orange River after the Dutch King William of Orange, and beyond the river they founded the Orange Free State. Some stayed there; some moved on northwards; and some moved eastwards and formed the Republic of Natal. But no sooner were these republics founded than they were seized by the British. Natal was annexed to the Cape Colony in 1845, to become a separate British Colony some time later; and in 1848 Sir Harry Smith (I was born in Harrismith) seized the Orange Free State and proclaimed the Orange River Sovereignty. The rest of the *Voortrekkers* moved further northwards beyond the Vaal River to found, or try to found, the South African Republic, with M. W. Pretorius as President. But in the beginning it was only a paper state, a creation of Pretorius and his followers in the Potchefstroom-Rustenburg district. In fact there were three other small republics north of the Vaal — Zoutpansburg, Lydenburg-Utrecht and Klip Rivier. (It was the religious strife associated with this political strife that was to bring my father's father from Holland to South Africa.) Eventually they all united enough to form the Transvaal Republic. At the Bloemfontein Convention in 1854 the British Government recognized Boer independence north of the Orange

River, as it had done two years previously with respect to the Boer-held territory north of the Vaal (the Little Englanders were in power, and they regarded imperialism as unprofitable). Thus it was that the Boers, who had hoped to establish one State, established two, the Transvaal (officially known as the South African Republic), and the Orange Free State. In 1854 the Orange Free State had 15-20,000 Whites and an unquantifiable number of Blacks. As an old friend, Leo Marquard, puts it: 'The Orange Free State was more fortunate in that it was closer to the Cape and in more continuous touch with the base of Western civilization. It drew many of its civil servants and judges, and its most statesmanlike President, from the Cape; and it attracted professional and commercial men, largely of British stock, to its towns and villages. The result was that the Free State became a settled state in a remarkably short time, while the Transvaal retained for many years much of its frontier mentality ... Another result of the close contact between the Free State and the Cape Colony was that, in 1848, English-speaking people settled in the Free State, particularly in the villages, where they started commercial and trading businesses or became estate agents and auctioneers; and banking companies from London and the Cape found it profitable to follow trade and commerce. These people identified themselves with the life of the Republic and played a considerable part in public affairs, particularly in local government .... They transacted a good deal of their business in English but usually spoke English and Dutch; and soon had their own churches. ... All these things counteracted isolationism and made for a more tolerant and progressive society than was possible across the Vaal River. ... In the Free State, Britons had settled and become part of a society in which co-operation between Boer and Briton had ripened slowly and naturally ...' [18]. Among those British who came to the Orange Free State were my mother's people.

In 1837, when my mother's grandfather, Charles Higgs, had either just arrived in Cape Town, or had been there since 1820, he married Sarah Ann Spiers, and they had a son, Charles John, in December 1837. She died shortly after, and some time before 1845 Charles and his son moved to Fort Beaufort, a little north of Grahamstown in the eastern Cape Colony, where he opened a hotel. Charles then married Katherine Emily Austen, who had been born in Grahamstown in 1820. They had ten children, all of them born in Fort Beaufort. My grandfather, Willam Edward, was born first — in 1845. His elder step-brother, Charles John, died in 1851. Some time after the last of the children, Percival Charles, was born in 1864, the family moved to Ladybrand in the Orange Free State. I don't know how Charles earned his living there. Perhaps he continued as an innkeeper, or took up trading. Certainly his son William Edward, and some of Willam Edward's sons, were traders dealing in horses, wheat and mielies (Indian corn), and selling blankets and simple goods to the Basutos. William Edward also rode transport by ox-wagon over immense distances, like the 900 miles from Cape Town to Johannesburg. I don't know how long Charles remained in Ladybrand, but I do know that his grand-daughter Mabel Constance, my mother, and six of her siblings were born there between 1876 and 1892. The family then moved southwards to Zastron, also near the Basutoland border, and to Mohales' Hoek just across the border.

The South Africa that my English and Dutch forbears came to was a wild and often savage country. Recently, reading about the country in the Rhodes House Library of the Bodleian Library, I was horrified to learn that the Basuto were cannibals as late as 1836, and the evidence is there to be seen to this day. If you look at a map of South Africa you will see Mensetersgrotte (Cannibal Caves) near Mohale's Hoek in Basutoland (now Lesotho), and a Menseterskop (Cannibal Hill) in the Orange Free State near the Basutoland border. The gentle, friendly, good-humoured Basuto live in Basutoland (in my day a British Crown Colony) and next door in the Orange Free State. They were of mixed origins, descended from refugees who had fled from ferocious tribes in the North to the shelter of the mountains of what became Basutoland, where they were united into one tribe by Moshesh. D. F. Ellenberger, a French missionary, who lived among them, tells how Motleyoa, driven from his home by invaders, 'gathered about him twenty-six broken men like himself, and having taken to cannibalism, at first from necessity, but afterwards from choice, they roamed about the country seeking whom they might devour.' From small beginnings cannibalism spread over the whole country between the Orange and Vaal Rivers. Those addicted to it formed secret societies. 'For all that it is improbable that the idea of eating fellow-men would have occurred to the South African Bantu had the example not been set by strangers from the north.' Late in life, in 1843, Moshesh admitted that he and his people were to blame for this. Around 1822-1823 Moshesh was weak enough to allow his brother Mohale to replenish his kraals with cattle at the expense of the Bafokeng, so the Bafokeng became destitute. On one occasion they captured passers-by, mainly women and children, and drove them to a cave near Leribe. 'Here, notwithstanding the children's cries and the wailing of the women, they slaughtered, skinned and ate them, without pity or remorse. They dressed the skins as they were in the habit of dressing the hides of animals, and made dresses for the women and breech-cloths for themselves.' Up to as late as 1836 the district of what is now called Bloemfontein, the Capital of the Orange Free State, was infested by cannibals, but these were Mahlapahlapa, not Basuto. Ellenberger tells how Mokapakapa and his family tried to escape with their servants from the cannibals, but 'Immediately the man-eaters were upon them, bound and gagged them, and drove them to their lair with shouts and blows, after the manner of cattle drivers. On their arrival they were received with shouts of 'Food! Food!', the children being alluded to as 'tender lambs', their mothers as 'cows', the servants as 'oxen', while the [surviving] narrator [Mokapakapa] was designated 'eland'. The family and servants were killed in his presence, skinned and cooked in earthen pots, or grilled on embers. He himself, owing to extreme emaciation, was allowed to live as a servant.' Ellenberger also tells about cannibals first eating the fatter of a number of captives, and making the leaner ones eat them too, to fatten them up for later consumption [13].

My Dutch grandfather, Petrus Arnoldus Conradus van Heyningen, completed his theological studies with distinction at the University of Utrecht, and was admitted to the ministry by the provincial church council of Gelderland in 1856, and appointed assistant minister in Hemmen. He was then called to South Africa by the Geestelike Commissie van Amsterdam (Spiritual Commission of Amsterdam). Shortly after his marriage to Boudina Ketel, and his ordination in the Nederduits Hervormde Kerk in February 1858 by his elder brother George Philips Kits van Heyningen, he and his bride, a lively, pretty, well-educated, Dutch-, French- and English-speaking girl, so it is said, studied a newly published map of South Africa. They were moved by the names of some of the towns that had been founded by the rather solemn, God-fearing *Voortrekkers* on their recently completed Great Trek into the hinterland. Thus there was a town called Weenen, which means weeping; another called Verdriet, which means sorrow; another called Ongeluk, which means misfortune, or unhappiness; even the town he had been called to was called Lydenburg, which means town of suffering. 'These are such a sad people, we must go and help them', the one said to the other. So off they sailed from Texel on 22 April 1858 on the frigate *Estafette* to Cape Town.

According to my Aunt Cara's *Orange Days* [34], the voyage took six months, the frigate having been becalmed several times, and having been saved from being swamped by my grandfather's warning the captain of an approaching cyclone. (My dear Aunt Cara — she was eighty three years old when she wrote her memoirs, and they were so inaccurate that when the historian Leo Marquard, an old friend of the family, was asked to write the foreword, he refused. They remind me of the young barrister who was presenting his first case, and was terribly muddled. At length the judge addressed him, saying, 'Mr Smith, in presenting a case it is a good idea to arrange the facts in some sort of order. Chronological is considered very good, but in your case alphabetical will do.' And yet these memoirs are not only delightful, they have their value, because they present a picture of the Orange Free State in the last two decades of the 19th Century that is so lively and so loving, that it gives a more vivid impression of the country and the times than many a more scholarly work could achieve.) In fact the frigate must have reached Cape Town in a little over two months, for the *Dictionary of South African Biography* states 'Van H. spent much of July in Cape Town, and arrived at Port Natal [Durban] on 28.8.1858' [12]. Aunt Cara goes on to say 'They travelled [from Cape Town] up to the Transvaal by ox-wagon, through the mountainous, rugged country of the Cape, through the long plains of the Free State, which was teeming with game and also hostile natives, to the Transvaal, which was surrounded by hostile native tribes in native territories, to the little frontier dorp of Lydenburg to preach the gospel to Boers in the little dorp surrounded by blue mountains, and there they established the first little Dutch Reformed Church'. What seems actually to have happened, according to the *Dictionary*, was that during the month of July which he spent in Cape Town my grandfather was admitted to the ministry, not of the Nederduits Hervormde Kerk to which he and his forbears had belonged in Holland, but to the Nederduits Gereformeerde Kerk that held sway in the Cape (and that was the start of a great confusion). He then sailed on to Port Natal, and it was from there that his trek into the interior began — still a long trek of about 400 miles, but not as long as the 1,100 miles from Cape Town. Actually the journey from Port Natal was interrupted for some time at Greytown, not far away, where my grandfather served his first South African ministry. (He was supposed to have been met at Port Natal with transport to take him directly to Lydenburg, but the transport was not there, so he took up the Greytown job for the time being. This caused some temporary ill-feeling betweeen the Lydenburg and Greytown communities.) The trek of several hundred miles into the interior, was presumably made by ox-wagon, over a rough road, if any road existed at all, through wild country filled with game and, if not actually hostile, not particularly friendly natives, remnants of the Zulu tribes of Tjaka and Dingaan, defeated by the *Voortrekkers* twenty years earlier. It must, as Aunt Cara wrote, have been a remarkable experience for this young Hollander predikant and his high-born wife to come from the sophisticated Europe of the Second Empire to an unruly society in an untamed country, after a long sea voyage (it may have been on a sailing ship as Aunt Cara says elsewhere, and the voyage could have been completed in two months under sail, but I note that the first steamship arrived in Cape Town in 1825).

My grandfather was inducted in Lydenburg early in 1859. He had been called there by the Spiritual Commission of Amsterdam to deal with a problem of religious strife that was taking place in the Dutch Protestant Church in the Transvaal at the same time as there was political strife among the four independent republics that had not yet achieved their intended ideal of a united republic north of the Vaal River. I must explain that at that time there were two Dutch Calvinistic Churches in South Africa. They were the established Church of The Netherlands, the Nederduits Hervormde Kerk, to which Hendrik, George Philips Kits and Petrus Arnoldus Conradus belonged, and the Nederduits Gereformeerde Kerk, a rather less rigid sect that had broken away in Holland in 1618, and had recently been introduced in the Cape by the predikant, D. Postma. There is also the very rigid Gereformeerde Kerk without the Nederduits. Nederduits means 'low German'; *Hervormde* means 'formed again'; *Gereformeerde* means 'reformed', but the difference is beyond me. Let us call these churches NH, NG and G. I don't think the G was there in my grandfather's day, but it was in mine. Its adherents were known as *doppers*, meaning 'baptisers', and those of the NG as *gaatjeponders*, *gaatje* meaning 'little hole', well, arsehole, and *ponder* meaning the short jacket they wore that ended above the *gaatje*. In 1854 the Lydenburg community had broken away from the NH, and was maintaining a fairly free association with the NG in the Cape, resisting all efforts to make the NH the established church of the Transvaal. My grandfather was called to put Lydenburg on the right NH path, but he made such a cock-up, it's almost interesting. It started as soon as he stepped ashore in Cape Town, where, you may possibly remember, he was admitted to the ministry of the NG, not the NH. When I went back to the *Dictionary of South African Biography*, I saw the light — I noticed that D.Postma (see above) had been a fellow-passenger on the *Estafette*. There was plenty of time on board; and I have no doubt it was he who persuaded my grandfather to change his allegiance. But then again, when he got to Lydenburg, my grandfather strived to get his congregation back to the NH fold, especially after Lydenburg rejoined the Transvaal Republic in 1860; and was even chairman of the general assembly of the NH for a short while. In 1863 he attended the Natal Presbytery of the NG as a representative of his congregation (at this stage NG ?), but the next year he and his congregation formally joined the NH of the Transvaal Republic, only to have this connection repudiated the next year.

No wonder the *Dictionary of South African Biography* states 'It is hard to assess the part Van H. played in Lydenburg, for at its last consistory meeting (5.12.1865) he persuaded the consistory to destroy all its documents which might in future give rise to dispute ... On his departure there was great confusion in Lydenburg, as he had clashed with leading personalities ... of the N.G.Kerk, and had frequently damaged relations between Church and State.'

My grandfather was soon to be translated from the troubled Transvaal to more settled and peaceful pastures, but even there he oscillated for a while between the two churches. In 1864 he was called to be first NG predikant in Kroonstad, in the Orange Free State, but by the time he got there in 1866 (his departure from Lydenburg having been delayed by his interest in his three farms), he was NH predikant in the same town. The next year, in 1867, he moved from Kroonstad to Winburg, also in the Orange Free State, where he lived until he retired in 1893. By 1881 he switched again, and was Moderator of the NG in the Free State. In the end he stayed NG, and in my family my father and his three sons were members of the NG, and my mother and her four daughters members of the Church of England, not that we were assiduous, my father having assured us there was no Hell, only Heaven. I get the impression that my grandfather was a liberal-minded man, and was thus drawn to the more liberal NG, and that his vacillations were due to his having been torn between that and his loyalty to the NH of his father and his elder brother. The *Dictionary* states: 'In his first years in the country Van H., being fairly young, was inclined to be frivolous and obstinate, and, in addition, rather negligent, unsystematic and discourteous. As a result he quarrelled with many Lydenburg inhabitants and so increased the tensions in the church.' I expect there was truth in that, but perhaps also some lack of understanding of a lively, educated, foreign spirit. He and Boudina were newly arrived from a far more sophisticated Europe, and must have seemed strange to the rough inhabitants of the primitive new country, and, with their High Dutch accents, snooty. And unconventional — she wore pretty coloured dresses, and was told by the women of the congregation that a married woman, especially the wife of a predikant, should wear black. She would ride about visiting the congregation wearing a divided skirt and sitting astride her horse. She was considered *'n koddige ding* (something comic) because she was *'n domme mens* (a stupid person), who did not know how to make soap and candles, or *biltong* (dried raw meat). And my grandfather must have seemed eccentric. Once, for example, when there had been a terrible drought for a long time, his elder suggested he should pray for rain. 'Ben je gek, man' he replied, 'het wind is in de west!' ('Are you crazy, man, the wind is in the west!') My cousin Marietjie Grosskopf told me that when he was asked by someone 'Meneer, is dans sonde ?' ('Sir, is dancing a sin ?'), he replied, 'In Zuid Afrika well, maar in Holland niet' ('In South Africa certainly, but not in Holland'). He used to buy thirty-six-yard rolls of German print, Horrock's calico, and pink flannelet cheaply at sales that were then made up into dresses and underclothes for his unfortunate daughters. The poor girls also had to wear atrocious *veldschoens* that he bought at bargain prices in assorted pairs. Soon after their arrival in Lydenburg they shocked the community when they took in ten little Black orphans and had them sit at the table with them for meals. On another occasion my grandfather invited two German missionaries to take his pulpit in the Lydenburg church, and he found himself confronted by a group of irate locals, threatening to beat the missionaries to pieces if they did so — they were not going to allow preachers to the Black heathen to preach in their church. It is not surprising that my grandfather's family were known as *'die trotse goddelose troep'* ('the haughty godless troop').

If my grandfather was perhaps not a success as a predikant in the eyes of the higher management of the church, he was recognized as having played a leading part in preparing the educational system of the Orange Free State. In Lydenburg he had been a member of an education committee set up by the Transvaal government, and in 1866 he was commissioned by the *Volksraad* (parliament) of the Orange Free State to produce a *Reglement op het onderwijs in den Vrijstaat* (Regulations on education in the Free State). It provided for a general schools commission consisting of five ministers representing the three Afrikaans churches, two lawyers and one teacher, with each district having its own school committee consisting of the magistrate, the minister and one other public figure. As a member of the Synod Commission, my grandfather put these proposals before the Volksraad as a basis for subsequent legislation. His bill for public education (of White children only, of course) was passed in May 1872. In Bloemfontein there is a van Heyningen Street, which I suppose is there to commemorate his services to education.

My grandmother Boudina had arrived in the Cape speaking Dutch, French and English; I don't know how fluent my grandfather became in English, but according to Aunt Cara he was a keen reader of Dickens (a liking I have not inherited), and he improved his English by reading his works over and over again. In the van Heyningen family in South Africa my grandparents spoke what was called High Dutch, while their children spoke the simplified variant called Afrikaans, which had begun to differ from Dutch early in the 19th century. In 1822 Lord Charles Somerset, Governor of the Cape, began an attempt to anglicize the Cape; but the Dutch language persisted, and at the same time it changed, acquiring a simplified grammar, a modified vocabulary, and to my mind a prettier sound. The attempt at anglicization eventually failed, and Dutch was admitted on an equal footing with English in the Cape Parliament in 1882. By this time it had changed so much that some people were beginning to write it and spell it as it was spoken. When I was at school in Keetmanshoop in the 1920's we spoke Afrikaans, but read and wrote in High Dutch, and I can remember the great day we officially changed to Afrikaans.

The van Heyningens settled down comfortably in Winburg after the strife of the Transvaal. Eventually there were ten children, six girls and four boys, one of whom was my father, George Phillipus Stephanus. Of my father's nine siblings, I knew only the four sisters surviving in my time, Mina, Marie, Ada and Cara. They lived quite well, and often had the great and the good to stay in the parsonage, including, many times, the brilliant President of the Orange Free State, F. W. Reitz. When my grandfather retired from the NG ministry in 1893 the President composed an illuminated *Afscheidslied* (farewell song) for him. It exemplifies the gloom of the Dutch Reformed Church that helped to put me off religion. Here is the translated first verse, sounding more like a funeral dirge, although my grandfather had another 10 years to go:

> The time is come the day has dawned
> Community and Teacher must part
> 'Tis hard to separate but we must take comfort in our loss
> One day there will be an end to sorrow and pain
> Rest! rest. Oh sweet rest!
> Above there in Heaven you will enjoy sweet rest.

When Oom Paul Kruger, the President of the Transvaal Republic, came to Winburg on a State visit, Cara was delegated to present him with a bouquet of flowers, which made no sense to her — what would a man want with a bunch of flowers? (This reminds me that many years later, in the 1920s, when the Prince of Wales was visiting South Africa, my sister Koekoe was delegated to present him with a bunch of heather; and that reminds me of a dinner forty years later in Magdalen College, Oxford. After dinner we retired to the Senior Common Room for port, and as I was talking I was interrupted by one of the Fellows, Sir George Pickering. 'Forgive me for interrupting you' he said, 'but your South African accent reminds me of the time when the Prince of Wales was visiting South Africa in the nineteen twenties. He was with a pretty South African girl [she might have been Koekoe], and as she was talking he said ''Forgive me for interrupting, but I love the way you roll your r's.'' ''Oh thank you, your Royal Highness'' she replied, ''it must be the high heels I'm wearing''.')

The older children in our family went to English schools in Bloemfontein, the girls to Eunice School and the boys to Grey College School, both of which still flourish today. The younger ones, Ada, Agatha and Cara, first went to Miss Jackson's one-teacher, one-room school, where English was the only language. Afterwards they went to the Government School, where they joined my father (who was always, for reasons unknown to me, called Ollie). This school was run after a few years by John Fivaz, who married my Aunt Boudina. In this school they had only English textbooks, and learned all their subjects in English, except High Dutch. It seems that my Dutch grandparents thought well of the British, and were determined that all their children should learn English from the start.

In 1887 my grandmother Boudina died. Aunt Cara tells the sad story of how my father, at that time a *landdrost's* (magistrate's) clerk in Fauresmith, was summoned to the funeral, and rode the 120 miles to Winburg on horseback through the night. He arrived there the next afternoon, in time to meet his mother's funeral cortège coming from the church on the way to the graveyard. In December 1893 my grandfather retired. By this time all his children were married, except Agatha, who had died young, and Ada, Cara and Ollie, my father. He decided to return to Holland with his two unmarried daughters. There Ada met Pieter van Braam, a student of classics, in a colony of intellectuals called 'Walden', after Henry David Thoreau's hut in the woods of Massachusetts, where they lived the simple Transcendentalist life Thoreau advocated. A few years later she married him (and according to a letter my father wrote to my mother, he left for America the same day for an appointment in Grinnell College in Iowa, where she joined him after some months). Later she returned with her husband to South Africa, where he was appointed Professor of Classics in the University of Stellenbosch. Their house in Stellenbosch was also called 'Walden', and I used to lunch there every Sunday when I was a student.

The Higgses and the van Heyningens arrived in the Orange Free State at about the same time, from the South and the North respectively. My mother's father, William Edward Higgs, married Cornelia Jones, the daughter of an 1820 Settler, in 1873. They had fourteen children, with astonishing regularity: one every even year, boys and girls in equal number; nearly alternating, but not quite. The second child was my mother, Mabel Constance, born in Ladybrand in 1876. She and her youngest brother were the only two to marry Afrikaners.

William Edward Higgs and some of his family moved at some time from Ladybrand further south to a farm called Boomplaats (Tree Plateau) in the Zastron district, and later into Zastron, while others went to Mohale's Hoek on the other side of the Basutoland border. (The curious name of Zastron was the Christian name of the wife of President Brand of the Orange Free State, which explanation does not make it any less curious.) In Zastron my father met Mabel Constance Higgs, usually called May. She had been educated at St Michael's School in Bloemfontein. I suppose he wooed her in English, but I have no doubt she could speak Afrikaans by that time, since she had been born in Ladybrand (another tribute to Zastron!), which was mainly Afrikaans, in 1876. They married in 1896, and from then on my father's home language was English. We never spoke Afrikaans in the family — and I remember always calling ourselves English — but outside the family we spoke more Afrikaans than English. We were all bilingual from the time we learned to speak, and could slip from one language to the other without noticing it.

In 1897 my eldest sister Boudina Cornelia, named after her two grandmothers, was born. At this time the clouds of the imminent Boer War were looming very dark. After the great diamond rush to Kimberley in the 1870s, and the far greater gold rush to the Witwatersrand of the 1880s and 1890s, the treaty of mutual assistance between the Orange Free State and the Transvaal Republic of 1889 was reaffirmed. In 1898 my Dutch grandfather, then in Holland with his two unmarried daughters, Ada and Cara, and fearing the threat of war in South Africa, left Holland with Cara to return to his family in South Africa, leaving Mina and Ada behind in Torquay with Mina's English husband Herbert Hoskyn. They settled in Fauresmith, first with my father and his new family, and later in a rented house. When the war broke out my grandfather summoned his daughter Boudina Fivaz and her three babies to join them, her husband John having joined the Boer Commandos.

The Anglo-Boer War broke out in October 1899. The quarrel was in the first place between the British and the Boers in the Transvaal; but the Orange Free State, bound by the re-affirmed Treaty of 1897, had to come in on the side of the Transvaal. It came in reluctantly, because its relations with the British had always been good. Much as I admire the British for their past and their present, I am bound to state that in this affair they were wicked — through their arrogance and their greed for the new gold in the Transvaal. I believe the Boers in the Transvaal would rather gold had not been discovered in their country which had been so peaceful that there were no policemen. In Johannesburg the Boers were literally outnumbered by foreign adventurers — the *Uitlanders* — mainly from Britain, but also from other parts of the world, seeking their fortunes, and being outraged by President Kruger's reasonable refusal to allow the young Republic to destroy itself by giving these outsiders the vote. After Jameson's scandalous and unsuccessful raid on Johannesburg on the pretext of rescuing 'unarmed [*uitlander*] men, women and children at the mercy of well-armed Boers' [18], the Transvaal sent an ultimatum to Britain demanding withdrawal of her troops on the Transvaal border. This was contemptuously and joyfully rejected by the British Governor of the Cape and Natal Colonies, Lord Milner (as great a scoundrel as Cecil John Rhodes), who had been seeking all along to bring about a war [24]; and now it was declared.

A Third of the Twentieth Century

When the war broke out, my father, who was by now Public Prosecutor, became a *Veldkornet,* that is, a field officer with the Boer commandos, but his job remained civilian, carrying on with his assistant-magisterial duties in the war-time administration of the Fauresmith district. Early in 1900 my sister Christina was born, and shortly after that, on 11 March, a British brigade under General Clements, in pursuit of the elusive Boer General de Wet, crossed the Orange River from the Cape Colony into the Free State. Lord Roberts had seized Bloemfontein in the meantime, and, to quote A.Conan Doyle's *The Great Boer War* (published in September 1900 [9]), 'Clements was despatched to Philipolis, Fauresmith, and other towns in the South-West [of the Orange Free State] to receive the submission of the inhabitants and to enforce their disarmament.' According to Aunt Cara, Fauresmith was soon retaken by the Boer commandos (presumably after Conan Doyle had sent his manuscript to the press ?), and then some months later retaken by the British, who this time sacked the town. My father was taken prisoner of war on 15 October 1900, at the age of thirty years, and my mother and her two babies, and my father's sister, Boudina Fivaz and her three babies, were taken to the concentration camp in Bloemfontein; and my grandfather and Aunt Cara were taken to the concentration camp at Norval's Pont in the Cape Province, just across the Orange River.

The Boer War was an inglorious chapter in British history, both military and political; and there were many in Great Britain, as well as the rest of Europe and the United States of America, who took this view. It was the beginning of the decline of the British Empire. Not only were the British wicked in provoking it, they were ludicrously incompetent in the waging of it. It took more than two and a half years (from 11 October 1899 to 31 May 1902) for 448,435 well-equipped British troops, with a large professional core, to defeat a fifth as many ill-equipped Boer farmers (about half of whom were away from the fighting at any given time, looking after their farms) [2]. After the fatuous General Buller's 'Black Week' of defeats in the early stages of the war, Lord Roberts was sent out to replace him, with Kitchener as his Chief-of-Staff, and subsequent successor. Kitchener was baffled by the Boers' unorthodox guerilla tactics. 'To end the war was Kitchener's overwhelming objective. But how to end it if the enemy refused to fight a pitched battle? It was the guerillas' refusal to play the game and fight like men that appalled Kitchener, not his doubts (though doubts he certainly had) about his own troops' ability to fight.' By March 1901 he 'decided to break the stalemate by a double sweeping operation to flush out the guerillas in a series of systematic 'drives', organized like a sporting shoot, with success defined by the weekly 'bag' of killed, captured and wounded; and to sweep the country bare of anything that could give sustenance to the guerillas: not only horses, but cattle, sheep, women and children. But where could the women be put, if removed from their homes?' [24]. The answer was tented *laagers* (camps), similar to those that accommodated the soldiers, but more crowded, less well provided, and with the inmates (who were frailer) staying there for longer than the troops, with no leave from time to time, with not enough food, and that provided not nourishing, and with no medicines. Kitchener's monument in South Africa is not his victories, but the unforgiven memories of his 'Concentration Camps', as they came to be called, long before the Nazis thought of them.

Sir John Broderick, Secretary of State for War, wrote from London to Kitchener: 'Pretty bad reports have been received here of the state of the Bloemfontein laager in January — insufficient water, milk rations, typhoid prevalent, children sick, no soap, no forage for cows, insufficient medical attention . . .' [24]. Kitchener remained indifferent, but not Emily Hobhouse (a name revered to this day by Afrikaners in South Africa). She pleaded on behalf of the women and children in the concentration camps, and caused Mrs Millicent Fawcet and her Commission to investigate the camps: 'They were impressed by Norval's Pont . . They were shocked by the state of the hospital at Bloemfontein Camp, where there were no arrangements to sterilize linen infected by typhoid patients. They were still more shocked by the camp at Brandfort, where an epidemic killed 337 (nearly a tenth of the inmates of the whole camp) in the first three weeks of October' [24]. Altogether there were 114,000 people, of whom 95,000 were women and children, in these concentration camps, and 20,000 of them died [2].

It was to the fearful Bloemfontein camp that my mother and her two baby daughters were sent at the beginning of the war, together with her sister-in-law, Boudina Fivaz, with her three babies. My Aunt Boudina died there of typhoid fever, and, since nobody knew where her imprisoned husband was, her three babies were offered to anybody who would care to adopt them. My mother and her babies were soon released from the camp through the intervention of her father, who was supplying mounts to the British army. My Aunt Cara and her aged father were imprisoned in the more humane camp at Norval's Pont, where they were treated with positive kindness by their jailers. My grandfather was sent a glass of brandy every evening by the officers, and Aunt Cara seemed to get on famously with them. In those days it was the fashion for young ladies to wear a silk shirt with a stiff collar and a tie. She got several of the officers to sign their names on her tie, and then she made the signatures permanent by embroidering them [34]. Since my grandfather was old and frail, he was released after a short time, on condition that he and his daughter went to Engand and remained there until the end of the war. This they did, staying with my Aunt Mina in Torquay, where they met much sympathy and kindness, and outspoken support for the Boers.

I mentioned the Nazi concentration camps, but the connexion I had in mind was purely etymological. I am quite sure the sufferings of the women and children in the British concentration camps were not due to deliberate cruelty on the part of the British — the camp officers were not hand-picked for cruelty, as in the Nazi camps. The sufferings of the inmates were due to the incompetence and muddle-headedness of the British, and in some cases, exemplified by Lord 'Bloody' Kitchener, total lack of concern. And there were many acts of decency and kindness on both sides, such as that shown to my relations in Norval's Pont; and on the other hand, when the Boers would sometimes refrain from firing on unsuspecting British Tommies from concealed positions because it would have been 'sheer murder'. And there was courtesy — when Queen Victoria died in January 1901, some of the older Boers wore black armbands as a mark of respect [18].

My brother Kits told me recently that my father was caught by the British trying to run money in an armoured train for the Fauresmith commandos. He was Prisoner of War, Number 14487, for nearly two years, from 15 October 1900, when he was captured, to a few days after 6 August 1902, about two months before he sailed back to South Africa from the Mount Lavinia

Transit Camp in Ceylon. The British had kept some of their prisoners of war, like my uncles John Fivaz and Cecil van Heyningen, in South Africa, while others were banished to far-away places under British dominion, like St Helena Island and Ceylon. I don't know what the basis of this distinction was. My Aunt Cara says it was because they were key men, but that may just be family pride. On our recent visit to Cape Town at the beginning of our tour of South Africa, I found that my niece Elizabeth van Heyningen, daughter of Kits, had the 94 letters my father wrote to my mother every Sunday during his imprisonment. They had been given to her by my sister Boudina, and I had had no idea of their existence. My niece had photocopies of them made for me, and of some other correspondence between my father and my mother after his return to South Africa, and with some other of his relations. Naturally I was moved in the reading of them, and touched by mother having kept them all, and regretful that my father had not kept the equal number of letters she wrote to him.

The first three letters are from a prison camp at Greenpoint, near Cape Town. On 19 October 1900 my father and his fellow-prisoners were marched the seven miles from Fauresmith to Jagersfontein, where they were imprisoned for two nights in the mine that was famous for its very small, very brilliant diamonds (the eyes of the heroines of novels at that time used to 'shine like little Jagersfonteins'). He tried, but failed, to get permission to see my mother and the two babies. On the 21st they were marched twenty-seven miles to Edenburg, and on the 24th they were shipped by train, presumably in open trucks because when they arrived at the Greenpoint Camp they were 'dreadfully sunburned'. His brother-in-law, John Fivaz, was with him in the camp. On 15 November he still had no idea where May and the babies were, and was greatly concerned about them. The next day they sailed on the S.S.*Catalonia* for Durban (leaving some, including John Fivaz, behind), now having been told to his bitter disappointment that they were on their way to Ceylon. When they reached Durban on 6 December, he learned in a telegram from May's father that she and the babies were now safe with her parents in Zastron. He wondered what happened to their furniture, little knowing that it had all been destroyed in the sacking of Fauresmith. On 9 January 1901 they arrived at the Prisoner of War Camp at Diyatalawa, 70 miles east of Colombo. He found the country lovely, their train having run for many miles through tea plantations, and alongside huge mountains and high precipices, and over deep ravines. There were dense forests, with roses growing wild, and beautiful scarlet oleanders, far superior to those of the Orange Free State. He was pleasantly surprised by the kindness they met from white and coloured people. Along the railway the Indians [*sic*] gave them fruit and cheered them, but seeing a little girl about Boudina's age calling 'ta-ta' made him unbearably homesick. They were comfortably housed in wooden huts and well-fed. (I have a photograph of my father standing with an insouciant air in a barbed-wire-enclosed prison camp with a couple of British soldiers on guard in the background.)

The remaining letters, with exceptions, follow a pattern. The first quarter consists either of anguished but unreproachful lamentation at not having had a letter from May for the last three weeks; or exclamations of joy at having received three or four letters in a bunch, this being due to the slow and irregular transport of letters the long way from South Africa by sea, and to their being censored. The second quarter is gossip about fellow prisoners, and an account of his monotonous day-to-day life in the camp, which he relieved as best he could by learning French, German, book-keeping and shorthand, and reading as many English books (e.g. Walter Scott, Marie Corelli) as he could find. The third quarter consists of expressions of great affection (constrained by the knowledge that every word would be read by the censor), and of enquiries about the children — would Boudina still remember him when he got home, had Christina cut any teeth yet? The last quarter expresses his longing to be home with his dear family, and how happy they will all be with the present misery in the past; his determination to be patient; and encouragement for May. For example: 'Yes, it would be grand if we could have a nice long chat with each other instead of having to be content with writing, which at the best of times is rather unsatisfactory — but when you feel that every letter you write has to be read by a stranger it makes writing well-nigh impossible. My poor old darling, you must not allow yourself to become so despondent. Just think of the happy time to come when we will be together again and be able to look back upon this misery as a dreadful nightmare . . . but you must know me well enough to know that I do not share your view as to the hopelessness of it all. What *would* become of us if we had not hope to fall back upon? Why life would be simply unbearable. If it were not for the hope of seeing you again I think I would go mad — but having that hope I try to remain as cheerful as possible in the circumstances, see?' Reading that I could damn well weep, because at that stage he had already been imprisoned for eighteen months and had a further six months to endure. It was bad enough for my poor mother, but at least she was unfettered, and had the solace of her children, her parents, and the rest of her loving family. And even when he got back to South Africa at last, settled happiness was to evade them for some time. And after those bad years they were to have only another fourteen years together before she died, and he was to have only another eight years after that.

For the first three months in Ceylon he did not know that May and the babies, and his other relations, had been in concentration camps. On 10 February 1901 he writes 'Andries van der Linde had a letter from Miss Spruyt in which she mentions that you also were a "prisoner of war!!" in Bloemfontein for a fortnight before you got parole. I was surprised as I thought you had been allowed to go to Aliwal North direct. Fancy Boudina and Christina being "Prisoners of War", isn't it too ridiculous for anything! One of our men got a letter this morning saying that everybody in Fauresmith except [indecipherable] and young Stokes had been sent away. Is that so, and where are Father and Cara? I am very anxious to know everything. Is Dina [Boudina Fivaz] still in Bloemfontein?' After seven months of imprisonment he writes 'Last week several of our men left for Africa. They took the Oath of Allegiance and so were allowed to go on "parole". Much as I long to be with you and the little ones, I would rather sit here another five years before I take that oath.' It amazes me and pleases me that in spite of the war between the Boers and the British, and of the imprisonment of my father and his relations, and of that sentiment just expressed, there was never the slightest hint of animosity between my father and his people on one side; and my mother and her people on the other. They all seemed to be fond of each other.

On 14 July 1901 he wrote: 'This time I have very sad news if you have not already heard it. Mrs Sennett wrote from Bloemfontein to her son here that poor Dina died in the Camp there of Enteric and that they were going around offering her little children to people as they did not know where Fivaz was. Wilhelm Bilso took Boo, but she does not mention what became of Doto and Madge. Later I heard from young De Villiers who had a letter from his sister from the Camp that Johnny [Fivaz] was coming from Greenpoint [the prison camp] to his children, I hope this is true. I feel very sorry for him. He will feel it very much. Oh my darling I am too miserable about the news for words. It came as a great shock to me as I had heard the day before from a friend that his wife had written to say that she and Dina were at Tempe together both doing well. Yesterday he had another letter from his wife saying that they had returned to the Camp and that Dina died the same day. How long, oh Lord how long?' My poor father was dreadfully sad about his sister's death, and about its effect on his father and his other sisters, and he wrote frequently about it. 'Oh my darling it is too terrible to think about poor Dina dying amongst strangers.' Aunt Cara, still in England, had written to Emily Hobhouse about Dina's children, and asked her to help her to get them to England, since John Fivaz had not been allowed to stay out of the Greenpoint camp.

In October 1901 he was transferred from Diyatalawa to the Krygsgevangenen Kamp (Prisoner of War Camp) at Ragama, 8 miles from the coast of Ceylon, near Colombo, and I was glad to read that he writes to ask whether May has received the 'lovely letter box' he had had made for her from teak, ebony and other precious woods, and had sent to her from Diyatalawa. I have that box now, and indeed it is lovely. It used to sit in the parlours of the various houses we lived in, and when we visited my dying beloved sister Boudina in Rhodesia in 1953, she gave it to me and I have treasured it since. On the ebony lid is carved an escutcheon which I presume to signify the Orange Free State since it has an orange tree; it also has a lion, and another, unidentifiable, animal; and below there is a *Voortrekker* wagon with the famous error of a double shaft, perpetuated also on some now very valuable coins of the old Transvaal Republic. The motto puzzles me — 'freedom, patience, courage' it says reasonably enough (in Dutch), but then 'emigration'. Surely a young republic would want to encourage immigration! On the underside of the lid is carved *Aan May van Ollie, Diyatalawa, Ceylon, Augustus, 1901*. In spite of his English wife and his friendly English in-laws, it seems that my father was damned if he was going to have the inscription in English. I like that, but perhaps he simply thought it would be tactless to use English in that camp of imprisoned Boers.

In February 1902 the slow beginnings of the end started coming into sight. 'Let us hope your father is right in thinking that the war will soon be over. What a loyal little darling Boudina is, kiss her for me and tell her she must always be her father's little Dutch girl . . . it is nearly seventeen months since I was taken. Wasn't that a miserable day? One thing consoles me is that those jingoes [English people living in Fauresmith when it was taken] who were so pleased then did not have a very happy time during those same seventeen months. One of them is dead — I suppose I ought not to be glad over their misfortunes but I get so bitter when I think of those people that I can't contain myself.' Almost every subsequent letter touches on the rumours of an end to the war, with the Boers finally defeated. And: '. . . since we were in gaol. It seems strange to talk calmly of the time one was in "gaol" doesn't it? I can't say that I'm at all ashamed of the fact that I was in gaol — in fact I'm proud of it. Give my love to Boudina and tell her she must get ready to take her father for a walk . . . tell her she must teach Christina to say *'Dag Papa'* when he comes home.'

By now my father seemed to be coming to the conclusion that after the war there would be nothing for it but to take the Oath of Allegiance, though not a moment before. On 15 June 1902 he wrote: 'We've been informed officially that Peace has been signed [on 31 May] so I don't suppose it will be long before they start sending us back', but he had another three and a half months to wait; in fact he seems to have been one of the last prisoners to be sent home. On 27 July he wrote: 'I have made application to be sent back with the first batch and told the authorities that I am willing to sign the oath of allegiance to England. I am quite convinced that we have lost our Independence and now there is nothing to be done but go back to South Africa and submit to the new state of things. I have not had a reply to my application yet and seven other men have been told off to leave for South Africa from this camp so I am afraid I will not get off with this batch. Don't you think it will be a good idea if your father were to use his influence there and ask the authorities to send me back as soon as possible? I wish you would ask him to do so — Will you my darling? I think the sooner I can get home the better chance I have of getting employment. I wonder what I shall have to do? I am ready and willing to do anything as long as it is honest work. Thank God I am still young and strong. Our future is not very bright but side by side we will help each other through our troubles, eh? As long as I have you to cheer me up and give me courage I am sure everything will be all right.'

By 15 August 1902 he was a free man in the Ragama Camp, able to write and receive uncensored letters — as long as the correspondents liked — and to visit Colombo and walk on the beaches. By 15 September 1902 he had been transferred to the Urugasmanhandiya Transit Camp, and on 1 October he wrote his last letter from Ceylon, in the Mount Lavinia Transit Camp. I don't know the date of his arrival in Basutoland, where May and the babies were staying with her brother Willie.

His longed-for return to his people was a terrible disappointment for my poor father, a disappointment he had foreseen in his letters from Ceylon, for there was no job for him, and no house to live in with May and the babies. Aunt Cara writes in *Orange Days*: 'Poor Ollie, before things were better for him, seemed the worst off of all of us. When he came back from Ceylon he looked like a skeleton and was far from well. His wife and children, who had been with her people in Basutoland, now joined him, but he had no billet [job] and no money; he could not get a billet; there were no billets; so my brother Cecil, who had a small billet in Winburg, offered him the farm, where he could get food but nothing else. He had to plant trees on the farm for Cecil. . . . One day Ollie came into the dorp (Winburg) looking most unhappy, tired and ill. He put his hands over his face and I saw tears in his eyes; he said, ''I have come to beg''. He had broken his teeth and had not the money to get them fixed. Is there a more heartbreaking sight than to see a strong man weep? — and that one's favourite brother? Hard to forgive and forget!' [34].

By mid-December 1902 my father had to leave May and the babies with her relations in Basutoland again, while he moved to Bloemfontein where he had got a temporary job in the office of the Registrar of Deeds through a fellow prisoner in Ceylon who was employed there. He wrote to May: 'Isn't it hard lines that we have to be parted again so soon. I hope however that this parting will be very short. As I wired you, I obtained employment in the Registrar of Deeds office at £12/10/0 per month. I will be able to make a few extra pounds by doing work after hours. This situation is only temporary for about 2 months. However, both the Regst of Deeds and the Asst. Reg. of Deeds know me well and told me it would become permanent and have a better salary. I am very confident of working my way up only being parted from you again is very hard to bear. . . . Do you people think I ought to keep this billet temporarily? I do, but then it seems so cool on my part to shunt you off on your father again, but it is impossible for you to come here on the very poor pay I am getting — please write me what you all think about it. It is so hard to be parted from you and the little ones again but what can one do? . . . I've got this temporary billet but it's only temporary and then such a small salary. We cannot of course think of living here on that. I am fortunate in getting a small room with young Boshoff for only £2/10/0 a month and I pay £5 for Boarding so I come off cheaply in comparison to what other men pay. But of course I can't keep on at this rate, because I can't expect your people to support you and the children for years. I did not marry you for that, did I my sweetheart? . . . That fellow Martin from Fauresmith (the brute who came to arrest you and Dina) had the cheek to want to greet me the other day: Of course I cut him dead.' He spent Christmas with May and her family, and his letter to May of 28 December 1902 on his return to Bloemfontein suggests that during his visit to her he must have told her that he had got a job on the railway, because he writes: 'I saw the Traffic Manager this morning also, and he is going down the line today and will look for the most suitable cottage for us and I will let you know later where to go — it will be somewhere between Bloemfontein and Springfontein I think. I will wire you as soon as I know, he says I can take the place as soon as I like.' Four days later he writes: 'Won't it be jolly when we are together in our own little home again? I went to Fichardt's [a department store in Bloemfontein] to see some furniture — the things are not so dear as we thought. I can get an English Pearl No 7 stove at Parker's for £11 with utensils. On Monday when the stores open I will buy the furniture we want.' So at last things began to be better for my poor parents. I don't know what the job on the railway was, or how long it lasted, but I think not long.

From information dug up for me in South Africa by Professor Arthur Davey, it seems that some time before July 1903 he had some sort of unestablished job in the office of the Resident Magistrate of Winburg (where his father used to be Predikant), and was about to be promoted to the established post of Dutch Interpreter and clerical assistant in the court when he resigned, apparently to take up a post in 1906 as assistant in the General Post Office, I don't know where. By August 1908 he was back firmly on his old career, as Assistant Magistrate in Smithfield, also in what was now, after the Boer War, no longer the Orange Free State, but the Orange River Colony. In 1910 he was transferred to Heilbron (at £350 a year), and in 1911 to Harrismith as Assistant Magistrate and Justice of the Peace. In 1913 he was transferred to Bloemfontein, earning £522/10/0 a year, and in 1918 he was appointed to the full Magistracy of Brandfort, still in the Orange River Colony, at £586/10/0, rising to the grade of Magistrate Grade II at £700/0/0 in 1919.

Nearly as soon as possible after my father returned to South

Africa they had five more children. My sister Ethel Marie, always known as Koekoe (pronounced Kookoo), was born in October 1903; my next sister, Gladys Mary, was born three years later. After such a string of girls, my brother George Phillipus Kits was born in 1909, and as he justly claims, he must have been very welcome. I was born in Harrismith on the day before Christmas 1911, which in my childhood had its disadvantages but some advantages, and my brother Petrus Arnoldus Conradus, known as Peter, was born three years later.

South West Africa

I have no memories of childhood in Harrismith or Bloemfontein, and only the dimmest of Brandfort. Brandfort lies at the dead centre of the Orange Free State, forty miles to the north of the capital, Bloemfontein. You may have heard of it, since Winnie Mandela, wife of the African National Congress leader now imprisoned at Polsmoor, was banished to the Native location there after the riots in Soweto in 1976, and would still be confined there had not her house recently been burned down by persons unknown — I believe she is back in Soweto. (At this time of writing, but things are coming to a head in South Africa.) I have a very faint memory of hearing that Uncle Harry, my mother's younger brother, had been killed in action in the Great War in Europe (at Arras in September 1917), and of standing in the main street lined with people celebrating the Armistice on 11 November the next year.

My mother died in May 1918, of Bright's Disease, I believe, officially, but her heart was in a bad state. I have photocopies of seventeen letters she wrote to my father in June and July 1917, while she was staying with her parents in Zastron. She was there trying to rest her heart. Like his letters to her fifteen years earlier, they are very loving, and brave about her condition. (There are two references to me: 'Poor old Willie, he does so hate the cold [it had snowed a little]. His feet get cold and then he just sits down and cries .... Willie is a dear little man, only he still wants to fight everybody.') For me those letters are painfully sad. They, and his to her, are really the only picture I have of my mother, except three photographs, the first when she was the prettiest, rather solemn twelve-year-old girl you ever saw, the second when she was an adorably beautiful young woman of about twenty, and the third probably when she was near the end of her forty-two-year life, looking sadly worn. I was six and a half years old when she died. I don't remember her dying, I don't remember being sad about her, or missing her. It is only now, having read those letters, and thinking about her as I write this, that I realise that I miss her, that I miss never really being aware of having a mother. I envy my children, as infants and as adults, having such a wonderful mother and friend, and my grandchildren for having such a wonderful grandmother. But then I remember that they have only one sibling each, whereas I had six. My sister Boudina, then aged twenty-one, took over her mother's responsibilities, aided by her three younger sisters. I think the loving and patient care we three boys had from our four sisters made up so much for the loss of our mother that that is perhaps why I don't remember my mother, or grieving for her.

My only distinct memory of Brandfort — I suppose it was 1920 — is of covering my face with mud because Rosalie Shields wanted to kiss me and I wasn't going to have any of it. She had her way fourteen years later.

In 1920 we left the Union of South Africa and moved to South West Africa, where my father had been transferred to the magistracy of Keetmanshoop and its district. South West Africa lies on the west coast of Africa. It adjoins the Cape Province on the south, with the Orange River as the border; Bechuanaland (now Botswana) and part of the Cape Province on the east, with no natural border; Portuguese Angola (now Angola) on the north, with the Cunene and Okavango Rivers as border, and at this border it extends eastwards in a narrow strip (the Caprivi Strip) reaching over the north of Bechuanaland to make contact with North and South Rhodesias (now Zambia and Zimbabwe) at a point near the Victoria Falls. In the past the Germans, like most European Powers, had large colonies in Africa — German East Africa (now Tanzania, or Tanganyika plus Nyasaland in my time) on the east coast, and Togoland (now divided into the Republic of Togoland and part of Ghana) and the Cameroons (now divided into the Cameroon Republic and part of Nigeria); and German South West Africa on the west coast.

The Germans took South West Africa in 1884 and claimed a Protectorate over it. They defined the District of Keetmanshoop, and appointed a *Bezirksamptmann* (magistrate) over it in 1895. When the Great War broke out in 1914, General Louis Botha (who had fought skilfully against the British in the Boer War) invaded South West Africa, and by 1915 it was surrendered. At the Treaty of Versailles in 1919 Germany lost all her African colonies; and in 1920 the League of Nations entrusted South

West Africa to the Union of South Africa as a C-Mandate under Article 22, to be administered as if it were part of the Union of South Africa.

My father's first duty was to take over from the Military Magistrate of Keetmanshoop as the first Civil Magistrate, on 12 April 1920. The Keetmanshoop district is enormous. I had previously guessed, from studying the map and remembering places my father used to go to, that it was about 60,000 square miles (equivalent to 250 miles squared), and on our visit to South West Africa in 1984 that was, in a way, confirmed by the present Control Magistrate, Mr Truter. The administrative area is about 25,000 square miles, but the Magistrate's juridical responsibilities extend to 60,000 square miles. That is about as big as the Orange Free State, or all of England and Wales. That area is now divided into three areas under five magistrates presided over by a Control Magistrate. In our day the Magistrate was the biggest shot in the district, a fact that I used to gloat over when I was a boy.

Strangely enough, at this point my childhood memories come sharply into focus. I can remember arriving in Keetmanshoop after an endlessly long (about 1000 miles) railway journey, during which we spent at least two days and two nights on the train. We were met at the station by the outgoing Military Magistrate, Major Manning. He wore a khaki shirt and shorts, and a *sola topi*. I can remember all that, but I can't remember leaving Brandfort only two days before.

I was enthralled by South West Africa from the moment we arrived there, and remained so all the time we were there, and am still so in retrospect. It was a strange, fiercely hot, fiercely arid, country. You needed to be tough to live in it, and so to me it seemed really and truly glamorous. Most will disagree, and find it barren and hostile. Keetmanshoop lies in the highlands of the southern, hotter, more arid part of South West Africa, on the western limit of the Kalahari Desert, which stretches eastwards into the northern Cape Province and Bechuanaland, and northwards towards the Caprivi Strip; to the west lies the Namib Desert, stretching further westwards to the cold Atlantic Ocean and then northwards towards the Cunene River. In the summer the temperature is usually about 125 degrees Fahrenheit, often higher, and it has been known to rise to 156 degrees. In the winter it is rather less hot, but not much less, and never cold, except sometimes at night. But the heat was always bearable because of the total lack of humidity. Your sweat evaporated before it became apparent, and this evaporation kept you reasonably cool; and then there were various home comforts that employed the absence of humidity to keep people and things cool, as we shall see.

The town was very small — a score or two of houses and other buildings on half-dozen wide streets, with the native servants living in huts in the 'location' at a prescribed distance from the town. But small as it was, it was administratively second only to the northern capital of Windhoek, though the coastal towns of Luderitzbucht and Swakopmund may perhaps have been a little bigger. In German times it was taken very seriously: 'There is one official out of every three [whites of course] in the population, and it is a great burden to the country. Take a place like Keetmanshoop. The town and country around can be compared with Uppington and the district [across the border in the Cape Province], where they have a magistrate and one or two clerks. At Keetmanshoop they have a Deputy-Governor with a secretary and about half a dozen clerks, in addition to ten or a dozen policemen who are also largely engaged in clerical work. Then there are the Law Courts, with two judges, a secretary, and half-a-dozen clerks' [8]. This was the administrative and judicial system that my father succeeded to, with an assistant-magistrate, a few clerks and a police force.

We lived in an official house, called The Residency, which I thought was the grandest address anyone could possibly have. It stood in an enclosed compound on one floor (as did every other building in town), with a veranda at the back, and a big square roofed-over terrace in front. Not that we ever called it a terrace — we called it a stoep, pronounced as a short stoop. (The Dutch introduced the same word to America when New York was New Amsterdam.) Apart from houses, I remember the Magistrate's Court, the Post Office, the Church, the Hansa Hotel, the butcher, the baker, and the one and only general store, called the UDFI, or Union Defence Force Institute, which I suppose was a kind of garrison shop still being run by the government. The most wonderful building by far was the Police Station, which was housed in an immense stone fort with crenellated walls, built by the Germans when the natives were still hostile. And what is more, the police rode about on camels. A few years later, when I took to reading P.C.Wren's *Beau Geste* and *Beau Sabreur*, it took on an even greater glamour because it looked like the North African forts of the French Foreign Legion portrayed on the dust jackets. Doubtless the Germans had got the idea from their

French fellow-colonists. I really felt privileged to live in such a romantic environment. The streets were nothing but several inches of Kalahari sand, and there were no pavements — no traffic, no need. I will never forget the strange sight I got used to seeing in those streets. The local dogs. You would see them lying in groups in little patches of shade, panting vigorously (their substitute for sweating); every now and then one of them would get up, standing irresolutely for a while summoning up its courage; then it would run frantically to join the dogs in the next patch of shade, yelping sharply all the way from the pain to its feet from the burning sand. This would happen all day long. We children never ran about bare-footed in the summer like our contemporaries in the Union.

The Blacks, or Natives, or Kaffirs as we usually called them, were mainly Hereros, Hottentots and a few Bushmen. The Hereros were the remnants of a tribe that had once been the most important indigenous tribe in German South West Africa. In 1904 the Germans opened the Herero War and destroyed 20,000 of them, '. . . probably half the entire race. The days of Herero lordship of large tracts of land and vast herds were terminated, and the tribesmen began to deteriorate. They abandoned their native dress and adopted European clothing' [8]. Their women were still wearing exactly the same European clothing when we got there in 1920. It was Victorian — a very tight bodice buttoned to the neck, with leg-of-mutton sleeves down to the wrists; several full skirts trailing in the desert sand; and a foot-high turban curving majestically forward, giving them great height and dignity. Lovely to look at, but not delightful to know at close quarters, for there emanated from them a dreadful, curious, *very* pungent peppery smell, never encountered by me before or since, and which I found hard to bear. Perhaps it was a body odour specific to them on account of their eccentric garments, which no doubt promoted the production and decay of sweat in that heat and were not often washed; but I think not, I am inclined to think it was an applied *parfum* compounded from local herbs. There is no accounting for taste. Like the women, the Herero men were tall, dignified and handsome, with acquiline noses and thin lips, so they differed a lot from the Bantu we were used to. The Bushmen were indigenous to South West Africa, but not the Hottentots who, I think, originally came from the Cape, whence they were driven northwards by the early Dutch settlers of the East India Company and their successors. They were small people who wore next to nothing and spoke with clicks, which I can imitate to the extent of saying 'I love you'. It goes something like this: 'tchk-eye tchk-oppee tchk-ngyahn see-yah', the click containing elements of the 't', 'ch', and 'k' sounds, and being attained by pressing the tongue hard against the palate and pulling it away instantly. Not that I believe that the Hottentots and Bushmen ever indulged in such sentimental talk — at best I think the expression must mean something like 'I am not unfriendly.' (This leads me to state that I don't believe a word of that nice man Laurens van der Post when he tells us on television of the wonderful philosophical thoughts being uttered by his Hottentot and Bushmen friends in the Kalahari. I don't believe they have these thoughts, or if they have them, that they would have the means of expressing them. And I don't believe that Sir Laurens can possibly be all that *au fait* with the language.) The Hottentots and the Bushmen in my day were never domestic servants or labourers, they were herdsmen on farms, or they lived wild. (I learned at school in Keetmanshoop that the Dutch for an exhibition of Hottentot tents — though I doubt that there ever has been such an exhibition — is 'Hottentottententententen-toonstelling'.)

Most of the Whites we first encountered in Keetmanshoop were Germans. I still remember the *Schweinefleisch mit Kartoffelen* we had with our first meal in Keetmanshoop, in the Hansa Hotel. In the Residency there were handsome heavy solid oak doors all over, with heavy brass fittings, and beer *Steinen*, and beautiful wine glasses with long pale green stems, all imported from Germany. The handsome young men who came to call on my sisters would bow from the waist and click their heels. It was my first taste of Europe, for we were living in a little transplanted Germany, where the culture was European, and exotic to the South African culture we knew. The lady in the butcher's or the baker's, when I went to buy something and thanked her on being given it, invariably replied 'Nichts zu danken, aber zu bezahlen'. At railway crossings there were signs saying *Halt wenn ein Zug sich nähert*, and I used to think that a Zugsich was a railway engine puffing away, zugsich, zugsich, zugsich. With so much contact with German, and with Afrikaans not being very far different, I was able to pick up quite a little German, which came in useful in later years, especially when I had to read many German scientific journals in Cambridge before the war.

The Mayor of Keetmanshoop was Herr Brandenburg. He had an Herero wife (another European idea), and I don't suppose she was ever called the Mayoress, but I expect she was allowed to live with him, and not in the native location outside town. Of course she could not accompany him on any official occasion, and so her absence did on one occasion present a social problem — a problem that my father with presence of mind solved. The occasion was a visit — a 20-minute stopover at the railway station — of the Governor General of South Africa, the Earl of Athlone and his wife, on their way to the capital, Windhoek. I remember both of them vividly. She died only a few years ago, not long after I had seen her on television, looking as lovely at an immense age as she did that day at the Keetmanshoop railway station sixty years ago. My father was there to meet them, and lined up at his side were my sister Boudina as the Magistrate's Lady, then the Mayor, then one or two other officials and their wives. But of course the Mayor's Herero wife could not possibly be presented to the Gubernatorial couple. The Mayor and his wife understood that as well as anybody. My father presented first his daughter, then the Mayor, then the others. 'Are we to meet the Mayoress?', asked the punctilious Earl. Awkward moment before my father leaped into the breech: 'She's a little off-colour today, Sir'. (This splendid occasion was nearly ruined for us. Just before the Governor-General's train came in, and everybody was already lined up, a scruffy shunting engine came along the line, and out of it leaned the grimy face of the black sheep of the family. I had only vaguely heard about him — a young Higgs who had gone wrong, I don't know how, and was now occupying the lowly station of shunting engine fireman — not, thank Heavens! stationed in Keetmanshoop but somewhere near. With a leer on his blackened face he called out 'Hullo Uncle Ollie!' My poor chagrined father looked uncomfortable and mumbled. I bet young Higgs sort of borrowed that engine and deliberately staged the meeting.

We lived comfortably in The Residency. There were plenty of Herero servants, and on Saturdays there were even more, because a gang of prisoners from the local jail, all Kaffirs of course, would come under a one-man armed guard to tidy up the compound and water the trees and plants and the vegetable garden. This wasn't a magisterial privilege — it was paid for, and any honest (and white) citizen could avail himself of the service. Many of the prisoners were in jail because they had been caught smoking *dagga*, which I learned many years later was cannabis. I can't remember any of our servants except one, a big man who worked in the kitchen. One day we were waiting at the dining table for him to bring in the apples. After some time Koekoe went to the kitchen to see what was keeping him. She found him spitting on the apples, then polishing them with a dirty cloth. She must have shown some consternation, because he gave her a big friendly smile and asked, 'Why you look so sour to me you bugger?'

Of course there was no electricity (at night we read in bed with candles on our chests), and no ice-boxes, let alone refrigerators, but like everybody else we kept perishable food cool in ingenious home-made cabinets that employed the heat and the dryness of the atmosphere to provide coolness. The cabinets stood outside on four legs in the shade of a pepper tree: they consisted of a box made with a frame of three by three-inch timbers, with a solid top and bottom, and one side hinged to make a door. Stretched on the inner and outer sides of the wooden framework were sheets of chicken wire, with the intervening spaces filled with walnut-sized lumps of porous coke. Thus you had a box, with a door, through which the breezes could easily pass. On top there was a zinc tray three inches deep, with the edges flush with the outer sides of the coke-filled walls. Around the periphery of the bottom of the zinc tray there were holes at half-inch intervals, with two-inch nails hanging loosely through them, and their points just reaching the coke below. A tap trickled water into the zinc tray as fast as it dropped out again along the nails to the coke. This water never reached the ground, because it evaporated so rapidly from the coke into the bone-dry air. Evaporation needs energy, and the energy was provided by the heat in the air in the box, so the heat went away and the air in the box cooled down, enough to keep the butter hard. Water was plentiful although it hardly ever rained. It came from copious sources not far below the surface of the ground, and was pumped into the town reservoir. Our drinking water was kept cool on the same principle as that of the cold boxes. It was kept in canvas bags that allowed some of the contents slowly to seep to the outer surface and so evaporate in the dry air. There were always plenty of them about, and we would take some with us on our excursions to the country. The same evaporative principle was used to keep us cool in, or rather on, bed on particularly hot nights. We all slept on the veranda that ran along the back of the house; the girls one one side of a bath full of water, the boys on the other, wearing night clothes, but with no covers on the beds except the bottom sheets. Every once in a while one or the other of us would dunk her- or himself in this bath, still wearing night clothes. Then the sopping dunker would stretch her- or himself on the bed and in no time the water would evaporate almost at once, providing delicious coolness.

When we arrived in Keetmanshoop it had not rained for five years, we were told. Two years after we arrived a small cloud appeared in the sky, no bigger, as they say, than a man's hand. I remember someone saying to my father, 'In two days it will rain', and in two days it did. It bucketed down, and within a few minutes the streets were running about two feet of water. There was nothing more delightful for us boys and our friends than to rush about in the flood. This happened only three or four more times during our stay in South West Africa. Every time it rained a miracle happened. Almost the next day, it seemed to me, the entire arid landscape turned green. This was due to the flat confluent growth of hitherto practically invisible thorn bushes. The next day, so it seemed, another miracle happened. The green was now copiously dotted with beautiful yellow flowers about a foot high. And within a few days all that lovely vegetation was dried up and gone, leaving nasty pea-sized thorns behind, each armed with many pricks that were a trial to a boy walking barefoot in the winter.

The landscape I remember was mainly almost bare earth scattered about with desiccated little bushes, tufts of white grass, some low thorny trees, and some taller camel thorn trees. In some parts even these evidences of vegetation were absent, and the earth was simply hard and bare, with occasional accumulations of black boulders. One day, walking with another boy through that landscape, we came upon the corpse of a man who had committed suicide by putting the end of his gun in his mouth and pulling the trigger by means of a bootlace attached to his big toe. It was the first dead person I ever saw. The back of his head was blown away; but what really shocked me was the filth of the foot that pulled the trigger. We ran off to report to my father, and were disappointed at not being allowed to show the police the way.

In other parts of the landscape there were sand dunes covered with ripples, and I used to dream of inventing a way of converting this easily available material into petrol, but I've learned enough chemistry since then to know better. I loved this arid landscape. I can't say why, except that my young soul found it heroic, and even today when I go through England's green and pleasant land I occasionally get fed-up with all the greenness and pleasantness, and long for some aridity. My friends and I would wander about the veld all afternoon, and as we started homewards at sunset we would often encounter a patrol of police on their camels looking for us at my father's behest. I never understood why he worried so. I always knew roughly what time it was and exactly where we were, and it was invariably when we were on our way home that we were intercepted. But it was nice to ride home on a camel.

The vanished dunes were the setting of my first religious experience; or non-experience. Nominally we were a church-going family, but I don't remember ever going to church. Very early on my father had stilled any fears I might have had by assuring us there was no Hell, only Heaven, without actually guaranteeing that we would get there. I went through a phase of thinking I *ought* to be religious. At that time there were plenty of stories going about of people suddenly Seeing the Light, and I thought that was the only way people got religious. But I received no call, so I thought I should try and encourage it. I would go by myself to the dunes and find some private hollow in them, and there I would fall on my knees and pray. I didn't know how to make up a special prayer to call for the Light, so I would recite the Lord's Prayer, in English, then in Afrikaans, over and over again. It always seemed to me that prayers were bound to be more powerful in Afrikaans, and still more so in High Dutch; and to this day I can't imagine the Apostles speaking anything but High Dutch. But the Light never came, and I don't suppose it will in the modest number of years left to me. If you will forgive me, I will now try and state what my feelings are about God. I don't believe that, 'There's a friend for little children, Above the bright blue sky', as we were taught in kindergarten. There is no God who loves us. God is a neutral IT, properly indifferent to us, disinterested and impartial. IT is the Origin of the Universe, or the Fact of the Existence of all things animal, vegetable, mineral and philosophical. IT is a mystery that will never rightly be comprehended, no matter how far beyond the Big Bang the astrophysicists may be able to reach one day; they will never know what triggered it. Therefore IT should be considered with respect, reverence if you like. I suppose the way to feel respect is to appreciate and respect our existence, and our environment, animal, vegetable, mineral or philosophical; to be aware of our faults; to be decent and kind. This of course is what all religions strive for in their different ways, but they do not take my view as to the disinterestedness of IT. Perhaps that makes me an agnostic rather than an atheist. Of course my views are not original, and I am sure are shared by many. On the other hand — and this is what most gives me pause — I am humbly aware that there are many, many people who are genuinely religious; and it this fact that most undermines my agnosticism.

Through the glorious South West African veld there would wander from time to time immense herds of game, and I would wonder what there was for them to feed on, and where they got water. There were kudu, gemsbok and springbok, sometimes being pursued by leopards. I often saw vast great flocks of ostriches, sometimes running at fantastic speed. There were jackals and hyenas, but you never saw them, you only heard them at night. There were lizards of every sort, and vultures. Once in a while there were immense clouds of locusts, a mile long and a mile wide they would say, and I don't know how deep, but enough literally to darken the sky. I was fortunate to be so familiar with all this wildlife, because you won't see it in the interior of South West Africa any more, only to the east in the Kalahari and to the north in the Etosha region, and then only in game parks, not in one's normal environment.

My friends and I would go off into the veld and camp for a night or two. We would each have a waterbottle — a proper metal bottle covered with felt and leather, but that was only for emergencies. We would camp out on the bed of a dried-up river (they were dried up practically all the time), and make a bivouac (for shade) from the branches from bushes growing on the bank or on the bed. For water all we had to do was to dig a hole about eighteen inches into the river bed, and the water would soon seep in. The water table is quite near the surface, as I have already pointed out; otherwise the Kalahari would be uninhabitable, and in the river beds it is even nearer. This underground water was very *brak*, or salty, so much so that when we returned to the Union after some years the water was so bitter we could not drink it unless a teaspoon of salt were added to a glass of it.

Camping on the river bed reminds me of a terrible, but temporary, disillusionment I suffered. My father once took me out with him on a trip to hold court at Aroab, a settlement about 100 miles due east of Keetmanshoop. We travelled in a Reo Speedwagon, which was a flat-bed American truck. It was the only motor vehicle in the District. My father, the driver and I travelled in front, while the Assistant Magistrate, a couple of policemen and a couple of Herero servants sat on ordinary park benches screwed down onto the flat bed at the back. The first night out we camped on the sandy bed of a dried-up river. As I lay in my sleeping bag (I suppose it was winter), listening to the jackals howling and the hyenas barking in the distance, I felt very happy. We were all so tough out here in the desert with the jackals howling. Then I heard the Assistant Magistrate say to my father, 'Would you like a night-cap, Sir?', and to my bitter dismay I heard my father eagerly say yes, please. My illusions of the tough life were shattered by this revelation that my father was sissy enough to want to wear a night-cap against the desert air. I took a long time to sleep, but the next day I learned the truth. It was a great relief to me, especially since whisky-drinking fitted the tough image.

The Reo Speedwagon did not remain the only motor vehicle for long. My father introduced the first motor car in the District. It was an American Willys Overland, with wooden spokes to the wheels, and of course a collapsible canvas roof plus celluloid side screens that were used far more to keep out the dust than the rain. It was considered very grand, and everybody in town and around wanted to be driven to their weddings by my father, which he did, but in time grumbled about. In those days, and on those surfaces, the tyres frequently punctured, and I spent a lot of my life helping to jack up the car, take off the tyre, remove and patch the inner tube, replace the inner tube and the tyre, and pump up the tyre with a hand pump. All cars had folding roofs in those days, naturally; I heard stories about Americans having limousines with metal tops and glass doors, but I knew they wouldn't last.

We were also the first to get a gramophone. A wooden wind-up one of course. Among the first records we had were Blue Danube, Valentia and My Brave Picador. I was thrilled by this one — 'My brave picador' it went, 'how proud am I to know tonight you fight for me.' It was only many years later at a bull-fight in Madrid that I was disillusioned, when I saw the sneaky role the seedy picador really played — riding a beat-up old nag covered with mattresses and carrying a long pic to stick into the neck muscle of the bull so that it would not be able to raise its head, and thus would be exposed to the final thrust of the matador. Many of our gramophone records perished in the sun after being left out projecting over the balustrade on the terrace. They would fold over like Dali watches.

I think my father was popular. At any rate he had a famous very loud sneeze, and every time he let it off in public the entire audience would clap. I was proud of him. He used to amuse or terrify the Blacks by suddenly pushing out his false teeth at them. I used to think it was a scream, but in retrospect perhaps a bit 'off'. Once he flew into a terrible rage with me, and it was a long time before I understood why. At lunch one day, talking about a boy I didn't like, I said he was 'an illegitimate son of a jew' — it was a term I had heard some grown-up use in a clearly disparaging way, and although I had no idea what it meant, it struck me as a good powerful term of abuse. My father roared at me, 'Go into the kitchen at once and wash out your dirty mouth with soap!', and into the kitchen I had to go and under his livid eye rub a bar of kitchen soap on my tongue. This insult reminds me of an exchange of others. Two of my contemporaries were working up for a fight, exchanging escalating insults. Then one came up with the penultimate: '*Your* father is an IDB!' He had gone too far. The other hurled himself at his throat shouting the ultimate, 'And *your* father is an Englishman!' In case you're wondering, an IDB was an Illicit Diamond Buyer. Diamonds were being picked out of the sand of the beaches of Luderitzbucht by teams of Black workers crawling forwards on their stomachs in rows, and from time to time one of them would be tempted to secrete one in his rectum and sell it to a White IDB, who made a great profit. My father often had to send IDB's to gaol.

Occasionally on Sundays, when the weekly train from Cape Town came through on its 4-day journey to Windhoek, we would have a treat. On the Saturday before, my father would send his official equipage, which was a four-wheel cart with a fold-down top, drawn by four black mules led by four white horses, up 50 miles north to the railway siding of Tses. The Hottentot driver would spend the night there, sleeping between the wheels, awaiting our arrival the next day. At noon on Sunday we would board the train and make for the dining car, where we would have a princely lunch, preceded by a whisky and soda, or two, for my father and lemonade for the rest of us. The train guard was always very friendly and helpful. I remember once my father's *sola topi* blowing off as he put his head out of the window, and the train being stopped while the guard trotted down the line to recover it. After an hour and a half we would reach Tses and board the waiting cart, and then spend the rest of the afternoon driving the 50 miles back, where we would arrive as the sun was setting.

The headmaster of the school was a dreadful little man called O. P. Tarr. I remember his name because I hated him so. I can't remember why I hated him, but it was not because he denied me my prizes for coming first in class. I always used to come first, and at the end of the year I would win a prize. But after a few years O. P. Tarr decided that other people should have a chance of getting the prize, so I was by-passed and the prize went to whoever came second. I didn't mind. I arrogantly agreed with O. P. Tarr's ruling. We always spoke English and Afrikaans in school, but we were not allowed to read or write in Afrikaans, because Afrikaans was not the official language. We had to use Dutch, which was always called High Dutch, because Afrikaans at that time was still called Dutch. I remember the day Afrikaans became official and High Dutch went out of my life. (When I go to Holland it is no use my trying to talk Afrikaans to the natives because they think it is laughable and beneath contempt. They pretend not to understand and reply, as practically all Dutchmen are able, in perfect English. On the other hand, the Flemings in Belgium understand my Afrikaans with ease.)

My sisters had a rare old time in South West Africa. Not Stinie, because she was not there most of the time. She had been very clever at the University of Stellenbosch down in the Cape, and after graduating there she won the Abe Bailey Scholarship, which took her to Somerville College, Oxford. My other sisters remaining in Keetmanshoop had many followers, and there seemed to be dancing on the terrace to the gramophone every evening. There was one strange fellow who took a fancy to Koekoe, who was the prettiest and the jolliest. I don't know where he came from, or what he did for a living, but he was, as far as the eye could see, a real American Wild West Cowboy, though he'd never set foot in America. He always wore a real cowboy Stetson hat, real cowboy sheepskin chaps, real cowboy high boots with long-pointed spurs, and he rode about on a horse with a real cowboy saddle with a high pommel and back, and big all-enclosing wooden stirrups. Nobody had ever seen the likes of him; and where he got his gear from I haven't the faintest idea. Even more marvellous was his banjo, and the way he played it. One day he invited me to a meal in his house to eat a marvellous dish I had never seen or heard of — potato chips the shape and size of matches. After the meal, he gave me his wonderful banjo for keeps, with a promise that he would teach me how to play it. Of course I was overwhelmed with joy. I floated home with the banjo. The elation lasted no more than five minutes: as soon as Koekoe saw the banjo, and learned how it had come into my hands, she flew into a great rage, chorused by Boudina and Gladys, and instructed me immediately to retrace my steps and return the banjo.

Around this time I got a hint of the possibility that grown-ups could be naughty too. One day I wandered out from a farm house where my father was on business, to a big water tank about half a mile away. As I came round it I came upon two grown-ups, a man and a woman whom I knew by sight. They looked mortified and guilty, and I just knew they had being doing something they should not have been doing. I had no idea what; but in my mind I connected it with the time two or three months previously, when I learned something about a difference between the sexes that I had not been aware of. On another farm we visited there were three little Black girls of my age playing in a tented cart resting on its shafts. As I approached, they giggled and turned their backs to me, lifting their skirts. They seemed to think they were doing something naughty, but I didn't know what — all I could see were bottoms, much the same as mine, only black. Then they giggled even more, turned their faces to me, and lifted their skirts again. This time I was amazed. I knew there were differences between males and females, such as breasts on women and bald heads and beards on men, but these girls had no penises! Just nothing at all as far as I could see, and I wondered how, indeed whether, they ever pee-ed.

Most of the farms we visited were owned by Germans. They were raising karakul sheep for their foetal fleeces, i.e. Persian lamb; and the fattest-tail sheep you ever saw, for wool and meat. All the farmhouses had rarely-used parlours, and in each parlour there would be a photograph on a little stand on an occasional table. The photograph was always pasted onto a rather larger army biscuit, thus making a double souvenir of the Herero War of 1904, when half the race was killed. The photograph showed how some of the killing was done — each had a dozen Hereros hanging in line side by side from an extended gallows.

My father also had to supervise wars against the natives. Six such wars. As far as I can remember, four of them were Hottentot Rebellions: two of the Bondelswarts (Bundel Blacks?), and two of the Veldskoendraers (Veldschoen wearers). The fifth was a Herero Rebellion; and the sixth the Rebellion of the Rehoboth *Basters*. These *Basters* were the bastard descendants of the offspring of early Portuguese sailors and indigenous Hottentot women who were descended from Cape Hottentots who had fled northwards. They were mainly settled in the Rehoboth District several hundred miles north of Keetmanshoop, but there was an enclave of them in the Keetmanshoop District. They were proud of being Bastards. Most, if not all, of these rebellions were in protest against the Dog Tax that had been imposed on these people. It seems to me now to have been entirely unreasonable, and must have seemed incomprehensible and oppressive to them, living miles away in the desert, minding their own business, which was using their dogs for hunting. I remember going with my father to the Keetmanshoop gaol to see some of the imprisoned Herero women. They had been attempting to commit suicide by running full tilt with their heads down into the walls of their cells; or trying to choke themselves by attempting to swallow their own tongues. At the time I thought it funny; ten years later I began to think differently.

I used to think that in all these wars there had been only one casualty — that of a White soldier accidently shooting off his toe while cleaning his rifle — but recently I learned with dismay from Marquard [18], and from an editorial footnote in Aunt Cara's memoirs [34], that more than a hundred Bondelswarts had been killed. I will come to this point again.

I wrote earlier that my father 'supervised' these wars. I don't know exactly what his role was, except that the happenings with the Hottentots, Hereros and Rehoboth Basters were in his district, and that he had to parley with the rebel chiefs before the military were called in from the Union. I will not forget one such parley, with the Bondelswart chief and his men. It was out in the open in front of the Magistrate's Court, my father and his men on one side facing the Bondelswarts on the other. I was looking on from the side. The Bondelswart Chief drew a line in the sand with his *knobkierie* (club) and said to my father, 'Cross this line and I will kill you!' Of course I was terrified, and of course my father stepped across the line without hesitation. The Bondelswart Chief raised his *knobkierie*, but one of his men restrained him. I dare say now that the police would have acted in any case. I can't remember what happened then, but I was terribly proud of my father.

On at least two, and I think three, occasions the Air Force came from Roberts' Heights (near Pretoria) to deal with the rebels. Their function, I believed (note past tense), was to demonstrate Government military power by dropping 2-pound bombs from their flying machines on to previously white-washed crosses marked out on the ground near the Bondelswart settlements, the Bondelswarts having been given ample notice. But they did also drop bombs to kill. I learned recently in the Rhodes House Library that the Bondelswart settlements in the neighbourhood of Karasburg were in fact bombed, and I think that is where all the killing took place. Karasburg is well to the south of

Keetmanshoop, and I would like to think that it was in the Warmbad magistracy rather than my father's.

For us, especially for my sisters, the Air Force coming to deal with these wars was great fun (I would certainly not think it fun today). If ever there were Magnificent Young Men on their Flying Machines, these were they. They were a fact, not a cliché, outworn since then. Their aircraft were canvas biplanes with two open cockpits, and the helmeted and goggled airmen were the most beautiful creatures any girl could wish for. To my sisters fell the duty of providing entertainment for these gallant heroes. Every night on the terrace of The Residency there was dancing to the strains of the gramophone, far into the morning. There had been nothing like it since the Ball on the Eve of Waterloo. The Departure of the Gods was even more glorious. The whole town would go to the area on the edge of the town where the airplanes landed and took off, and when the Magnificent Young Men finally took off, they would circle over the town several times; then, as they left, they would drop three-yard-long red, white and blue streamers that would drift down slowly. At the ends of these streamers there were canvas pockets containing notes wrapped around a lead bar. The notes were thank-you notes addressed to my sisters.

We went on holidays in what was always called The Union [of South Africa] from time to time, several times to visit our Higgs relations in the Orange Free State, and to Somerset West near Cape Town, where I saw the sea for the first time, and there's no better place to see the sea than from the Cape. (This reminds me of an encounter a friend of ours had in the Drakensberg Mountains between Natal and the Orange Free State. He had motored inland from the Natal coast, starting early in the morning. By noon he was high up in the Drakensberg, with the valleys below filled with mist. He came upon a car stopped at the side of the road, and an elderly couple sitting on a rock, gazing down. He stopped to ask if they needed any help, but they replied thank you, no; they had come from the Free State to see the sea, which they had not seen before, and there it was, they said, pointing to the mist-filled valleys, wasn't it wonderful?) We also saw the sea at Swakopmund and Walvis Bay on the Atlantic coast of South West Africa, west of Windhoek, with the train stopping on the way at stations with strange beautiful names — Brukkaros, Usakos, Okahandja, Okazizi, Karibib. We went on board a Woerman Brock ocean liner anchored in Walvis Bay. This was a wonderful new experience, but most remarkable of all was an English boy on board. He was about my age, but quite unlike any boy I had seen before. We gazed upon each other with reciprocal wonder. I found him beautiful, with his white, white skin, his pink cheeks and his golden hair; and I suppose he thought I must be a little brown African monkey wearing clothes.

In 1926 my father was found to have cancer, on his cheek for all to see. It rapidly got worse, and he was sent to Cape Town to have it excised by Professor Saint. We received a telegram from Stinie, 'Saint as good as his name'. But that was over-optimistic; my father came home a broken man. I can't forget the sight of him weeping as my sisters led him into the house. I did not know that he was dying, but I did a month later. Boudina gave me a letter in an unsealed envelope and asked me to take it to the post office, buy a postal order for £2, enclose it with the letter and post it. On the way to the post office I read the letter. I wished I had not. It said, 'I am sorry we have been so long in paying this bill. My father is dying, and we have had many things to deal with.' I never told my sisters, let alone my brothers, that I had read that letter. I did not react in any way to that dreadful news. I have found in my life that I do not react immediately to bad news (or to an insult). It's as if I haven't heard it.

As a result of his illness, my father was transferred from Keetmanshoop to Bethulie, a little town in the Orange Free State, where his duties would be less onerous. That is how it came about that we left South West Africa. I hope you can see how much I loved it; and why, when I had to make a very important speech in Oxford fifty-three years later, in the presence of Sir Harold Macmillan, Chancellor of the University of Oxford, and former Prime Minister, I started with the words, 'When I was a small boy in the Kalahari Desert'.

The Orange Free State

Bethulie lies near the southern border of the Orange Free State, not far from Norval's Pont, where my grandfather and Aunt Cara had been imprisoned during the Boer War. We were not there for long, and I have practically no memories of it. I wonder whether that is because my father died there, just as I have no memories of Brandfort, where my mother died. I don't remember our house, or the Magistrate's Court, or the school. I don't remember whether my father was fit enough to work. I suppose he must have been, otherwise he would have been pensioned off. My father's dying was secretly very painful for me, because I used to sleep in the room next to his, and I could hear him groaning with pain during the night. I couldn't tell my sisters — and certainly not my brothers — about it, what would have been the point? Late one afternoon I was about two miles away from the town cycling in the countryside, when two men approached me in a car. They looked at me strangely and told me they had come to take me home, they would not tell me why. Early the next morning Boudina came into the room I was now sharing with my younger brother Peter and told us our father had died. She asked if we wanted to see the body, and I said no, feeling ashamed of myself. My father was too young when he died, only fifty-six, and I was too young too, only fourteen. I very vaguely remember the funeral service in the Nederduits Gereformeerde Kerk, but not the burial, and nothing more about Bethulie.

Nothing more except Latin, and the man who taught it, Mr Bedford. Bless Mr Bedford. He was enthusiastic about Latin and he taught me to like it and respect it. He took a lot of trouble, and would catch up with me in the street to discuss tricky points that were likely to come up in the forthcoming examinations for the Junior Certificate. I passed those examinations in the First Class with an A for Latin. I wish I could have learned more of it. I couldn't have started any earlier, because they didn't teach it in Keetmanshoop. I would like respectfully to suggest to school Latin teachers (if there are any left) that they abandon translating from English into Latin, and double translating from Latin into English. I detested translating English into Latin because I never saw the point of it, since it did not help me to understand Latin; and I would never need, or want, to translate into Latin in later life. I could see the sense of learning the language of a people long since dead, but could see no point in translating into a language not understood by the living, except for serious Latin scholars. If I had not wasted so much time on translating into Latin I would be better now at translating from it, and at understanding English and French words. I wish I had an inkling of Classical Greek, but I haven't.

While my father lived we were fairly comfortably off, even though we were a large family. (Once, snooping in his office in Keetmanshoop, I came upon a paper which informed me that his salary was £900 a year. When I wrote this originally, it seemed an enormous sum — say £60,000 today — but in fact the pound in 1925 would be worth only £19.04 today, still giving my father the equivalent of £17,136, more than I ever earned.) But when he died there was no widow, no pension, and nothing saved up; and suddenly we were very poor. Koekoe and Gladys were independent, having started school-teaching jobs; and so was Kits, having started his first job at what seemed to me to be a terrific salary of £300 a year, getting on for a pound a day! So it fell to Christina to support Boudina, Peter and me. She had a job teaching in a school in Gwelo in Southern Rhodesia, and now she moved to an appointment in the Government Secondary School in Reddersburg in the Orange Free State — I bet she was the only B.A. Hons.(Oxon.) ever — so we moved there late in 1925.

Reddersburg (Savioursburgh) was (and still is, as Ruthie and I confirmed on our visit in 1984) a small, crummy, hick town forty miles south of Bloemfontein. We lived in a crummy little house, and we were very poor. At one time all I had to wear on my feet was a couple, not a pair, of boots. They looked the same from a shortish distance, but one had lace holes all the way up and the other had four pairs of hooks instead of the top four pairs of holes. I hoped that nobody would notice, but if they did, they would tell me, because I didn't want them to talk behind my back. Reddersburg lies in a flat featureless plain in the most boring part of the Orange Free State. And it was an oppressive place to live in, because of the dominant Dopper church. Dancing was frowned upon, and the predikant would prowl about peering into windows to detect sinners; so we always had to pull the blinds down if we wanted a little hop. The nearest town was Dewetsdorp, if possible even more hick. I bring it in because it came up at one of the most agreeable luncheon parties I have ever enjoyed, about forty-five years later. I had got to know Lord Caccia, the Provost of Eton College, and his wife invited us to lunch in the Provost's Lodgings on a Sunday at the beginning of spring. I had never visited Eton College, and we drove there on a lovely bright morning, filled with pleasurable expectation of things to come. There were drinks first in the drawing room, where we met Lady Caccia and her son and his ravishing newly-wedded wife, and marvellous Celia Johnson and her husband Peter Fleming. Then we went into lunch in a beautiful panelled room, lined with a double row of portraits by Lawrence and the like of distinguished eighteenth century leaving Etonians. Lady Caccia sat at her end of the table, with me on her right, and her ravishing daughter-in-law on mine. I was in an exhalted state. I turned to her and said, 'As I sit down here in this dining room of the Provost's Lodgings at Eton College, I am giving thought to the little school that I went to in a little town that God forgot in the middle of the Orange Free State, called Reddersburg'. 'For God's sake,' she cried, 'I went to school in Dewetsdorp!'

New boys at the Reddersburg Government Secondary School had to undergo initiation by the other boys at a pool in a little stream just outside the town. The pool was called the Wolwas, because at one time wool was washed in it. We were thrown into it and the initiators would leap on us, push us to the bottom and stand on us until the instant before the point of expiry. How they judged it, I do not know. Then we would have to lie on the ground side by side on our bellies, and the chief inquisitor would poke a stick into the rectum of the boy at the end on the left. He was the lucky one, and I was not he, for the boy on his right had then to pull out the stick, suck it, and insert it in his own rectum, and so forth. Then we were chased around naked by our inquisitors with gravel scooped up in their hands, with which they would seize our testicles with a nasty excoriating twist.

The school itself was not too bad. As a matter of fact, although the schools I went to in the Kalahari and the Free State may have been primitive in comparison with the schools in England today, and more Afrikaans was taught in them than English, it seems to me I was taught better English in them. The English that is spoken and written in England today is not only ugly, it is often downright wrong.

There was one oafish teacher called Grobbelaar. I can't remember what he taught, but it was not, and could not possibly have been, English (which Stinie taught anyway), and I can't remember on what pretext we needled him on English spelling, but we did. We would ask him how to spell wagon (or waggon), quivering with gleeful anticipation of his answer, and he fell for it every time. 'One yee or two yees, yes as you please' he would answer. He never understood why we rolled on the floor in delight. Many years later I was to carve a wee niche for him in the Hall of fame, as we shall see.

Every year, when the watermelons were ripe, we would have a Watermelon Feast. We would pull a wagon (one yee) around the town and solicit fruit. Everybody would be waiting for us with generous contributions of watermelons, grapes and peaches. At the school teachers' houses, one or the other of us would be deputed to make a speech of thanks. Mine happened to be the Headmaster's, who was also the Latin master. He had made a particularly fine contribution, and I proclaimed 'Timeo magistros et fructos ferentes!' Simple enough, but it pleased him. Those watermelon feasts were bliss, because of the girls. We'd go on our laden wagon, now drawn by a small team of oxen, out into the country and have a wonderful time in some shady place. We'd play tug-of-war, one boy and one girl. I was small, in fact I was called *kleinman*, which I hated; and they always got big girls to pull against me, and the big girls always pulled me over the line. Secretly I liked that. Then in the gloaming we'd slowly go home on the wagon. I was really interested in girls by then, and I would seek out the object of my heart's current desire, and we'd sit side by side on the wagon rail, exchanging exciting *double entendres* in the form of the first lines, generally by Irving Berlin, from our favourite gramophone records. She might provoke me with 'You Forgot to Remember', and I would respond with 'What'll I do?'; she'd say 'All Alone' and I'd reply 'You're Always in my Arms, Sweetheart'. The bliss was quite unalloyed.

Not all my outings with girls ended so pleasantly. The trouble was the nightsoil wagons. Each house had a privy at the end of the back yard, backing onto an access lane. The privies had a wooden seat with a hole over a very big bucket, which would be removed at short intervals and replaced by an empty one. This exchange was effected in the dead of the night by a team of Blacks equipped with an ox-wagon. I would go out with some desirable girl, and around midnight I would take her home, strolling slowly down the street in the moonlight, with me, and possibly her, feeling beautifully romantic. Then my heart would shatter, for I would hear the dreaded distant crack of a whip, inevitably followed by a creaking of wagon wheels and the subdued shouts of the *equipe*; and then there would diffuse over us the advance wafts of a dreadful mephitis; and finally the nightsoil tumbril would slowly come into sight, and even more slowly pass us by, creeping like a languorous snail. Romance had flown at that first crack of the whip, but bitter disappointment at its flight was not the worst. The torture seemed without end. The worst was the painfully prolonged embarrassment, because in those days one did not overtly recognize the existence of the unspeakable — you didn't imperturbably shout 'Here comes the stinkwagon!', and make jokes about it; you pretended it wasn't there, and tried desperately to find some other subject of conversation, but when you were young that didn't come so easily.

I participated only once in the traditional but rapidly dying-away form of courting (not necessarily with a view to matrimony). It was done by the light of a *vrykers* (pronounced fray cares), or love-making candle. That was two or three years later, when I was spending holidays from the University on Boudina's farm. I went about twenty-five miles, on horseback of course, to another farm, where lived a dear girl. I arrived at nightfall, to be greeted by her and her parents, while a Black servant looked after my horse. After supper the parents went to bed, leaving me and my girl in the sitting room. Her mother had provided us with a vrykers, which I was pleased to note was pristine and long, showing that she liked me. It was an absolute rule, never, *never* broken, that when the candle burned out you went home. It was also an absolute rule that you did not cheat by blowing out the candle for a while. So by the light of the candle you made conversation and love — nothing serious, certainly no sex, only hugging and kissing, and the occasional tentative and seldom successful fumble. It was lots and lots of fun, probably more fun than the real thing. When the candle burned out I rode off under the shining moon and got home about two in the morning.

Boudina had married a very nice man called Jack Coetzer, an Afrikaner who under the influence of our family became more and more anglicized. He was a farmer, and they lived on their farm, Bougainvillea, eleven miles from Reddersburg. Bougainvillea became home to us, and Boudina continued in her role as mother to us. We were all very fond of Jack. He was a sheep farmer, and he had a hard struggle, because from time to time there would be the most terrible droughts that dried out the vegetation his sheep grazed on. Sometimes it was so desperate that he would have to trek his sheep, many hundreds of them, over the Drakensburg Mountains to grazing land in Natal. Dear old Jack was hopeless with machinery, so his motor car was always broken down, and we would go to town on a horse-drawn cart. The horse was always inclined to take its ease, indifferent to strokes of the whip. The only way to get any acceleration out of the beast was to poke the whip shaft into its rectum — then it would snort, gallop a hundred yards, and forget all about it.

There were many Basuto servants on the farm, living in mud and straw *pontoks* (huts) a few hundred yards from the house. The men worked on the farm, and some of the women worked in the house. Boudina would make her own soap for washing clothes and floors by boiling up sheep fat and caustic soda, as had the *Voortrekker* women.

There was, so it seemed to me, a mutual liking between the

Blacks and the Whites. I once gained fame by playing a trick on the men, the women being excluded, you'll see why. I had by this time learned enough chemistry at the university to know that if you made a mixture of sodium peroxide and iron filings, then poured water on it, it would burst into flames, due to the sudden production of oxygen and heat, and the consequent ignition of the iron filings (yes, iron burns — try lighting a small scrap of steel wool with a match). I stole some sodium peroxide and iron filings from the laboratory and brought them to Bougainvillea one holiday. One evening when all the servants had gone to their pontoks I mixed the powders and covered them with sticks in the back yard. The next morning I invited the men to come and witness an event, telling the women to stay away. When the men were all gathered around me, I pee-ed on the sticks and they burst into flames. Naturally, the men were amazed, and convinced that I was powerfully endowed.

Not all the Free State was so drear as Reddersburg. My Higgs relations lived on farms in the the Zastron and Thaba 'Nchu districts, and we would spend many heavenly holidays with them, particularly with our beloved Uncles Willie and Jock. They were great horsemen, and did their best to make me reasonably proficient. When I came to England I couldn't help being amused by the stiff and stilted way the English ride, deliberately and laboriously lifting their bottoms every time the horse's back goes up while trotting. To the English, horse riding was a recreation, but in South Africa it was a means of transport. When the horse trotted you just naturally went up and down with it without exerting yourself. (And when I got to America I felt the same about the Americans' comportment on bicycles — they used them then for recreation rather than transport.) The sad thing I can't forget about horse-riding in South Africa, but it was a dreadfully sad thing, is that my sister Koekoe, who was always the jolliest of us, was severely thrown from her horse at Boomplaats and badly lacerated by a barbed wire fence. She never recovered properly from it, developed a bad heart, and died far too prematurely, after I had come to live in England.

My Higgs relations all spoke the Basuto language, Sesuto, as if it were their own; and I believe they enjoyed the company of the Basutos more than that of many of the Whites. Once I was sitting with Uncle Jock on the veranda when an old Basuto gentleman came by. Uncle Jock invited him to join us, and he told Uncle Jock something that amused him. He had passed by

Uncle Jock's mielie (maize) field, and found it so beautiful, 'I stood there and laughed for a long time.'

In Oxford on 3 October 1966, I read in *The Times* that there was to be a service the next day in the Roman Catholic Westminster Cathedral to commemorate the translation of the Crown Colony of Basutoland into the Constitutional Monarchy of Lesotho within the British Commonwealth of Nations. (The Roman Catholics had long been active as missionaries in Basutoland.) This was clearly something I should attend; and besides, I wanted to have a good look at the inside of the Cathedral, which I had not yet done, and wanted to, because it was a marvellous Victorian building, and the interior was said to be most beautiful too. The next morning I took the train to Paddington, the tube to Victoria Station, walked up Victoria Street, and turned right into Ashley Place, the little square in front of the Cathedral. Across the square I saw a little group of Black gentlemen on the steps of the Cathedral, wearing cut-away coats, striped trousers and top hats. So I did the polite thing. In Basutoland, if you see somebody in the distance, stranger or not, you give a hail of recognition. So I shouted the customary call-sign across the square: 'Eh-eh-eh-eh-heh'. Back came the same cry, signifying 'I am receiving you!' 'Dumehla morehna!' ('Good Day, Sir.') I cried. 'Sahpeeleh?' I continued, meaning 'How are you?' 'Eh hahntleh ah hooloo!' ('I am fine,') followed by a short pause, followed by a polite 'High ketsibi wehnah.' ('But I don't know how you are.') 'Eh hahntleh ah hooloo!' I replied. By this time the passers-by were looking startled. Then the Basuto speaker — he was the Lesotho High Commissioner in London — beckoned me to join them, and invited me to sit with them in the front row in the Cathedral. I was very happy to be so honoured, and to see the interior of that beautiful Cathedral in such exhalted circumstances.

Towards the end of 1928 I sat for the Matriculation examinations and passed first class, thus gaining a scholarship for further study. With the help of this, and a grant from the Freemasons' Lodge in Heilbron, I was able to go to university; so early in 1929 I went to the Cape Province to enter the University of Stellenbosch, where, as with all South African academical institutions, the academic year runs with the calendar year.

The Cape Province

To be translated in an overnight train from the dreadful provincialism of dreary Reddersburg to the abounding beauty of the Cape, and to all the new and broadening excitements of university life, was like being wafted from Hades to Elysium by the wave of a wand. The Cape landscape was physiographically so rich, with beautiful mountains and valleys, and so verdantly abundant. The first thing that struck me was a ditch near a railway siding full of beautiful white trumpet-like flowers which I was told were weeds called *varkblomme*, or pig flowers, but which I later learned in England were arum lilies, available only to brides with rich parents. There were great orchards and vast vineyards, which I'd never seen before. Thirty miles from Stellenbosch lay Cape Town, and its sea-side suburbs stretching north and south of it. All this, and the climate, were going to come to my mind again when I first saw the French Riviera twenty-five years later.

The town of Stellenbosch (Stel and Bosch) is the second oldest town in South Africa, having been founded by Simon van der Stel (whose wife had been a Mejuffrouw Bosch) in 1679, shortly after he became Commander of the Dutch East India Company's settlement in the Cape. The gunpowder house and the little church he built are still there, and the centre of the town is still largely composed of old Cape Dutch houses built not long after. The streets are lined with oaks, and the pavements are separated from the streets by deep wide stone-lined gutters carrying water from a reservoir, each household having its share of time for the water to be diverted to its garden by little sluice gates. It is just about the prettiest town I have ever seen, dignified by its age and seemliness. The country around is covered with vineyards producing excellent wines, although they were pretty dreadful when I tasted them thirty years ago. Since then the vintners have learned to reduce the temperature of their vats during fermentation.

In the town were three of my father's sisters: Marie Bauman, who was widowed, and who thought I was a scientific genius because I showed her (but could never teach her) how to switch on her bedside lamp by making sure the the wall switch was not off when she switched on the lamp switch, and vice versa; Mina Hoskyn, who was widowed, but had her two daughters with her, Boudina and Margaret — they had lived a long time in the Philippines and then in Torquay, before returning to South

Africa; Ada, married to Pieter van Braam, Professor of Latin in the University, and their daughter Boudine. I used to lunch with the van Braams almost every Sunday, and there was always red wine, which I'd never tasted before. I don't know whether it was domestic or imported, but I detested it because it tasted like ink. Aunt Ada was rather terrifying, at first. When the predikant called on her, and gave her a harrowing account of the Crucifixion, she is said to have said (but maybe others have said it too) 'Ag Meneer, dit is so ver verlée en so lang gelede, laat ons liewer maar vergeet'. ('But Sir, it was so far away and so long ago, hadn't we better forget it.') When I visited Stellenbosch in 1938 after an absence in England and the United States I took her for a drive in the country. We came to a very rough stretch of road, and Aunt Ada got irritable. She leaned out of the car and shouted to a terrified little picaninny, no more than eight years old, 'Hoekom is julle paaie so sleg?' ('Why are your roads so bad?'). The van Braams lived in a house called Walden, after the settlement they had lived in for a while in Holland, which was named after Thoreau's Walden. Next door lived Professor Berthault de St Jean van der Riet and his large family. I mention them in the context of my relations because they were practically relations. Harry van der Riet married my cousin Boudine van Braam on my father's side, Frank van der Riet married my cousin Mavis Morgan on my mother's side; and Professor van der Riet taught me organic chemistry, which made him practically an uncle to me. Mrs van der Riet was a very sweet woman of remarkable but unstudied gentility — one evening she had a number of the girls gathered about her in the drawing room, and in the course of conversation she said to them, 'Last night when — if you will excuse me for being so blunt — I was having my bath.'

For my first three years at Stellenbosch I lived in a student house called Wilgenhof (Willow Court), where one of my contemporaries was Danie Craven, the famous rugby player, and probably South Africa's greatest hero. He was intending to be a *tokkelok*, or theological student, and believed firmly that the earth was flat. Naturally, this idea offended me, and I would argue with him far into the night, but he remained firm. He countered all my arguments with the incontrovertible one that the Bible said the world was flat. But I liked him, and when I visited Stellenbosch in March 1984, and he was probably the most idolized man in a South Africa where rugby football is taken very seriously, I took up the matter again.

At Wilgenhof they had the horrible custom of initiating first-year men that is still practised today, and was indeed the subject of a scandalized article in *The Times* on 5 March 1985. It lasted for about three weeks, and was perfectly dreadful. We would be woken almost every night by a party of initiators wearing grotesque masks and speaking in high squeeky voices. They would insult us in various ways, then paint us with house paint, which we would have to spend the next hour scrubbing off under the cold shower. During the day one might be summoned at any time by any group of seniors who would humiliate one, for example by demanding that one told a joke, immediately; and if you don't think that is unfunny, just imagine yourself in a similar situation. Every once in a while we would be ordered to go out to the vineyards before dawn and steal grapes, and more than once did I hear the irate farmers' buckshot whizzing past my ears. (*The Times* refused my letter on this aspect of the initiation.) Then there would be a sadistic final ceremony, when we were tortured and insulted in various ways. Naturally, when I became a senior I delighted in having my turn at the torturing. Indeed I invented a torture which I now shiver to think of, since I might easily have killed someone. From the laboratory I borrowed a transformer for lowering the mains voltage progressively from 220 volts down to anything I wanted. From this I led two wires, one attached to a metal bicycle trouser clip and the other to a large zinc bath filled with water standing under a branch of a big oak tree in the courtyard. A pulley was attached to this branch, by means of which the victim was lowered into the bath, with the electrified bicycle clip attached to his arm. We started at a low voltage, raising it in steps until we judged the victim's cries were sufficiently anguished. I'm ashamed.

At the University I read Chemistry and Geology for the final examinations for the B.Sc. degree. If you read Chemistry for three years you had to read Physics for two years, and if you read Physics for two years you had to read Mathematics for the first year, all very logical; in addition you had to read one Arts subject for the first year, and I chose English. The lectures were given in English or Afrikaans, according to the preference of the lecturer. Thus I learned hard rocks in English, soft rocks in Afrikaans; algebra in Afrikaans; geometry in English; physics in Afrikaans; inorganic and physical chemistry in Afrikaans (except for Gibbs' Phase Rule in English); organic chemistry in English, with dearly beloved Professor Berthault de St Jean van der Riet. I loved it. And I loved examinations. I was a ghastly prig about them, but

I do think I kept my priggishness to myself. The fact was, I used to look forward to them, and on the first morning of the examinations I would wake up with a feeling of pleasurable expectation, like somebody looking forward to a tennis match; because to me the examinations were a contest, and I knew I was going to do well at them. Generally there were five questions, and we would have to answer any four of them. I would answer all five, and I would finish long before the others, being quite certain that I had done well. I would hang around for a while before leaving the room, not wanting to be too ostentatious about finishing so soon. My class mates would agonize afterwards over how badly they had done, but not I. I was insufferable. I didn't actually say I was sure I had done well, but I just couldn't pretend not to have, so I said nothing. And I had done well — I generally got, if not 120%, more than 100%. So I took my B.Sc. *cum laude*. The next year I worked for my M.Sc., specializing in research in organic chemistry under Professor van der Riet. He was very keen on the essential oils of the bushes growing in the surrounding mountains. He would take a tin still out there and steam-distil the oils out of them over a wood fire. He put me on to a study of a compound called diosphenol from the essential oil of the Buchu plant, Barosma betulina. I showed that it was not a phenol, but an enol, and I read a paper on it, the first one in my life, to the Cape Chemical and Technological Society, suggesting that since diosphenol, so called, did not come from a Diosma, but a Barosma, and was an enol, not a phenol, it should be called barosmenol. I don't know whether it ever took on.

One day we read in the *Cape Argus* that George Bernard Shaw, who had been visiting South Africa, and whom Professor van der Riet had met, was sailing back from Cape Town to England the next day in one of the Union Castle liners. It was also stated that he was suffering from a cold. So Professor van der Riet asked me to go to Cape Town the next day and give him a little bottle of Buchu oil, with the suggestion that if Mr Shaw would sprinkle some on his handkerchief, it might relieve the congestion he was no doubt suffering in his nose. So off I went the next day to the ship, asked the purser the number of Mr Shaw's cabin, knocked on the door, and there was George Bernard Shaw, beard, knee breeches, squeaky voice and all. 'Compliments of Professor van der Riet of the Department of Organic Chemistry, University of Stellenbosch, Mr Shaw,' I said, 'he suggests that if you would sprinkle some of this Buchu oil on your handkerchief it might relieve the congestion in your nose.' 'Thank you young man,' said Mr Shaw, 'and please thank the Professor.' Many years later Ruthie and I went to a party in London at Douglas Fairbanks Junior's, and as I was signing my name in the Visitors' Book, I found by my side the most beautiful, the most gloriously charming woman in the world. She was quite bewitching, and the fact that she was eighty-eight years old did not diminish her wonderful aura at all. I asked Douglas who she was, and he told me she was Cathleen Nesbitt, who had been a friend of Shaw's. I made it my business to find a seat beside her and said to her 'I do believe, Miss Nesbitt, that you and I are the only people in this room who have spoken to George Bernard Shaw'. 'Oh did you?' she exclaimed with courteous rapture, 'do tell me about it.' Like a fool, instead of asking her tell me about her encounters with him, I told her about my trivial experience.

When I went into the room for the final M.Sc. examination, there was no examination paper, but a statement written on the blackboard. It was brilliant; but it could not be done more than once a decade: 'Ask yourself three questions and answer them.' I loved it. Obviously you couldn't ask yourself easy questions, and I supposed the examiners would judge the questions at least as seriously as the answers. I took my M.Sc. *cum laude*.

All those four years I was having a lovely time with the many lovely girls you'd expect in a university town, until I fell deeply in unrequited love with Valerie Wilcox, who was not particularly beautiful. One reason why she did not reciprocate my love was that she was deeply in love with a poet (whom I liked), and her love in turn was not requited. So she turned to me for some kind of consolation, as from a fellow club member. It wasn't much, sympathising with each other, in fact it was painful, but it was inescapable, and it was something. I always did everything wrongly. One holiday she came to stay with us at Bougainvillea, and on the first day she told me that I must not mind if she was irritable. I must stay away and not ask questions; things happened to girls. I hadn't the foggiest idea what she meant, but I stayed away until I couldn't bear it any longer. When I approached her, she flew into a rage, telling me she had warned me. I said I didn't understand; she said I was a stupid ignorant fool. I still didn't understand what she was talking about, but knew I couldn't ask her, so was all the more miserable.

I continued to make ignorant mistakes with Valerie. Some time later I learned there was going to be a dance in Bloemfontein, tickets half a guinea. Valerie lived in Bloemfontein, in fact her father was Administrator of the Orange Free State, so I wrote and asked her if she would come to the dance with me. To my joy she agreed. I went up to Bloemfontein, and collected her at the Administrator's Residence, whence we were driven by his chauffeur to the hotel where the ball was. I was feeling quite rich, because I had twenty-five shillings in my pocket, more than enough for the ticket and the five-shilling supper. Then disaster struck. When I produced my half-guinea I was told that I needed two such for two people. In my limited provincial experience of these affairs hitherto, the price given for dances was always the price for two. That meant I had only four shillings left, not nearly enough for the supper, which of course was ten shillings for two. Valerie was furious with me for being such a yokel, and we spent the rest of the evening in silence, hers sullen, mine sad.

A year later Jack Coetzer's sister Betty came to me one day with the newspaper in her hand. 'Did you see this?' she said, giggling all the time. Valerie Wilcox had been killed by lightning riding her horse in the Drakensburg Mountains. Somehow I had the wit to understand that Betty's giggles were nervous.

The Transvaal

Soon after I took my M.Sc. I got a job on a Geological Survey team with the West Witwatersrand Areas, Ltd, a subsidiary of New Consolidated Goldfields. They were in the early stages of opening up the new gold-mining areas in the general neighbourhood of Welverdiend in the western Transvaal. The engineers had already triangulated the area with their theodolites; that is to say, they had divided the area into ten-mile triangles, as I remember, with beacons on all the intersections. Our job was now to go around these areas with plane tables and alidades and plot the contours every ten feet, filling in the more important geological features on the way. We had a great lorry for carrying us and our equipment and our household goods to our shifting camps. These camps were very comfortable. We each had a tent with a duckboard floor and a comfortable bed. Our meals, and enormous they were, were prepared by Black servants, and so were the improvised showers when we got home in the evenings. We walked about twenty, sometimes thirty, miles a day, making our measurements, and I would be amazed at our accuracy. For example, we would go up one side of a hill topped by a triangulation beacon and determine its height at, say, 5345.3 feet above sea level, and then approach the beacon from the bottom of the other side of the hill and find it at 5345.8 feet. The beacons were marked with big white-washed crosses for the aerial survey, but the cattle used to lick off the whitewash, there being a deficiency of calcium in the soil, so one of our responsibilities was to put barbed-wire fences around them.

After a few months I was transferred to a geophysical team doing a magnetometric survey. The gold-bearing conglomerate reef is underlain, or overlain, I can't remember which, by a stratum of magnetic iron ore, and our job was to go about and measure the declination of a compass needle mounted to swing vertically (rather than horizontally, as with an ordinary North-pointing compass) — the more sharply the needle pointed down, the closer was the magnetic iron ore, and therefore the gold-bearing reef. We were followed by the people putting down drill holes in order to take samples of the various strata underground. Their drill-rods were put together in twenty-two-foot lengths, as I remember. These would be pulled out and stacked every evening. As spying aircraft would fly over and count them, because the price of gold shares on the Johannesburg Exchange would depend on how deep the boreholes were, they had to be hidden.

It was a happy time. We enjoyed the entirely male company, and the energetic life combined with making precise measurements; we enjoyed the enormous meals we had when we got back to our camp; and we enjoyed making fun of a rather wet member of our team. We put out a story that on a visit to a nearby farm he had broken the farmer's plough, and so had been made to marry the farmer's daughter. We were too young to think of drinking. But after about six months I saw a chemical job advertised in the newspaper by the newly-founded Fuel Research Institute of South Africa in Pretoria, and I applied for it because I regarded myself more as a chemist than a geologist. I got the job, as Junior Research Officer, and went off to Pretoria. It was interesting work, not all research, more of it routine. I enjoyed the routine work, which in the laboratory consisted mainly of doing analyses and making tests on samples of coal gathered from various sources; but it would probably have become tedious in the long run. What I enjoyed more was the routine work outside the laboratory, collecting the samples of coal, for which purpose I was armed with an impressive Governmental Certificate empowering me to take coal samples from any face in any mine, and from any railway truck. I had two Black assistants who I am sure thought I must be mad, or sadistic. I would commandeer a very large sample of coal from a coal face or a laden truck, say about two hundredweight, and the trick then was to bring away a sample of only about five pounds. But the smaller sample had to be an accurate representation of the larger. This was achieved by getting my men first to break up the large sample into walnut-sized pieces. They would all be heaped up into a cone, and I would then get them to divide the cone into four equal parts by bisecting the cone, and then the two halves, so there would be four clumps arranged in a rough square. I would then get them to pull away two diagonally opposite clumps and discard them. Then we would mix the two remaining clumps into one cone, and repeat the process, and so on, until I was left with a conveniently sized sample. Naturally they thought I was mad — why not just take the first five pounds that came to hand? Within a few months our Director invented a far more satisfactory method, which also made more sense to the Blacks. He enclosed all but the bottom inch of the four-foot length of a one-inch bit of a power drill in a tube, with a side tube near the top end. This side tube was connected by means of a rubber hose to the collecting-bin of a vacuum cleaner. So I would take this contraption on to the top of a truck of coal and push it down, quite easily, to the bottom; or I would push it horizontally into a coal face down in a mine, and come away with a beautifully powdered half-pound sample of coal. Tests showed that this was in fact a more representative sample than that got by the more laborious method. I loved doing this, especially down in the mines, feeling important.

The reseach was to do with investigations into the possibility of liquefying coal underground by hydrogenating it and so turning it into a kind of petrol. We didn't make much progress, in my time at any rate. It was a process invented by the Russians, and I believe they are still working on it.

To my amazed joy in June 1934, I was informed by the University of Stellenbosch that I had won the Sir Donald Currie Memorial Overseas Research Studentship. It was awarded to the best M.Sc. student in the three years comprising my year, the preceding year, and the following year. That is why I heard the good news more than a year after I left Stellenbosch. I had had no idea it existed. It was worth a total of £450, to be spent over two or three years. I decided immediately I was going to do research on the Cause and Cure of Cancer, and I was going to do it in Vienna. I chose Vienna because I had learned from novels that that was where the great men did medical research. I had no conception of how little I knew about medical research, or about any kind of research, or about the world of learning.

It happened that at that time I was friendly with a girl whose mother was postmistress of Onderstepoort, the great Veterinary Research Institute a few miles away from Pretoria. At that Institute there was a Dr Claude Rimington, who was spending a sabbatical year from the Sir William Dunn Institute of Biochemistry at University of Cambridge; and who, the postmistress knew, had spent some time in Vienna. She told him about my intention to go to Vienna, and he invited me to come and see him. He told me the best place for me to go to was the Pearson Stiftung for cancer research. He arranged for me to go there, and to be enrolled in the University. The University sent me a list of student lodging houses, and I ran my finger down the right hand column of prices until I came to the cheapest, and I chose it. It was the Pension High Life in the Ringstrasse. Of course I was in heaven. My friend Mello MacRobert, a law graduate, and his cousin, young Adams, were going to Cambridge, so we arranged to travel together early in September in the Italian liner *Duilio*. The *Duilio* sailed from Cape Town to Genoa, touching at Dakar in Senegal, Gibraltar, and Marseilles on the way. For £22 they would deliver you, third class, to any city in Europe. Thus, if you were going to Paris, you disembarked at Marseilles and took the train, the *PLM* — the *Paris, Lyon, Marseille* — to Paris; if you were going to London you stopped in a hotel in Paris overnight and continued the next day by air from Paris, Le Bourget to London, Croydon; if you were going to Vienna you disembarked at Genoa and took the train. All this, including the hotel bill, for £22.

On 25 July Dolfuss, the Austrian Chancellor, was murdered in an attempted Nazi coup in Vienna. The Austrian Consul in Johannesburg telephoned me. 'Vienna is zee powter-keg of Europe!' he said; it would be madness to go there. So back I went to Claude Rimington. Why not go to Cambridge, he suggested, to the Sir William Dunn School of Biochemistry, under Professor Sir Frederick Gowland Hopkins? Cambridge! I couldn't possibly go there on £150 a year! And who was that stuffy old Sir Frederick Gowland Hopkins anyway? — I'd never heard of him! Claude Rimington explained and gently persisted, bless him. If I did well enough I could take a Ph.D. in Cambridge in two years, and so have £225 a year. So, having learned that Uncle Pieter van Braam was willing to lend me some money, I decided on Cambridge. But how to get in at this late stage? Rimington would try Caius College, because they had a medical tradition. Weeks passed, and Caius said no. So then Rimington suggested we try his College, Emmanuel. I was determined to sail with Mello MacRobert and young Adams on the *Duilio* on 6 September (I think it was), but there was no hope of hearing from Emmanuel before that date; so Rimington arranged for them to send me their answer to intercept the ship at Gibraltar. If it was yes, I would get off at Marseilles; if it was no I would sail on to Genoa for Vienna, powter keg or no.

So I left Pretoria for Cape Town at the end of August. I went to a party on my last night in Pretoria, and who should I meet there but Rosalie Shields, looking prettier than ever! She remembered my muddied face of fourteen years ago in Brandfort and forgave it, and we soon made up for that evaded opportunity.

2
CAMBRIDGE

Mello MacRobert, young Adams and I boarded the *Duilio* at Cape Town on 6 September 1934, and since the ship was not full, we were each given a second-class cabin for our fare of £22. We shared a table in the dining saloon with an American student, the first American I ever cast my eyes upon. I was fascinated by his way of speaking, and even more by a good-looking compatriate of his. Eleanor Knight she was, from California. She would come to me while I was leaning on the ship's rail smoking and say, 'Say honey, would you give me a drag?', which drag naturally I was always pleased to give. The sea voyage was unalloyed bliss from beginning to end. Our first port of call was to be Dakar, the capital of the French African Colony of Senegal, and I looked forward to my first sight of a foreign land. Our Italian waiters would tell us at every meal about the terrific girls they would get for us in Dakar, and we jollied them along. When we went ashore at Dakar I received a cultural shock, for there were those Blacks speaking fluent French! Damned cheek! For the first time in my life I began to realise what my sister Christina was talking about when she came back from Oxford with the strange idea that Blacks could be civilized too. It was very good for me.

The four of us at our table went ashore as quickly as we could, so that we could get away from the Italian waiters, because we were in fact scared stiff of the idea of the girls they threatened to get for us. We wandered about our first literally exotic city — and it really was something out of the world we were used to — marvelling at everything we saw, and after a few hours set off to return to the ship. As we neared it we were dismayed to be waylaid by our waiters, reinforced by some sailors. They hustled us with them to the whorehouse, dragging us there by the arm. When we got to it, it was set in a shady garden with a high wall on the street, just like the tropical whorehouses I had seen at the movies. We went in. We were greeted by the Madame, and she summoned her girls. In they came, white, and, I was dismayed to note, in equal number to ours, clothed (if that's the word) in minimal garments. The waiters and sailors took their picks. Then the American, after agonized hesitation, took his too. That left Mello, young Adams and me in the salon, with three young ladies, who seemed not to understand our reluctance to do business. We were just waiting for our friends, we said. One of them leaped onto Mello's lap. He was terribly embarrassed, but terribly polite. 'Oh no, no, please. No, please don't, please', he muttered frantically. I got up. 'It's time to go', I said as coolly as I could, 'let's just run like hell.' So we just ran like hell, down the shady garden path, with the ladies shouting behind us — rather angrily I thought. We leapt in unison over that six-foot wall, God knows how, adrenalin I suppose, then sat on the edge of the pavement in the broiling tropical sun, waiting for our American friend. He was the first to emerge, looking terrible. 'Oh God', he said, 'I'm going to get the claps', and I didn't care to ask him what the claps might be.

The lovely voyage continued northwards. People would ask me where I was going, and I'd reply I didn't know, maybe Cambridge, maybe Vienna, I really didn't know, but I'd tell them after Gibraltar. So we got to Gibraltar, and there I got my letter from Emmanuel College, Cambridge, telling me I would be admitted. I could hardly believe it. Everything that was happening to me was unbelievably marvellous. And what nicer companions could I have for my entry to Cambridge than Mello and young Adams! We saw everything there was to see in Gibraltar and sailed on, soon to dock in Marseilles. I fell in love with France instantly, and have remained so ever since. Le Vieux Port that I saw then was Le Vieux Port that I saw many years later in films of Marcel Pagnol's plays, *Fanny*, *Marius* and *César*. It was a real working port then, and not the shelter for pleasure craft it is now. All we had time for was a brisk walk up and down La Canabière, that runs from the port into the downtown city. It was to be a long time before I saw Marseilles again. We took the PLM to Paris, and spent the night in an hotel somewhere near the Gare du Nord. We spent a few hours wandering about the neighbouring streets looking at the sights, which in that area were neither interesting nor beautiful. I assumed that all Paris looked like that, and was disappointed.

The next morning Mello and young Adams went off to Le Bourget to take the flight to London, but I could not go with them. Owing to the uncertainty of my destination when we sailed from Cape Town, the flight was no longer open to me, and I had to take a cross-channel boat. As I was waiting in the front of the hotel a man with a briefcase came to me. 'You are Monsieur van 'Eynighen?', he asked. He explained that he was an agent of Italian lines, and had determined that I could fly after all, so if I would come immediately we would take a taxi to Le Bourget and I could join my friends. What service! For £22! So I got to Le Bourget in the nick of time, and there was the beautiful aircraft. The biggest aircraft I had ever seen! Imperial Airways' Handley-Page *Hengist*, an immense biplane made of horizontally corrugated aluminium, with four great engines in two pairs, one above the other. It was the sister ship of *Horsa*, and *Hannibal* (and an augury for the future? For I have been living in North Hinksey Village, Oxford, since 1955, and Hinksey is derived from the Anglo-Saxon *Hengest eg*, pronounced Hengist aye, and meaning Hengist's island). Tea with scones and cake was served by a steward, no air hostesses in those days, and we sat on padded wicker chairs at a wicker table. I was astounded at my first sight of England, and that from the air, divided as it was by hedges into thousands of minute fields; and as we circled in to land at Croydon, then Britain's premier airport, our circles seemed to be centered on a helmeted British bobby, exactly what I expected. We took a train from Liverpool Street Station to Cambridge, and when I arrived at Emmanuel College I was directed to my lodgings in Lyndewode Road; and was handed a note from Lady Hopkins, inviting me to tea the next day, Sunday, at Saxmeadham in Grange Road.

Professorial Sunday Afternoon Teas in Cambridge were grand affairs in those days. There were Sir Frederick and Lady Hopkins and their daughters, Barbara Holmes and Jacquetta Hawkes, and Sir Charles and Lady Martin, and a number of others, including a rather solemn agreeable young man, not much older than me, recently arrived as a refugee from Nazi Germany, called Hans Krebs. Lady Hopkins presided at her tea table, while we young men made ourselves useful. Hans Krebs handed around a silver *etagère* loaded with cakes, and I followed with a sugar bowl. Nobody took any of my sugar, and what with being overwhelmed by my first encounter with Knights and their Ladies, and not knowing how to address the Ladies (I thought I should use their first names too, but didn't know them), I concluded that having the sugar passed, but not accepting it, was the vestige of some ancient politeness, like saying, rather than asking, 'How d'you do', and I felt reluctantly obliged to go without sugar myself. After tea Hans Krebs took me to the Sir William Dunn Institute of Biochemistry, and I had my first sight of the inside of a real research laboratory. He showed me Warburg manometers containing very thin slices of animal tissue waving like corn in a field, and spoke to me about metabolism, glycolysis, and respiration. I hadn't the foggiest idea of what metabolism and glycolysis might be; and as to respiration, how could little slices of tissue in Warburg manometer vessels respire? I thought you needed lungs to respire.

The Sir William Dunn Institute of Biochemistry was at that time, and for many years to follow, the foremost biochemical research laboratory in the world. (Thank Heavens for the post-mistress's daughter at Onderstepoort!) Two members of the Institute had already won Nobel Prizes — Sir Frederick Gowland Hopkins for discovering the vitamins, and Albert von Szent Gyorgyi, who had left for America by the time I got there, for his work on Vitamin C. (After I left Cambridge, six more members of the Institute were to get it: Hans Krebs, Dick Synge, Fred Sanger (twice!), Roger Porter, Ernst Chain and Peter Mitchell.) And of course there were countless Fellows of the Royal Society. Hoppy told me once about how, when he was a newly qualified doctor at the London Hospital, he had seen his first case of Vitamin C deficiency, without realising it at the time, since he had not yet conceived the idea of vitamins. A sailor lay dying of scurvy, and his wife and children came to visit him for the last time, bringing with them an orange. After they left, the sailor ate the orange and almost immediately got much better; but as quickly relapsed and died.

The only member of the Laboratory that I in my ignorance knew anything about was J. B. S. Haldane, because he was quite famous, and I had read some of his essays. He had not long left the Laboratory, and I was amazed to hear Marjory Stephenson speak about him as if he were an ordinary person. (There was a story going about that some French Letters had been discovered in his bedroom, and he had been had up before the disciplinary body called the Sex Viri, who referred to these devices as 'erotic machines'; and because of the mirth that followed, that august body decided to enlist another member, so that they could change their name to Septem Viri.) Besides Marjory Stephenson (whom I mentioned on page 1) there were many other people on their way to distinction, including Robin Hill, Malcolm Dixon, Norman Heatley, Ernst Chain, Bill and Tony Pirie, and Joseph and Dorothy (or Dophi) Needham, and some other couples (in fact the Laboratory was known as 'Professor Hopkins' Matrimonial Agency', and indeed that is where I met my Ruthie just before the war, as I was to inform the Prince of Wales nearly half a century later).

I knew absolutely no biochemistry at all — my idea of biochemistry at that time was roughly what I now see as pharmaceutical chemistry, a kind of glorified pill-rolling. I was so ignorant, I didn't know how ignorant I was. I was so ignorant the people in the Biochemical Laboratory couldn't conceive how ignorant I was (and as a matter of fact that I can now admit, that ignorance never quite deserted me — I somehow managed to rub along for the rest of my scientific life without people really plumbing my ignorance).

On my first morning in the Laboratory, when I expressed to Professor Sir Frederick Gowland Hopkins my innocent determination to do research on the cause and cure of cancer, he listened to me with imperturbable courtesy, then suggested that perhaps I should have some experience of biochemical research before I embarked on the cancer problem. The best thing for me to do, he told me, was to start by working with Dr Dorothy Needham on the biochemistry of muscle. This was undoubtedly the best advice I have ever had in my life. That, and Claude Rimington's advice in the first instance to go to the Sir William Dunn Institute.

So I took Hoppy's advice, and went to work with Dorothy Needham on the biochemistry of muscle, with Hoppy as my research supervisor, which I took, and of course still take, as a great honour. I won't try to explain the work Dophi did, except to say that it was at that time one of the best routes to the understanding of many very important biochemical principles. We worked with frog muscle, and I worked hard, with great enjoyment. For the first time in my life I was doing real *research*. Many people nowadays, especially people in the advertising business, tell us about the research they do, but it is not research they do, it is making enquiries — they would probably call it research if they looked up a number in the telephone directory. But real research is a much more noble enterprise — it is using your head and finding out something important that was *not known before*.

I made it my business to get to the laboratory long before Dophi; so that by the time she came in the muscles were dissected out and ground in a mortar with a pestle, to make a muscle *brei* in order to study the chemical reactions going on in them. We worked together very well, and soon published a preliminary note in *Nature* (13 April 1935) on 'Linkage of

Chemical Changes in Muscle'. This was my first scientific paper, and it drew a pleasing response. For one thing, I received a request, *in Latin*, for an off-print of it from the Medical School of the University of Padua (the oldest Medical School in the World, but not the best); for another, I received a letter from one of the leaders of research in muscle biochemistry, J. K. Parnas of Lwof in Poland, inviting Dophi and me to a meeting in Brussels. Suddenly I was plunged into all this. It was glorious. Dophi and I flew in a little aircraft from a little airport in East Anglia (I think it might have been Stanstead) to Brussels. I don't remember much of the scientific proceedings (since most of them were over my head), except meeting the great and amiable J. K. Parnas, but I do remember the bidet in my bathroom. I had never seen or heard of one in my life, and I assumed, since we were on the Continent, that it must have something to do with sex, but I couldn't quite see what.

Dophi and I published a full paper in the *Biochemical Journal*, and then I went to work for a few weeks with Hans Adolph Krebs; and in those few weeks I did a lot of work, because Krebs worked one hard. He put me on to studying the inhibition of respiration in tissue slices by cyanide, and I worked from about 7 a.m. to 7 p.m., sometimes later. That resulted in another paper in the *Biochemical Journal*. Then I went to work with a very nice German refugee called Ernst Friedmann. It was hard work too, and it was organic chemistry, not biochemistry. One afternoon when I was alone in our laboratory a fire broke out. I managed to put it out, but burned my hand quite badly; and when dear old Friedmann came back to the laboratory and saw there had been a fire, and my hand was bandaged, his first question was, bless him, 'But did you save our product?' We published three not very interesting papers in the *Journal für praktische Chemie*.

Life in the Biochemical Laboratory was very pleasant, and always inspiring. We all had tea together in the Common Room every afternoon, presided over by dear old Hoppie; and on Tuesdays we'd have a 'Tuesday Tea', which was a meeting after tea, when a member of the Laboratory would give a paper on his work. Occasionally these were dull, but Hoppy had a genius for detecting some good in any paper, and would lead a lively discussion on it. He always brought out the best in everybody. He was a truly great man, and it followed as night follows day that he should be President of the Royal Society. I'll never forget one Saturday morning. I came out of my laboratory into the corridor, and there I saw a most wonderful sight. It was the slight figure of Hoppy, shuffling (as he always did) towards me. He was wearing shiny black shoes with big silver buckles, long black silk stockings, black velvet knee breeches, a kind of tailcoat with lots of embroidery on it, and a cockaded hat under his arm. With his silvery hair combed down the sides of his distinguished head, he looked perfectly splendid. But his face wore a worried expression. As soon as he saw me it lifted, and his face lit up. 'Ah, van Heyningen' he said, 'I'm so glad to see you — just the man I wanted to see. What shall I say to the Russian Ambassador this afternoon?' It's not every naive young colonial of twenty-four who's asked by the President of the Royal Society what he should say to the Russian Ambassador. I thought I must rise to the occasion, and asked him to outline his problem.

He was on his way to a reception in Buckingham Palace in his capacity as President of the Royal Society (hence the court dress, which the PRS used to wear in those days). He was bound to meet the Russian Ambassador there, and the Ambassador was bound to bring up the question of Professor Kapitsa's apparatus in the Royal Society Mond Laboratory. This was the time of the Kapitsa Affair. Kapitsa was a distinguished Russian physicist who had come to work in Cambridge, apparently for good; and the Royal Society had built him a special laboratory, the Mond Laboratory, in the court of the Cavendish Laboratory. It can be seen there today, with a handsome crocodile carved in the brick by the entrance, as a tribute of esteem and affection to Kapitsa, who was known to his friends as 'Croc'. Kapitsa had gone back to Russia for a holiday; but while he was there, the Russian Government had stopped him from returning to England, because they needed him in Russia.

As events were later to show, this turned out to have been a very good move on their part, because he did them great service during the War, and subsequently won the Nobel Prize; but at the time there was a great outcry about it. After some time the situation was accepted and the dust settled down. The Russian Government then began to negotiate with the British Government over purchasing Kapitsa's eguipment in the Mond Laboratory. Hoppy's problem was that he was afraid the Russian Ambassador was going to buttonhole him in the Palace and ask him what the Royal Society was doing about the negotiations, and he didn't want to discuss the matter without His Majesty's Foreign Secretary and the Royal Society's Foreign Secretary by his side. So what should he say to the Russian Ambassador that afternoon in Buckingham Palace?

'Well, Professor,' I said, 'why don't you tell him exactly what you've just told me?' A look of great relief came over Hoppy's face. 'What an excellent idea, van Heyningen!' he said, 'I can't tell you how much you've relieved my mind. I knew you'd be able to help me!' And off he shuffled, leaving me bursting with pride, and loaded with enough self-confidence to sustain me the rest of my life.

The three people in Cambridge who most affected my life at that time were Joseph and Dorothy Needham, and Marjory Stephenson. Joseph was, and still is even more so, an extraordinary man, filled with a vast and catholic range of restless interests, incapable (for example) of sitting down and reading a novel, let alone doing nothing at all (as I often do), yet blessedly endowed with a sense of humour. He was Reader in Biochemistry, and had published several books on philosophical topics, some of them to do with religion, and three fat volumes on Chemical Embryology, which was the subject of his research in the laboratory. He loved his food, and at breakfast would have at least half a dozen packets of different cereals on the table, and while he ate them, he would be tearing off the stamps from all the letters that had come in, and systematically arranging them in categories. He never wasted a moment. If he had to wait in the hall while Dophi was putting her hat on, he would make good use of the time by doing something that needed doing, like sorting out his card-index. We would drive around the country in his big open Armstrong-Siddeley looking for a nice tea-shop where we could get good scones and cakes. We used to go out with one or two other people to bathe in a water-filled gravel pit somewhere in the country, and the first time we went they all, except me, went in naked. I was secretly intrigued and pretended it was something I was perfectly used to. They urged me to take off my bathing trunks, but I pretended I needed them for retaining my cigarette case. On subsequent occasions I was not so shy, but terrified of my excitement becoming apparent.

Joseph and Dophi are somewhat older than me, and Marjory Stephenson was about fifty years old at the time; very handsome, and unmarried. She was an outspoken woman with a nice sense of humour, and quite well-off, with a beautiful house. She was a very distinguished scientist, having more or less invented the science of bacterial chemistry. Later she and Kathleen Lonsdale, the crystallographer, made history by being the first women to be elected, in the same year, Fellows of the Royal Society. (Queen Victoria had been a Fellow, but I doubt if she was elected, since you can hardly subject the Monarch to *election*. In Oxford we don't give Honorary Degrees to Heads of State — we can't presume to *honour* such personages — we give them Degrees by Diploma.)

While I was having a delightful time in the Laboratory, I was also having a lovely time in College, and in Town. During my first year I lived in lodgings in Lyndewode Road, a rather crummy street near the station. I was dismayed by the houses in this street, and in the suburbs of Cambridge — they all looked the same. Blocks and blocks of them, detached and semi-detached. Even worse were the long rows of terraced houses. I had never seen anything like that in sparsely populated South Africa, where all the houses had been separate and different from each other. It seemed to me that there was something unedifying and almost degrading about this sameness and lack of individuality of these English houses, as if their inhabitants had no imagination or souls of their own. I took me some time to get used to them, and now of course I like them. In my lodgings in such a semi-detached house I had, like all students, a sitting room of my own as well as a bedroom, and a landlady who brought me my breakfast, and my supper when I was not dining in Hall in College. I fear I may have been rather beastly to her. I remember complaining to her once about something in my room being dirty, and she told me she didn't see what I had to complain about; her last gentleman had been a prince and he never complained. It turned out it was an Indian prince, so I, being a not yet completely reformed South African, sneered and said well he wouldn't have known any better, would he.

In my second year I moved to a set of rooms in the oldest (late 16th century) part of Emmanuel right by Christopher Wren's beautiful chapel and cloister, and there I lived like a prince. When I tell today's students how we lived in College in those days, they don't believe me. I had a tiny bedroom, in the monkish austerity of which I revelled; a gyp room with a sink, a draining board and a gas-ring; and a large living room with a coal fireplace and a floor that sloped at a marked angle. In the mornings I would be woken up by my bedmaker, who would leave a copper ewer of hot water outside my bedroom. I would shave, walk down two flights of stairs in my dressing-gown, across a quadrangle (or court, as we call them in Cambridge), down a tunnel under the road to another court, across that court and into the bathroom where there were a dozen or more immense baths. I would go to a bath filled with hot water, with a college servant waiting for me beside it, with a large towel over his arm. After my bath he would hand me my towel and I would dry myself and walk back to my bedroom to dress. Then I would go into my sitting room, where a fire would be roaring in the grate, and my breakfast would be waiting for me, porridge, eggs and bacon, or a kipper, under a huge silver-plated cover, toast, marmalade and coffee, and the *News Chronicle*. Then I would go off to the Laboratory. If I were to come back within an hour I would find the room all cleared and cleaned and fresh coals in the grate, waiting for a match. If I wanted to, I could invite people to breakfast, lunch or dinner. For these latter meals I would consult the chef about the main course, but always the butler for the pudding and the wine. In those days there used to be a lot of entertaining at breakfast, and dons would often have their pupils.

I have been fortunate in having had the best of both worlds – the New World of South Africa and the Old World of Europe. It was far more exciting to come to the Old World at a modestly mature age, and in a fairly unsophisticated state, than to have been born there, used to it all. I was astonished and delighted by the antiquity and the beauty of the buildings of the Colleges and the University. They were blackened by centuries of soot, which seemed to enhance their authority. This was my first experience of the beauties of artifice and the majesty of antiquity.

At the backs of these buildings there flowed the River Cam, and on the banks of the Cam there lay the beautiful meadows and gardens of the Backs. And the autumn, 'Season of mists and mellow fruitfulness, close bosom-friend of the maturing sun', especially a mild autumn with an occasional nip in the air, was the best time for a young colonial to arrive in England for the first time. There was a gentle, cosy, feeling of mellowness and calm in the air, spiced with hints of indefinable pleasurable expectancy. I was being subjected to a continual series of delightful and inspiring amazements. And there was an astonishment of another nature, within three days of my arrival: I was taken to see an intercollegiate rugby match, and as we arrived at the playing field I was startled, and the shades of my *Nederduits Gereformeerde* ancestors outraged, by an immense full-blooded upper middle class roar: KILL HIM JEEZE-ZUZ!!! – I didn't know there was a college called Jesus.

And there were social pleasures. Cambridge was full of ravishing girls, every one of them desirable. Many of them served in the numerous cafés and teashops where we spent much of our time, to their satisfaction as well as ours. They were all middle-class girls, serving in a delightful tearoom called The Waffle on Petty Cury, and in The Whim on Trinity Street, and in Tullivers Tea Room on Pembroke Street; or if you wanted music, there was the Dorothy, with its four-piece orchestra, but the waitresses were older, there for the job, not the boys. These delights don't exist any more.

I also had a social life outside Cambridge, owing to the kindness of Lady Frances Ryder and Celia MacDonald of the Isles. They were concerned to maintain the bonds of the British Empire, and their way of doing this was to see that Cambridge students from the Empire overseas should receive hospitality from the gentry in the neighbourhood of Cambridge (I don't know whether they also operated in Oxford at that time). We colonials would be invited at first to a grand tea party in the house of one of these ladies at Trumpington on the outskirts of Cambridge, and this would then lead to our being invited individually to spend week-ends in the country houses of the gentry. They were kind to us, and I enjoyed myself, except that I was never sure that I was wearing the right clothes, and would hope they would not notice that the tweed coat and trousers I was trying to pass off as a suit did not in fact match exactly. The only thing I can remember about these house parties is being taken out in a car with several other people, and being rather squashed in the back. Our host shouted over his shoulder to ask if my legs were comfortable, and I shouted back, 'Oh yes, thank you Lord Soandso, especially the left one'. It was at one of these house parties that I met Barbara Hunt, and I took a fancy to her, and she perhaps to me, and we went with a party on a skiing holiday in the Bavarian Alps in the winter of 1935, and held hands all night in the train coming back.

Towards the end of 1936 all kind of things happened. I submitted my thesis for the Ph.D., was examined *viva voce* by Hans Krebs and Barbara Holmes in the gardens of Downing College, and got the degree. I applied for a Commonwealth Fund Fellowship and got it. These were very grand Fellowships, America's answer to the Rhodes Scholarships, and I don't mind admitting that I was very lucky indeed to get one. I was never so rich again. The Fellowship was for two years in America, and carried a stipend of $3000 a year, at that time worth £600 a year (say £15-20,000 today?), more than twice my income in Cambridge. In fact I still have the receipts of the various bank draughts I sent from New York to Uncle Pieter van Braam in Stellenbosch in 1938 in repayment of the money I had borrowed from him to go to Cambridge. In addition, the Commonwealth Fund had the thoughtful notion of giving us each £60 to buy a complete new set of clothes before setting off; and of advising us not to wear heavy clothes on arrival in New York, since it was likely to be hot. As soon as I heard that I had won the Fellowship I rushed off to book myself a third-class passage from Southampton to New York on the brand new *Queen Mary*, then the world's biggest ever ocean liner; but the Commonwealth Fund told me to cancel it because I was to travel first class, not on the *Queen Mary* out of Southampton, but on the *Laconia* out of Liverpool.

That was not the end of the excitements that year. Marjory Stephenson invited me to go with her and Dophi Needham on a tour of the Union of Soviet Socialist Republics, at her expense. I felt a bit of a kept man accepting this generosity, but Marjory convinced me that I would be useful to them, and that she could easily afford it. So off I set with these two splendid women, at the end of Trinity Term, 1936. We went by train, via Berlin and Warsaw, first to Kiev, then Kharkov in the Ukraine. In Kharkov we visited a distinguished physicist in his high-energy laboratory, at that time producing a higher voltage than any other high-voltage laboratory in the world. As we sat in his office, I looked out of the window to a muddy field where there was a very ragged peasant urging his donkey to pull a two-wheeled cart through the mud, and as I looked, a wheel fell off. The combination of this dejected peasant scene and the world-record high voltage epitomised Russia for me. After Kharkov we went to Rostov and Ordzhonikidze, then southwards to Tiflis in Georgia and Erivan ('in the shadow of Mount Ararat') in Armenia, and finally to Moscow. Of course it was intensely interesting, and we enjoyed ourselves, especially since we were among the earlier visitors to the Soviet Union, but I do not seem to have anything to add to what many travellers have already recorded. We returned to England via Warsaw, where Joseph joined us on the train. He was full of news that had, not surprisingly, escaped us in Moscow, that Stalin had just embarked on the first of his bloody purges.

After our return to Cambridge, and very shortly before I sailed for America, I saw Barbara Hunt again. I was still quite soft on her, and invited her to come to breakfast in my rooms in Emmanuel (nowadays students invite girls *to stay* for breakfast). That breakfast ended on a fine note, for just as it was about to end there was a tap on my door, and in came the Master of

Emmanuel, Tim Hele, to invite me, there in front of Barbara Hunt, to put in a thesis for a Research Fellowship of the College. Subsequently I put in for that Fellowship and did not get it, but what did that matter later, compared with the circumstances of the invitation to apply?

3
AMERICA

I sailed from Liverpool in September 1936, with several other Commonwealth Fellows, and some of the Boston gentry, in particular some Cabots (who spoke only to God, and to whom only spoke the Lowells). Before getting to New York we were going to call at Boston. The voyage, as testified by the crew, was exceptionally rough, but that did not bother me, since fortunately I have good sea legs; but it bothered some of the passengers, so much so that they were convinced we were about to sink, and begged the Captain to admit it, so that they could put true conviction into making their peace with their Maker. However, we reached Boston safely, and I viewed it from the ship's rail with interest, because my destination, Harvard University, was in Cambridge, Massachusetts, just across the Charles River from the city of Boston; but first we had to go to New York City to be inducted by the officials of the Commonwealth Fund.

The pleasures of my life continued to multiply. Nowadays it is granted only to seamen on cargo vessels and rich people on cruise liners to sail into New York harbour, but in those days everybody who went from Europe to New York did it, and there were few finer experiences. If you are in New York, it is an experience you can reproduce in a passable fashion by taking the ferry from the foot of Manhattan Island to Staten Island, and back again to Manhattan. For many years, and even when I last took the trip about six years ago, it was the biggest bargain in America at a mere nickel, five cents; but I believe nowadays it may be as much as a dollar, still an excellent bargain; but still not as good as the virginal experience of sailing into New York harbour from abroad for the first time. I had that wonderful experience. And at that time skyscrapers were a wonder, largely confined to Manhattan Island, at any rate certainly not to be seen and wondered at anywhere else but in America. Skyscrapers are to be seen all over the world now of course, but most cities don't look any the better for them. The reason for that is that the skyscrapers rise in scattered isolation above their lower neighbours like so many sore thumbs. But Manhattan, and a few other cities, like Chicago and Hong Kong, are magnificent, and the reason for that is that their skyscrapers are grouped closely together, making their own elevated skyline. This has led me to formulate a Principle of Categorical Propinquity, which states that every skyscraper must be built next to, or across the street from, another skyscraper. To this I would add the rider that such a skyscraper city should preferably lie on the edge of an expanse of water, as do Manhattan, Chicago and Hong Kong.

In New York City we met the officials of the ever-generous Commonwealth Fund at their headquarters on East 57th Street, and were taken to lunch at Giovanni's on East 55th Street. Lunching well with the Commonwealth Fund at Giovanni's was subsequently to be a frequent pleasure. Back at headquarters it was explained to us that the reason why the Fellowships were for two years was that it would take us the best part of the first year to get to understand and know America and the Americans, so the second year was there for us to profit from this understanding and enjoy ourselves. We were also told, and it amounted to an order, that we were expected to travel all over the United States in the long vacation between the two years, and it was suggested that this was best done in a second-hand automobile.

After two or three days in New York I went to Harvard University in Cambridge, Massachusetts. I arrived there wearing an Emmanuel College blazer with its rampant lion on the breast pocket. This was slightly embarrassing, since banners bearing this same device were fluttering all over Harvard, for they were celebrating the Tercentenary of their Foundation by John Harvard, an Emmanuel man, whose rooms are still to be seen in Emmanuel. Harvard has a number of Houses, comfortable to live in, but little more than places to live in, whereas the Colleges of Oxford and Cambridge are self-governing republics, independent of the University, yet working with it.

I had been assigned to John Winthrop House, and had generously been given the Visiting Professor's set of comfortable rooms, with my own private bathroom of course (shades of the Emmanuel's distant public bathrooms!). Almost immediately I made a fool of myself: a man was putting my name on a board carrying the names of the inhabitants of my staircase, and he had me down as W. E. van Heyningen. 'I am *Doctor* van Heyningen' I told him haughtily. He gave me an old-fashioned look. 'Have it your own way' he said laconically, and added the Dr. It was only some days later that I learned that at Harvard *nobody* called themselves Doctor, or Professor, and that I was already being honoured by having the first initials placed before my surname rather than after, as was the case with all the other inhabitants of my staircase.

I had chosen Harvard because I had not abandoned my intention of doing research on the cause and cure of cancer; and having learned some biochemistry, I was now prepared to take it up. By that time I had learned that certain types of cancer could be caused by carcinogens — cancer-producing substances. The best-known of these carcinogens was methylcholanthrene, which had a cyclopentanophenanthrenoid structure. In a simpler word, a steroid structure. (Please don't be put off by these unbeautiful words — I have to use them, but I think you will be able to follow my drift without understanding them.) Some of the sex hormones also have a steroid structure, and I had developed a theory that as one aged, and if one were so unfortunate, the good steroid sex hormones might be converted in the body to evil steroid carcinogens. I had postulated an intermediate compound between good and evil, and my reason for choosing Harvard was that Professor Louis Fieser worked there, and he was a great steroid expert. My intention was to synthesise my postulated intermediary in his laboratory, and then treat it with animal tissues and see whether it would be converted into a carcinogen. When I arrived at Harvard, there was a chemical laboratory waiting for me in Fieser's Converse Memorial Laboratory for Organic Chemistry in Cambridge, and a biochemical laboratory in Professor Joseph Aub's department in the Cancer Hospital, then hard by the Harvard Medical School in Boston.

I started in the Converse, with Fieser's wife, Mary, keeping a helpful eye on me. I made the first step on the way to my hypothetical intermediate, but couldn't get it to crystallize, so Mary came to my aid. She dissolved my amorphous material in benzene, cooled the solution in ice, and out came enormous great crystals, and a triumphant smile on Mary's face. I had a problem. How to remind Mary that benzene itself crystallized on cooling? Nothing daunted, Mary started again, this time dissolving my amorphous material in acetic acid. On cooling, out came enormous crystals and another smile on Mary's kind face. Same problem, how to remind Mary that acetic acid also crystallized by itself on cooling? In the end I managed to make my material come out in very small crystals, but failed in all my attempts to take it to the next stage. It seemed to me then that that instead of guessing about how steroids might be metabolised in the body, I should first learn something about the metabolism of steroids, and there was nobody better qualified to guide me on these lines than Rudolf Schoenheimer in the Department of Biological Chemistry at the College of Physicians and Surgeons of Columbia University in New York. So with everybody's agreement I arranged to be transferred to his department, and sometime about the middle of 1937 I sailed for New York.

Indeed I sailed. In those days it was cheaper to travel from Boston to New York by boat than by train, and it was much more fun, and more comfortable, and it saved time because you did all your travelling during your night's sleep. I boarded the boat at Boston at about 11 pm, spent the night sleeping in a large comfortable cabin, sailing across Cape Cod Bay, through Cape Cod Canal and Buzzards Bay, and down Block Island Sound and Long Island Sound. I woke up somewhere near the East River, had a large breakfast and the choice of the *New York Times* (for Democrats) or the *New York Herald Tribune* (for Republicans), all included in the price of the fare, and stepped ashore at the foot of Manhattan Island at about 9 am, with the full day ahead of me. I was lucky — you can't travel between New York and Boston that way any more.

I made my way up to the College of Physicians and Surgeons at 630 West 168th Street, down from the corner with Broadway, on the left bank of the Hudson River near the great George Washington Bridge at the upper end of Manhattan Island. I was going to live for the next few weeks in Bard Hall, a hall of residence of the College, across 168th Street. The College was an immense complex of skyscrapers, and indeed I moved more vertical than horizontal distance from my room in Bard Hall to my laboratory. I was happy to be in New York City, and quite correct in thinking that I was going to enjoy myself all the time I was there.

Rudolf Schoenheimer had recently gained well-deserved fame through his use of isotopes in the study of intermediary metabolism. Forgive me if I explain metabolism and isotopes. Metabolism is the process by which the animal or vegetable organism, or the cells in these bodies, or unicellular organisms like microbes, build up nutritive material into living matter, or break up living matter into simpler substances; intermediary metabolism is the individual steps in this process. Up to Schoenheimer's time the way these processes were studied was, roughly speaking, to provide a more than usual amount of substance A to an experimental animal, or a tissue preparation derived from it, and see if a more than usual amount of substance B was produced. (When Schoenheimer's former chief at Freiburg University, dear old Ludwig Aschoff, came to visit us, Schoenheimer explained this principle to him. 'Yes I see,' nodded Aschoff sagely, 'when you put a penny in a slot machine and a bar of chocolate comes out, you conclude that copper is converted into chocolate.') Isotopes had been discovered by Frederick Soddy in Oxford (where he was a friend of Ruthie's uncle Noel Garrod Thomas) in 1913, and he had been awarded the Nobel Prize in 1921. They are forms of individual elements (such as hydrogen, oxygen, carbon, lead, etc) having identical chemical properties, but different atomic weights. (Some of the isotopes are radioactive, such as that of lead.) The isotope Schoenheimer was using was the hydrogen isotope, deuterium, the recent discovery and concentration of which by Harold Clayton Urey at Columbia University had won him the Nobel Prize in 1934. It is one of the three isotopes of the element hydrogen (H), which is a mixture consisting of protium (P, atomic weight 1), mixed with a small amount of deuterium (D, atomic weight 2), and an even smaller amount of radioactive tritium (T, atomic weight 3). Hydrogen being the lightest of the elements, the difference in atomic weights of protium and deuterium and tritium is the most marked. Thus it is that the specific gravity of 'heavy water' is quite a lot higher than that of plain water, so much so that while one cubic centimetre of plain water (H_2O) weighs one gram, one cubic centimetre of 'heavy water' (D_2O) weighs 1.1074 grams. Heavy water was being obtained at that time from Det Norske Hydroelektriske Aktieselskab at the price of $35 per gram (or put it another way, $38.76 per cubic centimetre), and the deuterium from it was being incorporated in various compounds of biological interest, and the metabolism of these was being studied. If you 'labelled' substance A with deuterium and fed it to an animal, and then isolated substance B from the animal, and found it contained deuterium, that was as good a proof as anyone could expect that substance A was metabolised by the animal into substance B. The deuterium in a substance was determined by burning the substance in a suitable apparatus, trapping the carbon dioxide and water that was formed, and very accurately determining the specific gravity of the water of combustion. The higher this was, the higher was the deuterium content. With the help of Fred Rosebury, the laboratory instrument-maker (who will appear again), I devised a means of accurately dispensing small drops of water for this purpose. Then, following a lead from a paper in a journal with the unpromising name of *Memoirs and Proceedings of the Manchester Literary and Philosophical Society,* I found a way of substituting a large amount of deuterium for the protium in fatty acids. The final test was to be done one afternoon when I was due to be with the great Peyton Rous at the Rockefeller Institute on the other side of Manhattan Island, so I jokingly suggested to Rittenberg that if I had succeeded in exchanging more than half the hydrogen atoms, he should telephone me in Peyton Rous' laboratory. That's exactly what happened — I'd exchanged 87.5% of them. I published this useful trick, with Schoenheimer and Rittenberg, in the *Journal of Biological Chemistry*; and after the war I learned from Rittenberg that during the war the U.S. Government, shutting the stable door after the horse had gone, had declared that paper to be an Official Secret, something to do with the Atomic Bomb (see below).

I was unable to incorporate deuterium in steroids in the same way; and so was unable to make any studies of steroid metabolism; and so it was that I gave up my ambitions to do research on the cause and cure of cancer, which, as far as my scientific career was concerned, was a blessing. But that did not stop me from having a profitable time at P & S (as the College of Physicians and Surgeons was called). The laboratory was filled with very clever and likeable young Jews, one of them, Conrad Bloch, a subsequent Nobel Prize winner. Apart from myself, the only non-Jew was the Chairman of the Department, Hans Clarke, a distinguished organic chemist who spoke English like an Englishman. One day he set off for the Rockefeller Institute, telling us he was bringing back the great Phoebus Apollo Levine (I *thought* those were his first names, but it was hard to believe, for P. A. Levine was just about the ugliest man I ever saw). Hans Clarke wanted all of us on our best behaviour. About ten minutes before they arrived, somebody dropped a glass flask containing a large amount of dimethyl sulphate, which is a very toxic substance. Frantic scrubbing ensued, and mopping up was still in progress as the great man arrived. Somebody whispered the news to Clarke. 'What's happening? What's happening?' demanded P. A. Levine. 'Oh nothing, nothing', replied Clarke, 'just some dimethyl sulphate dropped on the floor.' 'DIMETHYL

SULPHATE? *DIMETHYL SULPHATE*!!' roared P. A. Levine. 'You do not drop a *BABY* on the floor!!'

The Heavy Hydrogen technique had its limitations, which were that unless the deuterium label were placed in certain unreactive parts of the molecule, well away from the more reactive parts, it would wander off. By this time another isotope was coming into use — heavy nitrogen; and heavy oxygen was hovering in the wings. The concentrations of these isotopes were determined by means of the mass spectrometer, an apparatus that had been devised in Oxford several years previously by another friend of Ruthie's Uncle Noel, Francis William Aston. There were not more than a dozen or so of them in the world, so we had to make our own at P & S. It incorporated an immense electromagnet by means of which the isotopes of an element could be pulled apart and separately measured with sophisticated instruments. My job in all this was to help hang onto the miles of copper tubing (through which cooling water was eventually to be passed) that were being wound into the enormous electromagnetic coil.

The use of the nitrogen isotope, and the prospect of other stable isotopes, greatly enlarged the scope of the isotopic technique, and led to fruitful results. Very soon after I arrived back in Cambridge, I was invited by the Chemical Society in London to take part, with G.von Hevesy, in a discussion on the application of isotopes to biological research, which was then a completely new subject in England, and I, I suppose, the only exponent of it. von Hevesy was to speak about natural radioactive isotopes, such as those of lead, which had rather limited biological applications, and I was to talk about the stable isotopes, hydrogen and nitrogen, and the hopes for others. I was also asked by H. Munro Fox, the Editor of *Biological Reviews*, to write a review on Stable Isotopes as Indicators in Biology [36]. In this review I naturally mentioned the limitations that were inherent in the heavy hydrogen technique due to the difficulties in placing the heavy hydrogen atoms in unreactive parts of the molecule where they would not wander away; and of course I discussed the other stable isotopes. Naturally I sent a copy of my typescript to Schoenheimer at the same time. Then Munro Fox told me that he had had a cable from Schoenheimer asking him to desist from publishing my review. Shortly after that I got a letter, not from Schoenheimer, but from Hans Stetten (one of his group), telling me I was a scoundrel. They were upset about my remarks on the limitations of the heavy hydrogen technique. I was dumbfounded. After all, I had often discussed these limitations with Schoenheimer and his colleagues at P & S, and there had never been any disagreement. My two years at Cambridge had taught me to believe that the best compliment you could pay a colleague was objectively to criticize his work, but now my faith in the acceptability of scientific impartiality was shaken. Munro Fox stuck to my guns, and the review was published without alteration.

A few years later there was to be a sequel to my experience with the nitrogen isotope and the application of Aston's mass spectrometer. During the war I was doing a war job in the Wellcome Physiological Research Laboratories in Beckenham. It is a component of the Wellcome Foundation, which embraces, among other institutions, the Burroughs Wellcome laboratories and factories in Dartford. I began to speculate on the future possibilities of using stable isotopes in biochemical research in Great Britain. It seemed impossible at that time for individual laboratories to have the costly facilities for concentrating and for estimating these isotopes, and I concluded that any project to make use of them should be organized on a centralized national basis. I went to my chief, J.W.Trevan, and suggested that the Wellcome Foundation should undertake such a project, since it was well-organized and efficient, wealthy and altruistic. The Burroughs Wellcome establishment would concentrate the isotopes by the Clusius diffusion method and incorporate them in suitable compounds; these would be provided, free, to suitably qualified applicants; they would then do their experiments, isolate the metabolic products and send them for free isotopic analysis to the Wellcome Physiological Research Laboratories, where a mass spectrometer would be installed. Trevan liked the idea and encouraged me to look into it in more detail. So I went to visit physicist friends in the Cavendish laboratory in Cambridge to get their advice on the Clusius process and the mass spectrometer. As soon as I mentioned the idea to them they shut their faces and shuffled their feet. They insisted that I suppress my plan and wait, because new developments would overtake the idea I had proposed. They refused to discuss the matter any further. I went away mystified and dejected.

A few months later the atomic bomb was dropped and their secret revealed. It was that in the development of the bomb methods had been devised to produce artificial radioactive isotopes of many elements, including carbon, hydrogen and oxygen (but not nitrogen). It was far easier to make these new radioactive isotopes than to concentrate the natural stable ones, and what was even more important, it was far easier and quicker to estimate them with Geiger Counters than with mass spectrometers.

After a few weeks of living in Bard Hall in the remote and dreary upper reaches of Manhattan Island, I moved downtown to Greenwich Village. I found a pleasant two-room apartment on the second (third in the States) floor of a small apartment house (now alas demolished and replaced by the New York University Law School) on the unfashionable South side of Washington Square, just off the axis of the triumphal arch at the foot of Fifth Avenue. There was a fine view of the the Square from my sitting room window, and of the arch and the handsome old and expensive houses on the opposite side. The apartment was unfurnished, but it was easy to buy all that I needed, and liked, at Macy's at a price I could readily afford. The old Brevoort Hotel, long since gone, was on Fifth Avenue just beyond the triumphal arch, and from time to time on a summer's evening I would dine there for seventy-five cents, in a hedged enclosure outside on the sidewalk, treating myself to a glass of Graves, imagining I was a man of the world. In the mornings I would take the 8th Avenue Express Subway a few blocks away at 14th Street, and get whizzed up to 168th Street and Broadway, right by the Armory Bar & Grill, in no time at all, ready to start the day's work in the laboratory by about 8.45 am. I led a double life that suited me well: during the day at P & S in the company of those bright and amiable Jewish scientists; at the end of the day down in the Village in the company of equally bright, less ambitious, Gentile non-scientists. There was an always out-of-work, always amusing actor, Gerrit Kraber. His last play had been 'Casey Jones', the railroad engineer, or engine-driver as we would say. He would play his banjo and sing us a long ballad that began:

> Come all you rounders, for I want you to hear,
> The story of a brave engineer.
> Casey Jones was the rounder's name,
> On a big eight wheeler of mighty fame.

Casey Jones dies trying bravely to prevent an accident, and the ballad ends:

> Mrs Casey Jones was a sittin' on the bed.
> Telegram comes that Casey's dead.

She says, 'Children, go to bed, and hush your cryin'
'Cause you've got another pappy on the Frisco line'.

He had another song I liked:

Whiskey! Rye whiskey!
It's whiskey I cry.
If a tree don't fall on me
I'll live till I die.

If the ocean were whiskey,
And I were a duck,
I'd dive to the bottom
And never come up.

But the ocean ain't whiskey,
And I ain't a duck,
So I'll play Jack o' Diamonds
And trust to my luck.

Whiskey! Rye whiskey!
It's whiskey I cry.
If a tree don't fall on me
I'll live till I die.

He had a beautiful wife, Willie, who was a truly devoted school teacher. There was a brilliant New York University economist called Patterson, and his wife, and a bevy of marvellously attractive and always beautifully dressed girls who had jobs such as being buyers for Lord & Taylor and Saks Fifth Avenue. I used to pinch myself and think about Reddersburg.

Halfway between uptown and downtown New York, in fact at 60th Street and Lexington Avenue, I had another friend, Margery Clarke, with whom I would spend many a happy Sunday afternoon in Hickory House, somewhere mid-town, sitting at an enormous oval bar that enclosed a band we admired. We would spend two or three hours there, and I suppose we must have had something to drink, but I can't think what — I certainly did not drink much alcohol in those days. And we would spend a lot of time in the cinema blissfully looking (three times round once) at Fred Astaire and Ginger Rogers. Margery was by then a very dear friend, so much so that she became the subject of an investigation in the New York Public Library twenty-eight years later, as we shall see eventually.

The time came for the mandatory tour of the United States of America. So sometime towards the end of summer 1937, another

Commonwealth Fellow, Gordon Stephenson, and I set off from Washington. Gordon Stephenson was an architect, then studying city planning at the Massachusetts Institute of Technology in Cambridge, Mass., now living in Perth, in Australia, after a career of great distinction. We started our journey from Washington, in his Ford V8 coupé with a rumble seat. While I was at Harvard, I had bought the car second-hand for $280, with a new set of tyres, and had sold it to him when I moved to New York. (In case you're wondering, a coupé [pronounced coop] was a two-seater with a folding roof; and a rumble seat was a folding-down seat behind the roof, exposed to all weathers.)

Our first night was in Wheeling, West Virginia; then we drove through Ohio, on red brick roads that curved over the rolling green countryside. Now, when I tell Americans about those red brick roads in Ohio, they simply don't believe me. We drove through Columbus and Springfield to Cincinnati (in Ohio, not Iowa). (A man once rushed to the ticket counter in Grand Central Station in New York, crying 'Quick! Quick! Give me a ticket to Springfield!' 'Springfield, Colorado; Springfield, Illinois; Springfield, Kentucky; Springfield, Massachusetts; Springfield, Minnesota; Springfield, Missouri; Springfield, Ohio; Springfield, Oregon; Springfield, South Dakota; or Springfield, Vermont?' asked the ticket clerk. 'Whichever is the cheapest' replied the man.) The reason why we went to Cincinnati was that Gordon Stephenson was interested in a new *avant garde* housing development there. It is to him that I owe my amateur interest in architecture and town-planning; and through him that I had the honour of meeting Walther Gropius; and because of him that I am so pleased now that both my daughter and her husband are architects of distinction.

The Americans are the friendliest people in the world, as I'm sure everybody knows; and at that time there was far, far less travelling about in the United States by Americans, let alone by foreigners. By the time we got to Terre Haute, Indiana, they were beginning to notice our Massachusetts number plate and say 'My! You folks have come a long way!' Gordon would say 'We've come further than that — from England!'; and I would say 'Further than that — from South Africa!' We generally stayed either in motels or in houses that had signs in the window advertising bed and breakfast. Motels were a new idea at the time, and not very plentiful. They were groups of single wooden structures consisting of a two-bed bedroom with a gas-ring or electric hotplate, a shower and an attached carport. There might be a gas station, but certainly not anything like a restaurant, and they cost a dollar a night for the two of us. The bed and breakfast (often plus dinner) places were far more comfortable, and no dearer. By the time we were in Kansas our kind landladies, as often as not, would protest on our departure in the morning, 'I can't take your money — you folks have come such a long way, and we were glad to have you'; but of course we paid.

In Kansas City, Missouri, I had a strange encounter. We had stopped at a garage for a wheel alignment, and as I was talking to the mechanic, he interrupted me: 'Stop! Where have I heard that voice before?' he asked. 'Don't ask me', I answered. 'That's the voice' he said, 'that made the Abdication Speech!' In Denver, Colorado, we had lunch with the Bishop of Colorado, under circumstances that are now far beyond me; and I was amazed, shocked and delighted by his very informal manner.

Over the majestic Rocky Mountains we drove, to Salt Lake City in Utah. We viewed the nail-less and screw-less Mormon Temple with appropriate awe; we floated without effort on the very topmost surface of the Great Salt Lake; and we drove our Ford V8 at its utmost speed (eighty mph?) on the Salt Lake Flats, field of Donald Campbell's triumphs. We went on to Reno, Nevada, which then was Sin City, where all the divorces and all the gambling (and many a rodeo) took place. 'The Biggest Little City in the World' it called itself then, but now it is almost forgotten, and its place taken by Las Vegas at the bottom end of Nevada, at that time a tiny unknown village consisting of a shack or two.

Over the Sierra Nevada we drove, and through the Sacramento Valley to San Francisco, then and still one of the most glorious cities in the world. Gordon Stephenson stayed with friends of his, and I went across San Francisco Bay to the university town of Berkeley, to stay with the Knights. Remember the Knights? She, Eleanor, the glamorous American lady on the SS *Duilio* on the way from Cape Town to Marseilles in 1934, who used to ask me would I give her a drag, honey — my first acquaintance with an American woman. He, M.M., was Professor of Economics at the University of California. The situation *chez* Knight became a little fraught, because he, for no good reason at all, began to think that Eleanor and I were having an affair. He didn't actually charge either of us with this, but during meals he would mutter inconsequentially and loudly, talking to himself, about people coming from abroad and having affairs with his wife under his own roof. Since the remarks were not addressed directly to us, it was difficult to reply, and we would carry on as if nothing had been said. Eleanor and I certainly got on very well, but that was all.

From San Francisco we went south, and spent the first night in a whorehouse in Monterey. We didn't know it was a whorehouse, but did wonder why there was a constant tramp of feet on the stairs all night. The next morning when we were having breakfast in a diner across the way, and happened to mention where we had stayed, the man behind the counter roared with laughter and explained that the establishment did sometimes take in the odd passing traveller on the side. (A 'diner', by the way, was in those days a pensioned-off railroad dining car permanently parked on a street on bricks instead of wheels, serving food in the form of excellent short-orders and coffee. Generally it had a large, terse, explicit sign over it that told you all you needed to know — EAT. I loved them, but you don't see them any more, except as degraded ghosts in structures vaguely — probably not even consciously any more — imitating them, but with no ancestry.)

We saw everything there was to be seen in beautiful, wonderful California: Yosemite National Park (not Yoh-sim-might but Yossemmity; but the Americans are not consistent — Yellowstone is pronounced as spelled, and not Yellostenny); the Mission Trail, San Luis Obispo, Santa Barbara; Los Angeles; Hollywood; San Diego. We crossed the Mexican border at Tijuana and went to Ensenada, where the Mexicans really looked like those in cartoons in the New Yorker, sitting on their bottoms on the ground, knees up, backs against a wall, blankets over their shoulders, sombreros tilted down over their eyes, sleeping out the day. We drove over the San Bernadino Range, through the Colorado Desert, and into Arizona, where we gaped with joy and wonder at the Grand Canyon of the Colorado River from both the North and South rims, with a mile-deep chasm between them, exposing five out of the thirteen geological systems that make up the Earth's crust, so separated that there are only red squirrels on the north rim and grey on the south (or vice-versa), and never the twain shall meet, unless some fool mixes them. We went on to another canyon, called Bryce Canyon by the Palefaces; but I wish I could remember the bisyllabic name the Indians give it, because those two syllables mean 'Bowl-shaped-canyon-filled-with-red-rocks-standing-up-like-men.' Such a terse language would surely be useful to Secret Service agents, or as a computer language.

We crossed into New Mexico, where we stayed with some Hopi Indians in their village called Oraibi. How we contrived that I cannot remember, but I do remember that they were very earnest, kind folk. Then to Santa Fe and Albuquerque; and then to Dallas, Texas. Dallas then was no more than a medium-sized town, with hardly a building more than three storeys high, bearing no resemblance at all to the city in that evidently perpetual television serial. The Pan-American Exposition was on at the time, and Gulf Oil had some large rubber prehistoric monsters on display, and I was wearing my Emmanuel blazer, which had a well-padded red rampant lion on the breast pocket. A pretty girl asked me what that signified, and I told her I was a Gulf Oil salesman. She believed me, thought it was cute.

On to the State of Louisiana and its capital, the French City of New Orleans on the Gulf of Mexico, at the mouth of the

Em eye es
Es eye es
Es eye!
peepee!!
eye!!!

River. I love the names of its tributaries, recorded in Pare Lorentz's *The River*, which he wrote for his motion picture of the same name that he had prepared for the Farm Security Administration of the US Department of Agriculture in 1938. It begins this way:

From as far West as Idaho,
  Down from the glacier peaks of the Rockies —
From as far East as New York,
  Down from the turkey ridges of the Alleghenies
Down from the Minnesota, twenty five hundred miles,
The Mississippi River runs to the Gulf.
Carrying every drop of water, that flows down two-thirds of the continent,
Carrying every brook and rill, rivulet and creek,
Carrying all the rivers that run down two thirds the continent,
The Mississippi runs to the Gulf of Mexico.
Down the Yellowstone, the Milk, the White and Cheyenne;
The Cannonball, the Musselshell, the James and the Sioux;
Down the Judith, the Grand, the Osage, and the Platte,
The Skunk, the Salt, the Black, and Minnesota;
Down the Rock, the Illinois, and the Kankakee
The Allegheny, the Monongahela, Kanawha, and Muskingum;

Down the Miami, the Wabash, the Licking and the Green
The Cumberland, the Kentucky, and the Tennessee;
Down the Ouchita, the Witchita, the Red, and Yazoo —
Down the Missouri three thousand miles from the Rockies;
Down the Ohio a thousand miles from the Alleghenies;
Down the Arkansas fifteen hundred miles from the Great Divide;
Down the Red, a thousand miles from Texas;
Down the great Valley, twenty five hundred miles from
 Minnesota,
 Carrying every rivulet and brook, creek and rill,
Carrying all the rivers that run down two-thirds the Continent —
The Mississippi runs to the Gulf.

From Louisiana we went back to New York through Memphis, Chattanooga and Knoxville, Tennessee; a corner of Kentucky; Roanaoke and Richmond, Virginia; and Washington, D.C. I think it can be said we saw more of the United States than most Americans have seen, having motored in our trusty 'coop' over 8000 miles through thirty-three of the then forty-eight States, all very much to our profit, and with gratitude for the wisdom and generosity of the Commonwealth Fund in ensuring that we made this great journey.

Back in New York I resumed my scientific life uptown, and my private life downtown and midtown. At P & S my older colleagues, like Erwin Brand, were wondering when I was going to decide what line of research I was going to take up as my life's work. So was Marjory Stephenson in Cambridge. She wrote to scold me for being so aimless; told me I was a butterfly that was not going to be allowed to land on any of the flowers in her garden of bacterial chemistry. I couldn't understand what the fuss was about. It seemed to me that I was doing the sensible thing, making up for my ignorance of biochemistry by taking my time looking around.

I continued greatly to enjoy my life in Greenwich Village, and my delightful friendship with Margery Clarke, which had grown very warm. But Margery was a sensible girl, and saw no future in me. About three months before I was due to go back to England, she suggested we go for a walk in Central Park, because she wanted to tell me something. So we went for a walk in the Park and she told me something. She told me in an utterly charming way that she had met a nice chap, and that our ways were to part. So we affectionately parted.

About this time I began to think of future employment in England, preferably in Cambridge, so I applied for a Senior

Studentship of the Royal Commission for the Exhibition of 1851, and got it, which pleased me, since there was much prestige attached to it, as well as a decent income, and the right to use it wherever I wished in Great Britain. Naturally I opted for the Biochemical Laboratory in Cambridge.

I was going to spend my last week-end in America in Ithaca, New York, with the nice Bartons, that is, my Greenwich Village friend, Willy Kraber, and her equally charming sister and her friendly parents, and was much looking forward to it. I was to go there on Saturday morning, come back late on Monday afternoon, and sail on Tuesday morning. Now in those days, before you could leave the United States, you had to get a certificate from the Tax office down in the Wall Street district to prove that you had paid all your taxes. When I telephoned the office from P & S on Friday afernoon at about 3.30, I learned to my dismay that they closed at 4.00 p.m., not 5.00 p.m. as I had expected. There was no hope of getting from 168th street to Wall street in half an hour. That meant my lovely week-end was off, because I'd have to go to the tax office on Monday. As I walked dismally across 168th Street to seek consolation in a cup of coffee in the Armory Bar and Grill, an ambulance came by. By the driver there was a friend of mine, an intern in the Columbia-Presbyterian Hospital. He asked why I was so glum. I explained. 'Jump in!' he cried, and down the entire length of Broadway, across Times Square, we raced, siren wailing, bell clanging. That was far more sensational then than now, when sirens and bells clamour without cease in New York City. I got to the tax office with seven minutes to spare, got my certificate, spent a lovely week-end in Ithaca.

So at the end of the academical year of 1938 I sailed from New York to Southampton, very pleasantly on the French Liner *Normandie*, of the Compagnie Générale Transatlantique. It had made its maiden voyage the year before, and was incontestably the must luxurious vessel ever conceived; decorated in the Art Deco style by Dunand, Dupas, Ruhlmann and their like. The year after I sailed in it, it was trapped in New York by the outbreak of the war, accidentally set on fire, and the hull eventually sold as scrap. All the other ships I had ever sailed in were sunk during the war.

4
THE WAR

I didn't settle in Cambridge immediately, but sailed for South Africa within a week or two for a short visit. It was not much changed, except that I encountered certain manifestations of awe, due to my having been abroad; and to Cambridge, Harvard and Columbia Universities to boot; and was addressed as Doctor. I learned that my family had not eaten any tomatoes for the last two years, because in a letter I had written to one of them before leaving for America I had happened to mention tomatoes and cancer in entirely unconnected contexts; but my family were convinced that tomatoes caused cancer. In the Orange Free State two Higgs cousins came on horseback to greet me, and when they observed that there was nothing special about me, they told me that on the way they had asked each other 'Kan 'n mens nog met hom praat?' — 'Can one still talk to him?' When I visited my Uncle Jock he called all his Basuto staff together and delivered an oration, or *ditoko* (pronounced dee-talk-awe), telling them what a clever nephew he had. When it was over, one of the men seemed distinctly dissatisfied, and when Uncle Jock asked him the reason, he complained that I wasn't wearing glass shoes.

On my return to Cambridge I soon settled in a brand-new just about perfect one-room flat in Causewayside, by Coe Fen, where Mrs Reaves came twice daily on her bicycle all the two or three miles from Girton to prepare my breakfast and clean the flat in the morning, and to cook me a beautiful supper in the evening. It was fine to be back again in Cambridge, of course, but Europe was not as fine as it had been before I went to America. The coming war was imminent, the fascists were having it their way, and the pogroms were raging in Germany. Soon after I arrived back, Neville Chamberlain went to visit Adolf Hitler at Berchtesgaden, on 15 September 1938, to be told by his host that he intended to take Sudetenland from Czechoslovakia. We were all convinced the war was going to break out within days, but a fortnight later, at that notorious meeting in Munich, Chamberlain agreed to that seizure, so the war was postponed for a while. Within another fortnight the Germans seized Sudetenland. In the meantime the Spanish Civil War, which had started shortly before I went to America, was nearing its end, with Franco and his phalangists on the winning side. So I was immediately plunged into the left-wing politics of Cambridge, that is the left-wing politics of the Cambridge University intelligentsia. I agreed with them then, certainly, but the fact is, it was not a subject in which I could work up much interest. Today I am slightly inclined to the right, largely because I am no longer inclined to the left, but it is still not a subject that interests me enough to discuss it. I joined the left-wing clubs, went to political meetings, went around collecting miles of pennies for Spain, but never knowingly came in contact with the Burgesses, MacLeans, Blunts, etcetera, that were later to gain so much notoriety — excepting one, a physicist called Alan May, or Alan Nunn May as he is known to the public, or was, because he's forgotten now. Alan May was (and I'm sure still is) a very nice, amusing man, and Ruthie and I were fond of him. He would come to us every Sunday morning for coffee. During the war he was engaged in secret work on the atomic bomb in America; and some time after the second atomic bomb was dropped on Nagasaki on 9 August 1945, when we were living in London, we heard he was in London, back from America. I telephoned to invite him to visit us. He was hesitant. He said perhaps we might be sorry we'd asked him, because he had something to tell us that we might not like. We had no idea what he had on his mind, but it didn't enter our heads to tell an old friend not to come. So he appeared on our doorstep that night in St John's Wood, literally, really literally, looking over his shoulder. He told us he was in trouble with MI5, and couldn't stay. He did not specify the trouble, and we thought it better not to ask. The next morning but one we were amazed to hear on the wireless that he had been arrested for giving away secrets about the bomb to the Russians. MI5 must have observed that visit to our house, and I have always wondered why they did not come to question us. I don't approve at all of what Alan May did, but I don't believe in my heart, or that in his heart, he was a villain, certainly not a self-seeking villain. I believe that under the emotionally highly charged circumstances then prevailing, he genuinely saw only Russia's immense struggle against the Nazis, without which we would have surely lost the war; and he did not realise that the nobility of the ideal of communism was already and inevitably being superseded by the ignoble reality of a compound of incompetence and cruelty.

In spite of the overhanging doom, life in Cambridge continued to be pleasant. I saw a lot of Dophi and Joseph Needham and Marjory Stephenson. One day Dophi told me that a Chinese girl was coming to work with her. She was said to be 'fair, fat and forty', and her name was Lu Gwei Djen; not Miss Gwei Djen, known as Lu to her friends, but Miss Lu, known as Gwei Djen to her friends. When she arrived, she turned out to be fair of face all right, but not of complexion, which was of a lovely slightly yellowish-brown shade, topped with raven black hair; and she was not fat, but pleasantly rounded out; as for forty, it seemed just possible but not likely. Her arrival was an historical moment, for it marked the very birth of Joseph's insatiable interest in everything Chinese, and his quite stupendously vast accumulation of knowledge of the history of science in China. Just as he taught himself Polish in 1936, Joseph now set about learning Chinese, and I count myself fortunate to have been there to witness the very beginning. The beginning was his compilation of a hand-written Chinese-English dictionary, since he was not satisfied with those available. He has a marvellously quick, neat, handsome, easily legible handwriting; and he is amazingly systematic; and so this wonderful manuscripted dictionary just grew and grew. For all I know, it is still growing, and I should think now it must be priceless. Joseph eventually gave up his research on chemical embryology, and devoted himself entirely to writing the history of science and civilization in China, and is still engaged on it, assisted from the beginning by Lu Gwei Djen, and subsequently also by streams of scholars from all parts of the world. The way he writes his history is remarkable. He doesn't scribble away at a frequently altered manuscript like most of us. He prepares everything he wants to say in his head; and when he's ready, he loads his typewriter with specially prepared sheets of foolscap, the bottom six or so centimetres of which are ruled off in one-centimetre squares. He then rapidly types out these sheets, which seldom if ever need any correction, but do need additions. All the Chinese names are typed in Western characters in the text, each with a reference mark referring to footnotes in the squared-off section below, where the names are beautifully handwritten in Chinese characters, one to a square. The sheets then go off to the Cambridge University Press without a further glance. His rooms in Gonville and Caius College (usually called Caius and pronounced Keys) were crammed with books, not only on shelves on the walls but on projections of these shelves into the room space. He was elected Master of

Caius in 1966 (the Sir William Dunn Institute of Biochemistry has produced five Heads of Colleges in Cambridge, viz. Tim Hele, Emmanuel; Frank Young, Darwin; Joseph Needham, Caius; Donald Northcote, Sidney Sussex; Hans Kornberg, Christ's; and one in Oxford, viz me, St Cross). On his retirement from Caius Joseph became founder and Director of the East Asian History of Science Library in Cambridge, which is even more jammed with books and well-organized filing cabinets bursting with material for his monumental *Science and Civilization* in China, which now runs to eleven large octavo tomes (in six volumes) averaging about 650 pages each, with no end yet in sight. He was head of the British Scientific Mission in China and Counsellor to the British Embassy in Chungking from 1942 to 1946 (and when he stayed with us in St John's Wood on his return from China, and we stood in a queue on the Edgware Road waiting for the Number 16 bus, he gazed sadly at our companions and muttered, 'They all look so *ugly*, after China!'). He was Director of the Department of Natural Sciences of UNESCO from 1946 to 1948. He has countless honorary degrees, foreign medals and decorations. He is a Fellow both of the Royal Society and of the British Academy, bestriding the worlds of Science and Arts, all this due to his insatiable interest in China and the Chinese. He loves knowledge the way a good person, say Mother Theresa, loves people. It makes no difference to him whether the knowledge he loves is confirmable or not; he leaves that for others to judge, since he is too objective (or not arrogant enough?) to be critical.

Back in the Laboratory I alighted on a bacterial flower, in spite of Marjory Stephenson's previous warning-off, but in my own allotment, not in her garden. I took an interest in the proteolytic enzymes of an anaerobic bacterium called *Clostridium histolyticum*. Enzymes are the basis of biochemistry. They are proteins that promote, or catalyze, all chemical reactions in all forms of living matter, animal or vegetable. Proteolytic enzymes promote the breakdown of other proteins. An anaerobic bacterium is one that will grow only in the absence of air, or rather oxygen. One group of these anaerobic bacteria belongs to the species *Clostridium. Clostridium histolyticum* is so called because it produces proteolytic enzymes that break down proteins in living tissues and so dissolve them. I published a paper on *Clostridium histolyticum* proteinases in *The Biochemical Journal*. It was not very interesting, but that doesn't matter. What mattered was that the appearance of that paper told powers that be that I had had some experience with anaerobic Clostridia.

On the third of September 1939 the war broke out. It occurs to me now that I had been in Britain only three years, and could easily have gone back to the safety of South Africa when the trouble started brewing, but it never occurred to me then that it was not my war, and that I need not stay in England. I considered, fearfully, the obligation to join up; but before I was able to stiffen the sinews, summon up the blood, and disguise fair nature with hard-favour'd rage, I was informed by the Governnment that as a scientist I was in a Reserved Occupation and must await instructions. I won't pretend I wasn't tremendously relieved, but at least I joined the LDV, or Local Defence Volunteers, which almost immediately changed its name to the Home Guard. I was in the Cambridgeshire Light Infantry. I didn't enjoy the prolonged ache of running crouched low behind hedges with a heavy rifle in my hand and heavy boots on my feet; and while I was supposed to be hurling hand grenades with *élan* into the local quarry, I was terrified that the unlocked spring of my grenade would force open my nerveless hand and cause the grenade to go off in it. So I would steal up to the edge of the quarry and ignobly jettison the grenade down it.

Early in the Michaelmas Term of 1939, attending lectures in the Biochemical Department, and casting an eye over the girls in the new intake coming to do Part II of the Biochemistry Tripos, I realised by the third lecture that one of them particularly appealed to me. I think it was her sweet brown eyes, like a mouse's, only bigger. She turned out to be called Ruth Eleanor Treverton, and because she dressed quietly, and didn't have a hoity-toity accent (like the girls I used to meet under the wing of Lady Frances Ryder before I went to America), I was inclined to think she was a poor scholarship girl from the north country. I was very pleased when I was asked by those responsible for her Part II teaching to give her tutorials on proteolytic enzymes. I was only just one jump ahead of her, knowing practically nothing more about proteolytic enzymes than what I had learned from my *Clostridium histolyticum* proteinase. So I had to swot up the other proteolytic enzymes, trypsin, chymotrypsin, pepsin, papain, cathepsin, the night before I was due to give her a tutorial. So I fell permanently in love with her, and one night on Coe Fen, walking on the tow-path by the Cam, I was surprised to hear myself proposing to her — it was the first and last proposal of marriage I ever made, because she accepted it, thank Heavens; thank Heavens even more fervently now. It turned out Ruthie didn't come from the north of England, but from Newport in Monmouthshire (now called Gwent) in South Wales, and had been to Cheltenham Ladies' College.

The Phoney War became real. On 14 June 1940 the Germans took Paris. The situation was perfectly dreadful, and I was afraid Britain would be overrun any minute. Ruthie was with her mother in Newport. I telephoned to tell her I was coming to Newport to marry her, and within a few days, on 24 June, I did marry her, in the Registry Office at Newport. It must have been a dreadful shock for her poor mother and her relations, because they knew nothing about me, especially since I came from the colonies. Ruthie's father had died early in 1924, when she was six years old, the same age as I was when my mother died. Her brother Garrod, who had been at Balliol, was at the time away in Hong Kong as Private Secretary to the Governor. Her mother's father had been a most interesting man, as is hinted at in the following Postscript that Ruthie wrote to her article on 'Sugar Alcohols — Galactose and Diabetic Cataracts' in a book on the eye and inborn errors of metabolism [35]:

> Finally, this is my chance in a lifetime to pay tribute to my grandfather. He was born in Cardiganshire in South Wales in 1853. He was christened Abraham, but in those parts children were, and perhaps still are, encouraged to choose a further name for themselves when approaching adulthood. He chose a name and, years later, I was told that it was the name of a doctor 'well known at that time'. He himself went to Edinburgh, trained to be a doctor under (Lord) Lister, and afterwards settled down in South Wales as a general physician and surgeon.
>
> In 1938 I went up to Cambridge and, reading biochemistry, encountered the then almost forgotten 'Inborn Errors of Metabolism' by Sir Archibald Garrod. Garrod was the name my grandfather had chosen for himself about seventy years before! Many years later it occurred to me that it must have been not Archibald but his father, Sir Alfred Baring Garrod, who inspired my grandfather. But it was no disillusionment. Sir Alfred was himself a distinguished clinician and pioneer in the application of chemistry to medicine. His son used to say with pride that his measurement of uric acid in the blood of patients with gout was the first quantitative biochemical investigation on the living human body.
>
> We continue to honour the name. My great-nephew is the fifth generation Garrod in my family.

Abraham Garrod Thomas' brother John also gave himself another name — Aeron, after the River Aeron in Cardiganshire in West Wales, which flows into the Atlantic at Aberaeron, where they lived and their father farmed ('aber' = 'mouth', see also Aberystwyth on the parallel River Ystwyth). Abraham Garrod had a busy and fruitful career. As a medical student in Edinburgh, he had studied under the great Joseph Lister, whose invention and development of antiseptic surgery had been the cause of the saving of countless lives. Ruthie still has the copy of the *South Wales Argus* that reports a most interesting and moving lecture that he gave on Lister. In addition to being a busy physician and surgeon, and founding the *South Wales Argus,* and being a Member of Parliament for Newport, he also more or less founded the Royal Gwent Hospital in Newport. He was knighted in 1912 for his public services. I presume George V commanded him to 'Rise, Sir Abraham', but he was always known as Sir Garrod. Ruthie's mother's siblings, Dora and Noel, were unmarried. Noel had read chemistry at Balliol, and was concerned with various chemical and near-chemical manufacturing interests. During the war he was Controller of Sulphuric Acid, which was a highly responsible job, since the production of sulphuric acid is said (or was at that time said) to be the best quick indication of a country's prosperity, sulphuric acid being used in so many industries. I wish Ruthie's father had survived. He had been in the shipping business, and was interested in art. I have good reason to know that he had a fine eye for a drawing, because the walls of our house are covered with nearly 50 remarkably fine drawings, aquatints and etchings that he collected, including those of Béjot, Legrand, Beurdeley, Muirhead, van Herkomer, Muirhead Bone, Paton, Legros, Bauer, Chachine, Helleu, Gibbings, Squirrel, Whistler, Pennel, and Holroyd. His brother Godfrey was a farmer in the Newport district, and his brother Guy was in shipping in Newport.

We returned to Cambridge immediately after the quick and muted wartime wedding. The Needhams were away at the time, and we spent our first night in their house on Owlstone Road. It was a bit off-putting to start with, because Dophi had left us a number of detailed instructions about where to find fire-fighting equipment and what to do in case of an air raid. But there was no air raid (they didn't start until 15 July), so everything was fine. I can't remember why we didn't go to my nice flat, or where we lived immediately after, but we soon found a delightful very narrow three-storey house, called the Half Moon House because it had been the Half Moon Inn in the past, and still had the half-moon sign hanging outside. It was on Little St Mary's Lane, that ran by little St Mary's churchyard opposite, from Pembroke

Street to the River Cam. Mrs Reaves continued to look after us. One night some months later, after the air raids had started, when we were sitting in the sitting room at the front of the house, and Mrs Reaves was washing up in the kitchen not more than about fifteen feet away at the back, the air raid warning sounded. After some time the droning of an enemy bomber overhead could be heard. There was little one could do about it but sit and wait, and as we waited Mrs Reaves came in. 'Excuse me for coming in here,' she said, 'but there is a German bomber over the kitchen.'

Back in the Biochemical Laboratory, Ruthie and I started doing war work. She was engaged with Malcolm Dixon and others on research into methods for combatting mustard gas and other forms of poison gas, and this was to keep her occupied until we went to London in 1943; but since it was secret work she was unable in the end to present it in a thesis for a Ph.D. Cantab. I received a letter from the Anaerobes Sub-committee of the War Wounds Committee of the Medical Research Council asking me, more or less commanding me, to act as a chemical collaborator with a Dr Jacobson in Cambridge on the bacteria-killing effect that he had just observed of certain cobalt co-ordination complexes on anaerobic Clostridia. The anaerobic Clostridia were feared in war wounds, since *Clostridium welchii, Clostridium oedematiens* and *Clostridium septicum* caused gas gangrene, and *Clostridium tetani* caused tetanus, or lockjaw. Tetanus was easily prevented by active immunization (which I'll come to), but gas gangrene was a fearful problem. It takes place as a result of the infection of deep penetrating wounds. The Clostridia evolve gases during their growth in the tissues, which get blown up hard as a drum, and then undergo a terrible gangrenous destruction and dissolution of the flesh, hence the name.

I knew Jacobson; he was a pleasant and competent German refugee biologist in Cambridge, and I was pleased at the prospect of working with him, especially since the problem seemed so worthwhile. But before I could get in touch with Jacobson, the German parachutists started descending on Holland and Belgium, sometimes dressed as nuns, sometimes landing their gliders on glass-houses mistaken for lakes. The Government promptly and reasonably rounded up all enemy aliens in Britain, including the blameless Jacobson, and incarcerated them in a camp at Hoyton in order to have time to sort out the few suspect from the many innocent. Jacobson's wife was understandably but unreasonably indignant, and would not let me have even a glimpse of her husband's laboratory notes.

Bacterial Toxins : Gas Gangrene

Hoping for my intended collaborator's early release from Hoyton, and not knowing anything about his work on cobalt co-ordination complexes, and knowing only *Clostridium histolyticum,* I started reading up the three gas gangrene clostridia in Topley and Wilson's magisterially authoritative *Principles of Bacteriology and Immunity*. I learned that they produced toxins, and that these were considered responsible for the lethal effects of gas gangrene in infected limbs. This interested me enormously, because in the same reading I learned that the other lethal anaerobe, *Clostridium tetani,* causes tetanus, or lockjaw, by means of a lethal toxin; and that soldiers could be protected from lockjaw by immunizing them in advance against the toxin. At that time this immunization was effected simply by the following steps: 1. growing the tetanus organism in a sort of meat broth until it had secreted enough toxin into the broth; 2. filtering off the broth from the organisms; 3. detoxifying the filtered broth by treating it with formaldehyde; 4. injecting about a cubic centimetre of this 'toxoid' into the arm three times, a second after four to six weeks, the third after six to twelve months. This anticipation of an infection rather than waiting for it is called prophylactic immunization. Immunization against diphtheria was also achieved in this way — why not try to immunize against gas gangrene in the same way? Tetanus and diphtheria toxins were proteins, and presumably the gas gangrene toxins would be proteins too, and these biologically active proteins would be comparable with enzymes, perhaps even be enzymes. This seemed exactly up my street. Since by this time it began to seem that it would be some time before Jacobson, as blameless as ever, would be released, I proposed to the Anaerobes Subcommittee that I abandon cobalt coordination complexes, and study the possibilities of immunizing against gas gangrene in the same way as lockjaw.

The Anaerobes Sub-committee agreed to my proposal, but not without a struggle, since I met with some scepticism from some of the old-timers. They didn't think that immunization against gas gangrene was feasible, because their toxins were not 'strong' enough for making toxoid. That is to say, if their culture filtrates were treated with formaldehyde in the way diphtheria and tetanus toxoids were made, there would not be enough toxoid in a dose-sized volume of 1 to 2 cubic centimetres to evoke an effective antibody response. It seemed to me that there were two obvious ways of dealing with this difficulty, preferably combined: to devise a culture medium in which the organisms would produce more toxin; and to concentrate the protein toxins in these more potent filtrates by precipitating them from the filtrates. They could be purified to an acceptable degree, and then dissolved in smaller volumes. The old-timers were inclined not to comprehend, and the reason for this is interesting. In those days medical bacteriology was in the hands of the pathologists (there were no Professors of Bacteriology in the Medical Schools of Great Britain; only Professors of Pathology, who took bacteriology under their wing; and in Oxford there still isn't one). And the pathologists, at least those I encountered, did not have a chemical outlook, not at all. To me these bacterial toxins were no more than chemical *things* dissolved in the culture filtrates. They should be handleable like any other chemical thing. To the pathologists they were not things, but intangible attributes, like good or evil. To them the 'toxin' was the entire culture filtrate. You could no more take the toxic principle out of it and hold it in your hand than you could extract and weigh the beauty in a flower or the sin in a sinner.

This introduction to bacterial toxins was a case of instant and intractable love at first sight. *Clostridium histolyticum* proteinase was nothing compared with toxins. There now opened before me a new and practically untilled field of proteins that were active in a different way — they were lethal by means as yet undiscovered. Lethality was much more exciting than mere proteolysis, or any other known enzymic activity. And this lethality could be countered through the anigenicity of the toxins, i.e. their ability to stimulate the production of antitoxins. Thus I had at the same time gained entry into the marvellously interesting field of immunology. It was a truly glamorous subject, bringing me into the field of medicine in time of war. I was inspired by the thought expressed in Topley and Wilson's *Principles* that 'only when the chemist has replaced the immunologist shall we be able to give an intellectually satisfying account of what happens when a particular parasite invades a particular host.' I felt I had the biochemistry of this virtually unexplored field of bacterial toxins all to myself; but fortunately I hadn't, because the Anaerobes Sub-committee had also invited B. C. J .G. Knight and Marjorie Macfarlane at the Lister Institute in Elstree and London to take an interest in the problem, and we agreed to keep in touch. I decided to work on the lethal toxin of *Cl. welchii* that was called *alpha*. My first culture produced no measurable amount of toxin, since one ml failed to kill a mouse; the second produced fifteen lethal doses per ml; and after a month, using a culture medium devised by Knight, I attained about 100 lethal doses per ml. The toxin could be precipitated and partially purified by the simple techniques then available. But toxicity testing by injecting into the tail veins of mice was terribly laborious, and one had then to wait for several days to get very inaccurate results. The lethal glamour faded, and I longed to be back with test tubes. If only, I thought, I could find some reagent that turned blue when toxin was added! I didn't find that, but Macfarlane and Knight found that a turbidity developed when the toxin was added to a solution of egg yolk, and went on by means of this to make history by being the first to define the biochemistry underlying the lethal action of a toxin. They showed that the toxin split lecithin in egg yolk in a certain way. In the meantime I found a way of measuring the turbidity it produced with egg yolk solution and so turning it into a test-tube method for assaying the toxin within a few minutes with an accuracy far exceeding that of the mouse toxicity tests.

In order now to put the problem of active immunization against gas gangrene on a war footing, Knight and I decided to move to the Wellcome Physiological Research Laboratories in Beckenham, a suburb to the south of London. This was, still is I suppose, one of the world's foremost establishments for research on and production of toxins, toxoids, antitoxins, etc. So on 3 February 1943 Ruthie and I moved into a house on Smith Terrace in Chelsea. From there I commuted the twenty-minute train journey from Victoria Station to Beckenham Junction every morning. There Knight worked on the large-scale production and purification of oedematiens toxoid, and I worked on the welchii toxoid. We made a purified gas gangrene-tetanus toxoid preparation that was acceptable for injection into humans, produced good levels of antitoxin in volunteers from the Metropolitan Police force, and protected guinea pigs against experimentally induced gas gangrene. These last tests were done in Cambridge by Muriel Robertson, an anaerobic-bacteriologist who had encouraged me in the early days; but she cheated, though I don't think deliberately. She published a paper in *The Lancet* on these findings without telling me she intended to do so, which was not proper, since I had started the work and had given her the toxoid. Now everybody thought it was all her work.

In the end the Wellcome Laboratories produced enough suitable combined tetanus-welchii-oedematiens toxoid for a trial with about 50,000 soldiers under battle conditions. We had intended to call it TWOT, but that turned out to be a rude word in American, so we had to use the Americanized spelling of 'oedematiens' by eliminating the 'o'. Thus it was TWET that went out to the British 21st Army Group. But it never got tested in battle. Little did we know that it was only a few weeks before D-Day, so there wasn't time to get it distributed. I believe that the doses were then sent to be tested in our soldiers in the Far East; but again too late, for little did those responsible know that the Americans were going to drop those two atomic bombs.

About the time we were sending off the TWET from the Wellcome Laboratories to the 21st Army Group, I had a visit from Gwyn Macfarlane and John MacLennan. They were officers in the Royal Army Medical Corps, and had been on service in North Africa, where they had seen many cases of gas gangrene. In these cases they had observed that the reticular collagen scaffolding that supported the muscle fibres was dissolved away, leaving the muscles destroyed, but with their fibres intact. Collagen is a particular type of tough protein, tough as old boots you might say, because it is the main component of leather; and it is qualitatively if not quantitively also an important component of muscular tissue. I was aware that a German scientist called Maschmann had in 1938 reported the occurrence of an enzyme with this property in *Clostridium welchii* cultures, and had given it the name of 'collagenase', but had subsequently withdrawn his statement without stating the reason. Macfarlane and MacLennan thought it might be a good idea for me to investigate this enzyme. (They also suggested that after the war, which we knew we were going to win, I should be sent off swanning in Germany to find out what Maschmann had been up to, but in fact he disappeared without trace.) So I tackled the problem. I purified the enzyme to a reasonably decent degree and studied its properties, but nothing particular emerged — except a letter from the Ophthalmic Surgeon of the Royal Netherlands Court. He wrote to ask me to send him some of the enzyme to treat the eye of one of the young Princesses; but I had regretfully to refuse, because I could not guarantee that my preparation of collagenase was free of lecithinase, i.e. the alpha toxin I had worked on until then, and lecithinase might have damaged the eye permanently.

London during the War

Life in London after we moved into 15 Smith Terrace in Chelsea at the beginning of February 1943 was not as bad as it had been before we went there; and things had begun to go badly wrong for the Germans on all fronts. On the Eastern front Paulus had surrendered Stalingrad to the Russians on 31 January; Rommel was retreating in Africa and the Allies were preparing to attack the soft underbelly of Europe in Italy; Berlin was being heavily raided by the R.A.F. It still wasn't much fun in London. The German air raids had been renewed in mid-January, but by the time we got to London they were not too bad, for the time being.

It was a pleasant little house on a pleasant little street off the King's Road, not far from Sloane Square. The daily commutating to Beckenham Junction station, whence I would bike to the Wellcome Laboratories, was entirely bearable, because I was travelling against the stream and always had an empty carriage. While I was at the Wellcome Laboratories, Ruthie was in the Lister Institute, by Chelsea Bridge, not far from our house. She was working with Walter Morgan on Blood Group Substances. He was, still is, a very decent, distinguished man, and he had the pleasant and sensible habit of addressing her man to woman as 'van Heyningen'.

In the Home Guard I was transferred from the Cambridgeshire Light Infantry to the Royal Artillery in London. I was attached to the secret Z-Battery in Hyde Park, near the Dorchester Hotel. The Z-Battery consisted of fifty-six guns; if you can call them guns, for in essence they consisted of two pairs of rails from which were launched a pair of rockets, which were still so new then that they were secret. Each gun was manned by two gunners, the one who aimed the gun, and the other who had to fetch the rockets from the adjoining trench and load them on the rails. Being an intellectual, I was chosen for the aiming job. Therefore I was attached to my gun by earphones through which I received my orders from the command post. These gave the elevation, trajectory, etc. I should set my gun at, and then the order to fire. The idea was that when enemy aircraft were overhead we would simultaneously fire all 112 rockets, thus creating a blazing 'box' above the Dorchester Hotel. The drill was easy to master, so much so that my mate and I were chosen to mount a demonstration drill before a visiting general. The opening feature of the drill was to be an officer barking an order to me, and then me barking back a repeat of that order to show that it had been received and understood. When the day came, there I was, proud as anything and ready to be a credit to my battery. The officer barked his command. Agonized silence from me. Ferocious glare from the officer. I knew I was doing something terribly wrong, but I couldn't think what. Too late — I had forgotten to bark back.

I have to admit now that never during my entire service with the Z-Battery did we let off a single rocket. But I used to ready myself for action always with a heavy heart, for two reasons. One was that our sergeant had insistently taught us to look out for rockets that fizzed on the rails without provocation. That meant they were about to explode on the rails, and we should dive into the adjoining trench. But this was going to be difficult for me, for I was attached to my rocket by my headphone, and my headphone was fastened to my head by the steel battle bowler over it. So I always mounted my gun with a big sheath knife in my belt to cut myself loose from the telephone. The other reason for my unease was that I knew I wasn't going to get a wink of sleep that night, because of the horrendous snores of my fellow gunners in our Nissen hut where we were supposed to sleep after we went off duty. But my one consolation was the sweet voice of the female officer who gave me my instructions over the telephone. Four or five days after D-Day I met that sweet-voiced female officer. It was a Saturday morning, and I was shopping in Harrods. At around eleven I went to the tea place to have a coffee. All the chairs were occupied, excepting one, which was at a table for two. A really *nice*, really good-looking ATS officer was sitting at it; and when she saw me she smiled so sweetly, and motioned me to the empty chair opposite her. 'Good Heavens, you're Mary Churchill' I said as I sat down. 'How on Earth do you know?' asked this terribly nice officer. 'Well of course I know who you are' I said, 'I've seen you many times in the newspapers and on the newsreels.' I was determined to speak to her in her own right, and not as the daughter of the great man. She was wearing the Artillery flash on her shoulder, and I told her that I too had the honour of wearing that flash, but only at night, and only once a week, in Hyde Park by the Dorchester Hotel. She asked me what number my rocket launcher was, and it turned out then that hers was that sweet voice that comforted me on the telephone. After some artillery talk we went on to other things, like how childen's names are a give-away of the year of their birth. I mentioned her father only once, at the end. Churchill had been threatening to visit the Normandy beaches, and everybody was alarmed. I asked her to urge her father to desist. 'Yes, Daddy's being a dreadful nuisance', she said.

Some time during 1943 the Government gave us a Morrison Shelter. A Morrison Shelter was a rectangular cage that in our case took the place of the dining table. It was made of heavy steel girders with a sheet metal top and heavy wire grids on the sides. The idea was that you put a mattress in it and sheltered in it when there was an air raid on, and slept in it at night. It wasn't supposed to save you from a direct hit, but it did at least save you from your collapsing house. It came in time, for shortly after I installed it in our dining room the air raids on London started again after some months of relative quiet.

Towards mid-December 1943 Ruthie went into the Westminster Hospital to have her first baby. She was in a small ward with six or seven other women. One of them was a nice woman whose husband was said to be an up-and-coming man in the Board of Trade, and up he came, for he was Mr Harold Wilson. In bed in Chelsea at about two on the morning of 17 December, I felt a terrible itch all over, and discovered that my entire body was covered with shilling-sized weals that were rapidly becoming confluent. I was alarmed, but felt I couldn't summon a doctor or an ambulance for something that wasn't an emergency. So I telephoned somebody who might know what to do, and would certainly be up and about at that time of the morning, to wit the matron in charge of Ruthie's ward. She told me it was nothing, it was always happening to her prospective fathers. Some hours later our son Simon was born, and mother and child were both doing very well. I had never been really keen on babies, but now I was converted, and began to think about them with some enthusiasm.

Things were rather miserable in January and February 1944. There was a lot of snow about, and very little coal. I'll not forget walking home from Sloane Square tube station one evening to find Ruthie pushing the pram through the thick bumpy snow, loaded with some coal she had managed to find. And pleasures were scarce, just about limited to the cinema, which we couldn't go to because of the need to keep an eye on young Simon. He developed some ailment once that necessitated his spending the night in the Chelsea Children's Hospital. This gave Ruthie and me the chance to make a dash for the nearest cinema, heartlessly joyful in spite of the illness of our only child.

One night the air raids were really terrible, so I decided that Ruthie and Simon should no longer be exposed to them. I telephoned a cousin of hers, Joyce Lewis, married to a farmer in the Hereford district, to ask them to take them in. In those days you had to get the operator to get you through, and I had to hang on to that telephone for two hours, really, to get through to the exchange. Joyce, of course, was very kind, and glad to have them. The next thing was to get a taxi to take them to Paddington Station. There were no taxis in the King's Road, and all the taxis going around Sloane Square were engaged. After at least an hour an unengaged taxi came into view and I hailed it; but no sooner had I hailed it than a bowler-hatted young man-about-town emerged from a block of flats, languidly raised his furled umbrella, and captured my taxi. I seized his chest and told him I would strangle him if he did not yield my taxi. I meant it, and perhaps could have done it. But he had sense. 'Let me come with you to Paddington first, and then I'll continue on my way' he said; and that's what we did. That incident with the taxi was to stick in my mind. Many months later, *bicycling* my way from Beckenham Junction Station to the Wellcome Laboratories, I saw a free taxi, and before I knew what I was doing, I found myself hailing it. A man on a bicycle hailing a taxi! The driver was furious and I was embarrassed, but there was no way of explaining my neurosis.

I used to go to the farm, Bishopstone Court in Herefordshire, once every five weeks to visit Ruthie and Simon. The peacefulness was unbelievable, and so were some of the people in the neighbourhood. They used to maintain that the Londoners deserved to be bombed. The train to Hereford went by Oxford, with a good view of the Gleaming Spires, and I would long to be there, not only because of the Spires, but because it was unbombed, and because I was beginning to get homesick for the academic life. Going back from those week-ends was always miserable. Particularly that evening in Paddington Station when I heard an overwrought woman scream to a station official, 'I hope *your* house gets bombed tonight!'

Lying alone in the Morrison shelter during the air raids I would remember ruefully the horror I had felt many years ago in South Africa, when somebody who had been in London during the first World War would tell us about the terrors of the Zeppelin raids on London, when as many as five or six bombs (five or ten lbs each?) would be dropped on the city. But I found a way of putting things in perspective, literally you might almost say. In my mind's eye I would look at all London from the air, from Woolwich on the east to Ealing on the west; from Walthamstow on the North to Crystal Palace on the South. Then I would look at Chelsea, then at Smith Terrace. It seemed such a tiny part of the whole that I would realise that the chance of being hit was small.

June the 4th was D-Day, and that more or less put an end to the air raids, but their place was taken by the Flying Bombs, the V-1s, that were launched from the ground at the Pas de Calais. That first night was strange. Aircraft seemed to be flying overhead, then they seemed suddenly to stop, and then there would be an explosion somewhere in London. In the end I got used to those little monsters, and during those cut-outs I would pray that the bomb would land somewhere else and not on me. By the time we got used to them, they were replaced, in September, by the even more horrible V-2s, the rockets, whose descending whistle you heard *after* their bang. I developed another neurosis. I would think I must move away from *this* place because a rocket is on its way to it; but then I would think I mustn't move to *that* place because the rocket's going to land there. The onslaught slowed down, and by October it was safe enough in London for Ruthie and Simon to come back. The rockets still came, but not in large numbers, and by 28 March 1945 the last of the 1,050 fell.

Life in London began to have its compensations. We met Hetta Crouse, a large, beautiful, jolly South African girl, married to William Empson, the poet, and author of the formidable and to me incomprehensible *Seven Types of Ambiguity*. We would meet all kinds of marvellously interesting and talented people in their house on Haverstock Hill, including, once, George Orwell, and once that glorious artist, Matthew Smith. William Empson's style of dress was hardly formal. Under his jacket there was usually a grubby pullover with a rather large hole in it. This pullover was tucked into his trouser tops, and under his braces, one of whose branches was attached to the trousers by means of a nail. William had returned recently from China, where he had taught English Literature in various universities, and was now Chinese Editor at the British Broadcasting Corporation. A colleague of his there was Francis Dillon, a most talented man with a sense of humour. He was producing a weekly programme called 'Country Magazine', which was a great success, because the farmers appeared to be discussing their affairs in a manner that was spontaneous yet well-organized. This was achieved by having them all meet in the BBC Parlour on a Sunday afternoon and relieving them of their inhibitions with generous potions, which were hard to come by in London at that time. Then they would repair to the broadcasting studio and talk freely; and a skilfully cut and edited recording of their discussion would go on the air. Now he wanted to do the same with scientists in a 'Science Magazine', and William Empson suggested that I might be able to help him. So Francis Dillon invited me to be Editor. My job (which was well-paid by my standards) was to suggest what subjects should be discussed, and which scientists should discuss them. It did not interfere with my work, since it took me only an hour or two a week, and some thought and planning in the evenings.

For the first programme I suggested, among others, Professor Sir Alexander Fleming of the Inoculation Department of St Mary's Hospital, London, who had discovered penicillin in 1929, but concluded that it was little more than a plaything; Professor Sir Howard Florey, of the Sir William Dunn School of Pathology at Oxford University, who had developed penicillin as an antibiotic in 1940 and reported its clinical efficacy early in 1943; and Dr C. P. Snow, a Cambridge physicist who had recently published a masterly novel about scientists called *The Search*, and was now doing an important job of recruiting scientists for the war effort (I think that was when the phrase 'head-hunting' was invented). The first few programmes were a great success, but the trouble was that dear old Francis liked his tipple, and was consequently inclined to be spectacularly forgetful. I would telephone him on a Thursday and ask if the agreed speakers had agreed to speak on the Sunday, and Francis would groan with dismay and tell me they had gone right out of his head. (When I was a bit bleak about this once, he stormed at me: 'You're so bloody pure, you smell of Lifebuoy Soap.') So I would suggest we'd better have C. P. Snow again.

I used to know Snow in pre-war Cambridge, not very well. He was still teaching and doing scientific research, and editing a popular science magazine called *Discovery*, which seemed to me always to contain nothing but articles on bird-watching, which of course is easy to explain to laymen, but gives them the wrong idea of what science really is. One day, as I was biking past his College, Christ's, I leaped off on an impulse and went in to tell him what I thought, in the good Cambridge direct, no-nonsense way. He was stuffy, and I concluded he was a stuffed shirt. Now, in London, I knew we could always get him at short notice, and he would come along and talk about 'Science as a Career'. Thus it was that I knew Snow and he knew me. I was meaner about him than he deserved. At the time I thought he was only an average scientist who turned to novel-writing as a solace, and I didn't realise that in fact he considered himself primarily a novelist — and a very fine novelist he was — who had to make a living in the meantime.

Years later in Oxford, after the war, and a few days before Christmas 1964, my son Simon came to me with his finger marking a place in Snow's latest novel, *Corridors of Power*. 'Have you seen what Snow says about you, Pop?' pages 270 and 271 a character goes to his habitual pub in London, to be greeted by the landlady:

> 'Do you know who that is?' she whispered reverentially, pointing to the far end of the bar. There . . . was a commonplace looking man in a blue suit. 'No', I said. 'That', said the landlady, her whisper more sacramental, 'is Van Heynegen's brother-in-law!' It might have sounded . . . as if Van Heynegen were a distinguished public figure. Not a bit of it . . . Van Heynegen had been, in fact, an entirely respectable South African, but an unfortunate one . . . he had been murdered for the sake of a small sum, about a hundred pounds. There had been nothing spectacular about the murder itself, but the consequences were somewhat gothic. For Van Heynegen had been in an amateurish fashion dissected, and the portions made into brown paper parcels, weighted down with bricks, and dropped, at various points between Blackfriars and Putney, into the river.

That afternoon I went to my then College, Exeter, and was greeted by the Rector with the words, 'What's Snow got against you?' So I thought I would tease Snow. I wrote to him care of his publishers, Macmillan:

> 24 December 1964
>
> Dear Sir Charles,
>
> My friends and my enemies have been pointing fingers at me since I appeared to appear on page 271 of *Corridors of Power*, with my name slightly mis-spelled as usual.
>
> I was once a (entirely respectable) South African and I am sure I am the only South African van Heyningen you could possibly have known. Since all the van Heyningens in South Africa belong to the same family, since I am the only male one of them (apart from my son) to have lived in England, and since your peripheral paths and mine have crossed (prewar Cambridge — the Needhams, J.D.Bernal, etc.; wartime London — BBC Science Magazine, Society for Visiting Scientists) there is no doubt that I am the man in your book.

I wouldn't mind at all if I didn't cut such a faintly ridiculous figure. I don't claim to be a distinguished public figure, but all the same I didn't like this notion being so vigorously denied. And I didn't enjoy the idea of being disposed of in quanta.

A fortnight later the reply came, with the words LORD SNOW typed below the signature Snow. I had not realised that he had gone further up in the world:

4th January 1965

Dear van Heyningen,

I am most apologetic. I remember you with affection and respect, and there was no connection in my mind with the unfortunate victim.

The name swam into my mind when I was searching around for a South African appellation. It might just as well have been the name of one of the South African cricketers that I have known, and if I had reflected, it probably would have been.

I am genuinely sorry that you should have been embarrassed. The only redress I can think of is to change the name in later editions. That could be done without much trouble particularly if you could produce for me one or two rather picturesque Afrikaaner names. What do you think?

I liked the bit about affection and respect. His suggestion that I produce a choice of picturesque Afrikaner names gave me to think, and I had an inspiration. What about Old One Yee or Two Yees! Remember? He was that teacher in that Hell-hole of a dorp, Reddersburg in the Orange Free State, on whom we could always rely for a giggle when we asked him how to spell 'wagon' (or 'waggon'), and he would reply 'one yee or two yees, yes as you please'. Grobbelaar was his name. So I wrote

15 January 1965

Dear Snow,

I don't know what to say. On the one hand, I don't like to take myself so seriously; on the other hand, I do feel slightly uncomfortable, mainly because of what people have said to me. Those who have guessed that we might have met have been inclined to wonder whether, and then why, a dig has been made at me. Of course I know it hasn't, but they are not so sure. Perhaps I should accept your kind offer to eliminate me (without comment) from later editions. (This should provide fine speculative material for future Ph.D's!)

van der Walt? Viljoen? Oosthuyzen? Potgieter? Odendaal? Grobbelaar, especially Grobbelaar? But if one of them should write to you please don't blame it on me.

Snow agreed:

19th January 1965

Dear van Heyningen,

I will certainly change the name in later editions. I think we are too late to catch the fourth edition, but in all subsequent ones and in the Penguins, Grobbelaar will duly appear.

And so today there are two versions of *Corridors of Power*, the Van Heynegen edition [30] and the Grobbelaar edition [31]. I don't suppose Grobbelaar ever dreamed of such fame, not that he deserved it. In the end I made photocopies of the correspondence and sold the originals to Bertram Rota, the London bookseller, for a mere £25. My object was not the money anyhow, but a step towards the fulfilment of the prediction in my second letter to Snow that one day an earnest Ph.D. student of Eng. Lit. would come across them and make their name in the literary world, and Grobbelaar of Reddersburg's.

It was through Science Magazine that I met the other two of the three penicillin Nobel Prize-winners, Alexander Fleming of London, and Howard Florey of Oxford. I already knew the third Prize-winner, Ernst Boris Chain, then also of the Sir William Dunn School of Pathology at Oxford, for he had been at the Sir William Dunn Institute of Biochemistry at the University of Cambridge before the war. I was to have much to do with all three of them after the war.

One day while we were living in Chelsea, our neighbour, who seemed to earn his living in some mysterious way, and always seemed to have plenty of consumers' goods that were unobtainable by most people during the war, came to me to beg me to get some penicillin for a close relation who was in some hospital on the point of death from a staphylococcal infection. The doctors had told him that only penicillin could save him, but penicillin was almost unheard of, and quite unavailable in that hospital. Well, what with being connected with the Wellcome organization, and my being moved by his plea in spite of my mistrust of him, I got him some penicillin. I told him that on no account would I accept any kind of reward from him, since the facts of my being able to procure penicillin and of his happening to be my neighbour, were purely circumstantial, and there was no virtue on my part, nor on his. A few days later there was a crate of whisky in our hall. I liked an occasional whisky, and would have given a lot for a bottle, but a *dozen*! A dozen was not twelve times as difficult to get but a 1000 times! I telephoned and told him to come and remove his goddam crate at once and never speak to me again.

Towards the end of 1944 the pace of the V-2 rockets had slowed down enough for Ruthie and Simon to come back to London, so they did, in November 1944; and shortly after that we moved to an agreeable house on Clifton Hill in St John's Wood that we had taken over from J.D. and Eileen Bernal. Some time before this I had become a member of the Society for Visiting Scientists, which had its quarters in Old Burlington Street, near Piccadilly. It was a sort of club for refugee scientists fron the Continent, but behind that facade there was a cloak-and-dagger organization for smuggling in scientists from German-occupied territories, mainly France. One of those who were engaged in this perilous work was Louis Rapkine, a Russian-born Canadian turned Frenchman, a gifted scientist and a very fine man with an equally fine wife, Sarah. I introduce them now because it was through him that I got to know the Pasteur Institute in Paris very soon after the end of the war.

That war, or at least the European side of it, ended, as everybody knows, on 8 May 1945. Oh what a wonderful release! Oh what a glorious day! Oh what a glorious night! That evening Ruthie and I abandoned Simon in St John's Wood (Heaven remembers who looked after him) and went down to the West End to assist in the hearty heavenly hilarious hysterical happenings until several hours after midnight. By then there was no transport, but we thought nothing of floating on our feet all the five miles back home.

On 22 July our daughter Joanna was born, also in the Westminster hospital. This time I was hardened, and was not subject to premonitory dermatological manifestions. On 3 August the atomic bomb was dropped on Hiroshima.

In the middle of 1946 things started to go well, indeed very well, starting with the Victory Parade in London. I knew, still know, an excellent man, a South African called Frans Cronjé, who was at the time Secretary of the International Wool Secretariat, with an office on the second floor of a building right on Trafalgar Square; and he invited me (poor Ruthie was very much baby-bound) to a party in that room to view the Victory Parade. There we drank champagne, and ate plovers' eggs from Fortnum and Mason. I believe they are a great luxury, though they didn't seem to me to taste like anything but hard-boiled ordinary hens' eggs, but I liked the idea. All this while we enjoyed a perfect view of the glorious hours-long Parade. I could have dropped one of those plovers' eggs on the Queen's lap as the Royal carriage went by. All the pain of the war was washed away that day. The only flaw was that Ruthie was not sitting in that window too. But at least she had her little Simon and her littler Joanna, and for Ruthie babies are supreme.

There was nothing to keep me any more in the Wellcome Laboratories, and I longed to be back in the academic life. I had met Howard Florey on 'Science Magazine' and admired him, so one day in the summer of 1946 I went to Oxford to see him in the Sir William Dunn School of Pathology on South Parks Road. It was a hot sunny day, the Dunn School seemed most handsome, and an elderly scholarly-looking gentleman wearing a Panama hat was walking in the shade of the lime trees on the pavement in front ot it. Somehow this tranquil scene increased my desire for the academic life into an imperative need. I told Florey that I would like a job in his Department, and that I wanted to work there on bacterial toxins. Florey took to the idea, and promised that he would look into the possibility of getting me the post of Senior Research Officer. This was a new kind of post in Oxford that had been brought into being through Florey's efforts. It was an established post at the same level as a University Lecturer's (except that at that time lecturers in the scientific faculties were called University Demonstrators). The idea was that Senior Research Officerships should be held by people doing only research and no teaching or College tutoring (in fact they were paid an extra £100 a year for *not* tutoring). Such a post would suit me absolutely right down to the ground, and I went back to London with very high hopes. I had not been back for much more than a week when I was offered a University Lecturership in Cambridge, in the other Sir William Dunn establishment, so much beloved by me, the Institute of Biochemistry. What a perfectly marvellous dilemma! Such delightfully agonized ponderings! Like choosing between Chocolate Chip and Walnut Ripple Ice Cream, but on a more elevated plane! In the end I chose Oxford, largely because it was all research and no teaching, and to tell the truth, I didn't think I knew enough biochemistry to teach it. The fact is I never caught up with biochemistry, or any other branch of science. In all my scientific life, the only subjects I have known anything about in any serious way have been those on which I have actually been doing research. Possibly that has not been a disadvantage; perhaps it focussed the mind.

Fortune continued to empty its cornucopia on me. Towards the end of our last year in London, the *Cinquantenaire de la Mort de Pasteur* was commemorated in France during the week of 18 to

25 November 1946. The great Louis Pasteur had actually died on 28 September 1895, but in 1945 France had not yet recovered enough to commemorate his death. It was a great affair, but not a big affair. There were fifty-one guests from abroad, and about an equal number of French scientists. The seventeen-strong British delegation included the three who had won the Nobel Prize for Physiology or Medicine for their work on penicillin, namely Sir Howard Florey and Ernst Chain from the Sir William Dunn School of Pathology in Oxford, and Sir Alexander Fleming from the Inoculation Department of St Mary's Hospital Medical School in London. The Cambridge contingent were all from the Sir William Dunn Institute of Biochemistry, namely Joseph and Dophi Needham, Marjory Stephenson and Ernest Gale; and amongst the London contingent were Gabriel Knight and, of all people, me. My surprise was even bigger than my delight, which was immeasurable. I supposed André Lwoff and Louis Rapkine were responsible, out of kindness rather than good judgement.

Up to then, apart from those few hours in Marseilles and the night in Paris on my arrival in Europe in September 1934, I knew nothing of France. It was no more than a marvellous idea, and in that week I found the reality no less marvellous. That feeling for France is still with me. I love France, I admire it, and I overlook its faults. We started in Paris, at the Pasteur Institute of course, on the rue du Docteur Roux in the 7th arrondisement. Naturally, it was exciting to see the inside of that famous laboratory, and to talk with the people working in it. They included André Lwoff and his wife Marguerite, Louis Rapkine and his wife Sarah, and two people I had not met before, Jacques Monod and Francois Jacob. Jacques Monod was an apparently perfect man. He was most handsome; he spoke perfect, polished English; he had been the hero of the Liberation of Paris; his virtuosity with the piano and the violin was such that he had nearly taken them up as a career; he had a sense of humour; and he was an exceptionally good scientist, like André Lwoff and Francois Jacob. Indeed those three were to win the Nobel Prize for Medicine or Physiology in 1965, and Jacques Monod was to become Director of the Pasteur Institute.

I was embarrassed by my total lack of French, but several of our hosts besides those I have mentioned spoke English, and our other hosts struggled gallantly at it. Later, with the influx of so many British and Americans, English was to become a much used language in the Institute. There were not only the laboratories, there was Pasteur's apartment preserved as he left it, and his tomb. I was moved by them of course, more even by the apartment than the tomb. There were many lectures, many of them at great length in French by Professor Pasteur Vallery-Radot, a relation and biographer of Pasteur. There was an amusing and stimulating press conference with a remarkably good-looking French newspaper woman. There was a tremendously grand *Séance Solennelle* in the Grand Amphithéatre of the Sorbonne, where the foreign guests and some of the French Good and Great were seated on the stage, and I found myself seated besides Georges Duhamel wearing all his gear as Membre de l'Institut Français. We were addressed by the Prime Minister of France, and when he left, very large men with bulges under their coats left with him.

In Paris we stayed in the since demolished Hotel Palais d'Orsay on the Left Bank of the Seine, opposite the Tuileries Gardens. Food rationing was still very severe in Paris, but we were given plenty of food coupons and ate very well in a roped-off part of the hotel restaurant. One night I was sitting by that rope when two evidently well-heeled Parisian men of the world took a table on the other side and ordered a meal. All it consisted of was a plate piled high with mashed potatoes and a bottle of wine for the two of them. I felt awful with my sumptuous dinner, but they ate theirs as if it were even more sumptuous than mine.

After Paris we went in a special train, a *rapide*, to Dole, 230 miles to the south-east in the Jura, where Pasteur had been born. When our train drew into the station, *Monsieur le Maire et ses Conseils* were lined up on the platform with their blue, white and red *tricolores* over their shoulders, and the band played 'La Marseillaise' with vim rather than virtuosity. We were driven in a cavalcade through streets lined with cheering Dolois. 'Vivent les savants étrangers!' they shouted. I was delighted. I'd never been called a savant before. We went to Pasteur's *Maison Natale* on the street that is now called the rue Pasteur. When Pasteur was born there it was called the rue des Tanneurs, and his father was one of them. The living quarters of the house were on this street, with the tannery below, giving, quite a way lower down, on to the Canal du Rhône au Rhin. Some rooms in the house had been inaugurated as *Salles du Souvenir* by the President of the Republic in 1923 on the occasion of the centenary of the birth of Pasteur, and now another room was to be inaugurated at the commemoration of the fiftieth anniversary of his death. We all signed a scroll of names of those present (and a quarter of a century later, when I visited that house again, with Ruthie, and

I showed the gardienne my name on that scroll now hanging framed on the wall, she wept with emotion, and told me that I was the first of the *savants étrangers* to revisit the house).

After the ceremonies we went to lunch in the local school. It lasted from 2.00 p.m. to 6.00 p.m. There was no rationing on that occasion, far from it. There must have been a dozen courses, every one of them glorious, and entirely strange to me. The wine from nearby Burgundy flowed unrestrainedly and uninterruptedly, followed by cognac, armagnac and *fines de Bourgogne*. I was of an age when I could take it all. I was gloriously happy, and I must suppose I was gloriously drunk.

After Dole we went to Arbois, twenty-two miles further south-west. Arbois is a pretty town, where Pasteur had what would now be called his *maison sécondaire*, where he spent his vacations, where he had a laboratory, where he made his famous studies on the disease of the grape, and where he died in 1895. Of course we visited that house, and that vineyard, and of course there was another gigantic lunch in the local school. It must have been the day after the previous one, but I don't remember any hardship.

Then we took the *rapide* back to Paris. I was sitting in a compartment alone with Sir Alexander Fleming. He was the first President of the newly-formed Society for General Microbiology, and I was its Meetings Secretary, so I knew him quite well, and liked him well. In came four or five French students who were acting as couriers; and this is how André Maurois described what then happened in his *La Vie de Sir Alexander Fleming* [19]:

> Il revint en France en Novembre 1946, pour le cinquantième anniversaire de la mort de Pasteur. Tous les savants invités se rendirent à Dole en train spécial. 'Dans le train', écrit le docteur Van Heyningen, 'un groupe de jeunes étudiants français vint à nous; ils dirent qu'ils étaient là pour nous servir de guides et d'interprètes. Ils s'agenouillèrent, littéralement, aux pieds de Fleming et parlèrent de lui comme de l'un des plus grands savants de tous les temps. ''Mon Dieu!'' pensai-je, ''voilà qui est bien embarrassant pour le pauvre Flem! Surtout avec un collège assis à côte de lui! Ceci est une épreuve, voyons comment il s'en tirera . . . .'' Eh bien, il s'en tira le mieux du monde, et je crois que cela donne le vraie mesure de l'homme. Il ne devint nullement pompeux; il resta ce qu'il avait coutume d'être et parla de cette manière truculente qu'il prenait parfois. Il décrivit à ces jeunes gens la recherche qu'il était en train de faire et qui l'intéressait beaucoup plus que ses découvertes passées. Il jouissait de cette vénération, mais sans orgueil; il collectionait les décorations comme un collégien

collectionne les timbres, heureux quand un spécimen particulièrement rare lui était offert.'

[He returned to France in November 1946, for the fiftieth anniversary of the death of Pasteur. All the invited savants proceeded to Dole in a special train. 'On the train', writes Doctor van Heyningen, 'a group of young French students came to us; they said they were there to serve for us as guides and interpreters. They knelt, literally, at Fleming's feet, and spoke of him as one of the greatest savants of all time. "My God!", thought I, "this is going to be very embarrassing for poor Flem! Especially with a colleague seated beside him! This is going to be a test, let's see how he carries it off . . . ." Ah well, he came out of it in the best possible way, and I think that gave the real measure of the man. He was not at all pompous; he remained as he always was, and spoke in that truculent manner he sometimes assumed. He described to these young people the research he was doing at the moment, and which interested him far more than his past discoveries. He enjoyed this veneration, but without conceit; he collected decorations like a school-boy collecting stamps, happy when a particularly rare specimen was offered to him.']

There are many people still who think Fleming was the greatest scientist of all time, and are shocked when I say he was not. He would frequently tell me he did not deserve the Nobel Prize, and I could never bring myself to disagree with him over that; although there were several occasions when I found myself on the point of agreeing, not to be disagreeable, but to be polite in acknowledging the truth of what he was saying. He never pretended with me, or with anybody else, that he was a great scientist. He would probably even have denied that he was a good scientist, but if he had, he would have been wrong, for he was an excellent scientist, who did not really appreciate the significance of the phenomenon he had stumbled upon. I will come to that in the next chapter.

Now I will explain how Maurois came by that little tale. When I first knew Fleming his wife was still living, but she was to die quite soon. A month before the *Cinquantenaire*, a Greek scientist came to work with him, Amalia Voureka she was, a most attractive woman with great charm, 'an Athenian Goddess', as she was called by one distinguished bacteriologist, and I would not quarrel with that description. She was not, I think, very sophisticated with regard to science, and quite genuinely considered Fleming a genius. Fleming's wife died in 1949, leaving him grief-stricken and listless for some time. But he recovered, and after some further time it became clear that heand Amalia Voureka were attracted to each other, so it was no surprise when they got married in 1953. He died in March 1955. Some time later, I was invited to give the second of six Almroth Wright Memorial Lectures at the Wright Fleming Institute (formerly the Inoculation Department, where Fleming had worked) at St Mary's Hospital Medical School in London. These were to be given at weekly intervals. I went down from Oxford to hear the first of them (actually the chosen lecturer was not able to give his lecture because he had arrived from America so drunk that he had to be wheeled off his plane and wheeled back on to it again in the same state two days later, so a substitute had to be found). After the lecture, Lady Fleming, Amalia Voureka, came to me and told me that André Maurois had been commissioned to write a life of Fleming, and since I had known him so well she wanted me to jot down some recollections of him, and bring them to her when I gave my lecture the following week.

I spent the week polishing my lecture and trying to think of something for Maurois to write about Fleming, but I simply could not think of anything that was worth recording. I went to St Mary's to give my lecture, and after it Amalia came to me to ask for my souvenirs of Fleming. I was embarrassed, and had to tell her I was terribly sorry, but I had not been able to think of a single thing to say. Her eyes moistened. 'You too loved Alec,' she said (she called him Alec, we all called him Flem), 'I understand; come with me, and we'll talk, just the two of us.' She was all, all woman (and a year younger than me), and quite irresistible. She led me by the hand to Flem's former office, which she had preserved as a shrine, with everything in it exactly as he had left it, for she sincerely believed that Fleming was a genius as least as great as Pasteur. She produced a tape-recorder, and said, 'Just talk to me about him'. I panicked. Nothing came. Then I thought about the *Cinquantenaire*, and that incident with the students on the *rapide* on the way back to Paris.

5
OXFORD

A day or two after New Year's Day 1947, I drove to Oxford in my ancient Armstrong Siddeley, leaving Ruthie and the babies behind in St John's Wood, for I had not yet begun to look for anywhere for us to live in Oxford. Tony Pirie, an old friend from the Cambridge days, and now working in the Nuffield Laboratory of Ophthalmology in Oxford, kindly put me up for a few weeks in her house in Museum Road. After that I took a room in Halifax House on the Woodstock Road, a sort of club for dons, mainly those who were not Fellows of Colleges, at that time occupying Buckridge's former Victorian Holy Trinity Convent, which today is part of St Antony's College. Those first few months of 1947 were desperately cold, and every night I froze in my austere unheated room. In May, Ruthie and the children joined me in a house the University Chest had provided at a very low rent. It was a very tall house in a terrace of tall houses, like a terrace of lighthouses, in Keble Road, opposite the immense side of Keble College Chapel, a few minutes walk east to the Sir William Dunn School of Pathology, and a few moments walk west to St Giles Street and downtown Oxford. Soon after I arrived in Oxford I received a letter from the University Registrar informing me that it was necessary for me to matriculate, in order to be given the degree of M.A. by Decree, so that I could become a Member of Congregation, the sort of University parliament, which I will discuss later. In order for me to matriculate it was necessary for me to belong to a College, because it was the colleges that presented people for matriculation. I replied with crass haughtiness that I would inform him what College I belonged to when I was elected a Fellow of a College. In fact, I never became a fellow of a College, except an Honorary Fellow, and that only after I retired in 1979. After waiting in the wilderness for about six months, I capitulated and sought refuge as a Member of the Common Room of Exeter College, because it, like most Oxford Colleges, has a *concordium amicabilis* with a Cambridge College, in this case with Emmanuel

College. I was fortunate, because Exeter was always good to me, and still is.

At the Sir Willam Dunn School of Pathology everything was ready for me, because Gordon Sanders, a Senior Research Officer, had already written to me while I was in London, giving me details of the generously large laboratory that had been allocated to me, and asking what I needed in the way of laboratory benches and furniture, plumbing, electric fittings and so on. I was impressed and heartened by such kind thoughtfulness and efficiency. The Sir Willam Dunn School of Pathology is housed in a handsome red-brick building on the edge of the University Parks (which is in fact a singular park, in more ways than one; the plural refers to Cromwell's Civil War gun parks). Standing as it does before this handsome park, it is often likened to a grand country house. It is one of the only two modern buildings in Oxford approved of by Christopher Hobhouse in 1939 [16], not that I necessarily agree with everything he says: 'The modern additions to Oxford's architectural riches constitute a tale that is quickly told, and the quicker the better. To begin in South Parks Road, the recent School of Pathology and the new Radcliffe Science Library have already been commended as seemly additions to the colony of scientific buildings.' My pleasure at having an appointment in a laboratory that was so scientifically distinguished was enhanced by its architectural distinction, not to mention the historical, intellectual and architectural distinction of the rest of the University of Oxford and its Colleges, and the convenient proximity of the town (later the city) to London on the east and the Cotswolds on the west.

Among the members of the scientific staff of the Dunn School (as it is usually called) were those who had collaborated with Florey on his exploitation of penicillin as a clinically effective antibiotic. They were Ernst Chain, who shared the Nobel Prize with Florey and Fleming; Norman Heatley, who should also have shared in the prize; Gordon Sanders and Margaret Jennings; and Edward Abraham, who had come in a little later, and had made a critically effective contribution. Some of us were Senior Research Officers, others University demonstrators. There was also Florey's indispensable technician, Jim Kent. Chain and Heatley I knew well from the pre-war days in the other Sir William Dunn institution, the Institute of Biochemistry in Cambridge. Chain would grumble to me because he was still only a University Demonstrator and not a Professor, even though he was a Nobel Prize-winner; and I would annoy him by saying 'But Ernst, the University *expects* its University Demonstrators to win the Nobel Prize!' I meant it, because brilliance was not supposed to be out of the ordinary in the University, and the University couldn't multiply the number of Professors *ad lib;* and anyhow, I was beginning to wonder whether Chain was as clever as he thought he was.

And now the time has come for me to discuss, as a disinterested outsider who came on the inside after the event, who was who in the penicillin affair.

Who Really Was Who in Penicillin

Penicillin did not suddenly and dramatically spring into being as the result of a single discovery by a single individual. The idea of a natural microbial product destroying another microbe came into being soon after Louis Pasteur developed the germ theory of (infectious) disease in 1861, four years after he had demonstrated that lactic fermentation was due to a germ. In 1877 he and Joubert noticed that if a culture of anthrax bacilli were contaminated by common bacteria from the air, the anthrax bacilli were killed; and if they introduced these common bacteria into the animal body at the same time as the anthrax bacilli, the death of the animal was sometimes prevented. Looking sixty-three years into the future, they stated: 'Tous ces faits autorisent peut-être les plus grandes espèrances au point de vue thérapeutique.' ['All the facts perhaps allow the greatest hopes from the therapeutic point of view.'] Vuillemin coined the word 'antibiosis' for this phenomenon in 1889, from which Waksman derived the word 'antibiotic' in 1945, the year Fleming, Florey and Chain were awarded the Nobel Prize for their work on the antibiotic penicillin. Before antibiotics were to come into their own, the treatment of infectious diseases had to go first through the stage of antiseptic prophylaxis, then of chemotherapy.

It was Joseph Lister (teacher of Ruthie's grandfather) who introduced antiseptic surgery, basing his work on Pasteur's discovery that bacteria were the cause of what have since then been called infectious diseases. He washed his hands with carbolic acid before surgery, carried out his surgery under a fine spray of carbolic acid, and applied carbolic acid dressings to the wounds. But this procedure, though highly effective in contrast to the generally septic outcome of surgical treatment hitherto, had the severe limitation that the carbolic acid was completely unselective, and destroyed any living matter, whether it was the germs infecting the tissue of patients or the tissue itself.

It was Paul Ehrlich in Germany who was the first to conceive the idea that it should be possible to find chemicals — 'magic bullets' he called them — that would destroy infecting microbes without destroying the tissues of the host that harboured them. The Badische Analin und Soda Fabrik synthesised a number of chemicals for him; and injection of one of these, an arsenical organic compound known as Salvarsan, or '606', killed the spirochaete organism causing syphilis. It was the first synthetic compound to be produced that had such a powerful effect on a systemic infection, that is, an infection within the body. This was the beginning of chemotherapy. But '606' had limitations: it was effective only against spirochaetes, and not against the far more common bacteria; and it was fairly toxic to the patient.

In the twenty-five years preceding 1930 the chemical firm I. G. Farben Industrie in Germany had, in their search for dyes for wool, produced a large number of azo-compounds containing the sulphonamide group; and in the early 1930s Domagk injected a number of these azo dyes into mice to test their ability to protect the mice against experimental infection with a number of pathogenic bacteria, on the principle that since these dyes dyed bacteria (for microscopic examination), they must attach themselves to them, and therefore might kill them. Some of these azo dyes had an antibacterial effect in these tests; and one in particular had a marked effect, and was not toxic to mice. This dye was called 'Prontosil'. It was a good thing that they tested its antibacterial effect in experimentally infected mice, because they would not have found any effect on the same bacteria growing in test tubes. In 1935 Tréfouël and his colleagues at the Pasteur Institute in Paris (he later became Director) showed that only the azo-compound containing the particular sulphonamide called sulphanilamide was active. Moreover, sulphanilamide was in fact the active part, which was split off in the animal body, and was active in the test tube as well as the test animal.

To return to Pasteur and Joubert's 'les plus grandes espérances au point de vue thérapeutique' for good germs destroying bad germs: some antibiotic manifestations had been observed even before Pasteur and Joubert observed theirs, and continued to be made at intervals afterwards, to the extent that by 1928 Papacostas and Gaté were able to publish a book on the now extensive subject of the inhibition of bacterial growth by other bacteria and by moulds.

In 1929 an almost unnoticed paper appeared in Volume 10 of

the *British Journal of Experimental Pathology,* namely one by Alexander Fleming 'On the antibacterial action of cultures of a *Penicillium,* with special reference to their use in the isolation of *B. influenzae*'. This was the paper in which Fleming announced his discovery of penicillin. The best (and the most enjoyable) way to set about learning how that discovery was exploited ten years later by Florey and his colleagues in Oxford is to read Gwyn Macfarlane's two excellent books on the subject. After the war (where we saw him deal with gas gangrene and other wound infections), Macfarlane went to Oxford, where he became Professor of Clinical Pathology and one of the only two scientific Fellows of All Souls College. On his retirement he wrote *Howard Florey: The Making of a Great Scientist* [21]. In his Preface to this book Macfarlane wrote: 'before beginning it I explored the prospects of eventual publication. The results were utterly discouraging. It was made only too plain to me that a biography by an unknown author had no attractions whatever for commercial publishers unless the subject's name — famous or infamous — was already a household word. I had supposed that Florey's name would be known to everyone, but I learned to my dismay that this was not the case. On the other hand, it appeared that everyone did know of Fleming, for reasons that I was later to discover, and one London publisher even suggested that it was his biography that I might write with profit. Nothing could have made me the more determined to produce a book on Florey.'

Five years later Macfarlane published *Alexander Fleming. The Man and the Myth* [22], and in the Preface he wrote 'In Oxford, we soon became aware of Fleming's rise to world fame and of the fact that it seemed, at least in the newspapers, to be based on the work that we had seen done by Florey and his colleagues. I must confess that it was with a lingering sense of injustice that I wrote the biography of Howard Florey some years ago .... The present book is, so to speak, the other side of the equation. And I should say at once that any resentment I might have felt for Fleming at the outset quite evaporated as I studied his life and work in detail. He was, I am sure, an honest, likeable and truly modest man, and a highly talented and original scientist who believed that he had sound reasons for what he did and did not do about penicillin. But when the antibiotic revolution swept the world it was Fleming who was carried on the wave of an enormous public gratitude. In the circumstances, it would have been almost impossible for him to have abdicated his position. And if he had, the credit for the new era in medicine might well have slipped away — not to Oxford, but out of Britain and across the Atlantic.'

I am in full agreement with Macfarlane — Fleming was always the first to say to his colleagues that his part in the development of penicillin was small; and he was a very talented man, and a very decent one.

It is a fortunate fact of medical history that Fleming was not a tidy worker, by which I mean a worker who would have his laboratory glassware washed up and tidied away immediately after he had no more use for their contents. In Fleming's case the glassware was Petri dishes. Petri dishes are flat circular open glass dishes about nine centimetres in diameter with vertical walls about a centimetre deep. They come in pairs, one with a slightly larger diameter than the other, so that when inverted it can form a lid for the other. These dishes are sterilized by heating under pressure in an autoclave, and autoclaved molten agar jelly containing nutrient material for bacteria is poured into the lower dish, which is then covered with the slightly larger dish. When the agar is cooled and gelled, bacterial cultures are streaked on the surface; and the dishes (or plates, as they are usually called) are then placed in an incubator at human body temperature until the bacteria have grown in colonies. When observations have been completed, the Petri dishes are usually put away in a bath of lysol to be sterilized before being autoclaved and washed up. But in Fleming's laboratory they would pile up on the bench in growing accretions for months on end. I know: I saw them there myself when I visited him in his laboratory at St Mary's Hospital, and being neurotically tidy in my own laboratory, I was appalled. One day in September 1928, Fleming began to tidy his bench, putting his discarded plates in the lysol bath. By a great stroke of good fortune, the number of plates was so great, and the level of lysol so low, that some of the plates were left high and dry. Fleming was having another look at these when he noticed that one of them had been contaminated by a mould that had somehow got in and grown into a large round colony on the surface of the agar. Around this colony of mould the staphlyococci that had been streaked onto the plate had disappeared. Fleming kept everything; and that plate, with the famous mould *Penicillium notatum* and the vanished staphylococci, is now preserved in the British Museum.

Fleming went on to culture the mould in a liquid medium, to filter off the mould, and to test the effect of the filtrate, which he called 'penicillin', on various pathogenic bacteria, and on the host's protective system against these bacteria. He found for example that while highly diluted penicillin still killed pathogenic bacteria, undiluted penicillin had no deleterious effect on the host's phagocytes, i.e. those white cells in the blood that swallow up unwanted bacteria and destroy them. Filtrates of cultures of many other moulds that he tested had no such effect. He tested the effect of penicillin on many (but not all) pathogenic bacteria, and found that most of the Gram-positive organisms and some of the Gram-negative cocci were killed, but none of the Gram-negative bacilli. One of these bacilli that was not killed was the so-called *B. influenzae,* mentioned in the title of Fleming's famous paper.

Since Fleming's *Penicillium* culture filtrates still continued to kill germs even when highly diluted, and since his young assistants, Ridley and Cradock, had rid the penicillin of protein and other irrelevant materials, and obtained a partly purified preparation of penicillin that was still active after diluting 1/3000, he naturally considered the possibility of using his penicillin in the treatment of infectious diseases and wounds (it was a weakness of Fleming that he did not include his two assistants as co-authors of his now famous paper). Such hopes as he had were dashed. He found that his penicillin preparations took four hours to act, and were inactivated by human serum, and he therefore concluded that penicillin would be no use systemically. But he still entertained hopes of using it as a local antiseptic. This hope too was dashed when he found that irrigation of an amputation stump of a hospital patient with a continuous flow of penicillin failed to check infection. He did have one clinical success, which he never recorded (clearly he was not an *ambitious* man): an assistant in the laboratory suffered a pneumococcal infection of the eye, and irrigation with a penicillin solution cleared it up almost at once. This did not seem to re-awaken his interest in the therapeutic possibilities of penicillin, and his main interest in it seemed to be its possible use in the preparation of a vaccine against *B. influenzae,* otherwise known as Pfeiffer's Bacillus. Since this bacillus was not destroyed by penicillin, it should be possible to destroy contaminating organisms in a culture of the Bacillus by treating the culture with penicillin, then to concentrate the bacilli, and so make a vaccine against influenza (such a vaccine would have been of no use, because influenza turned out not to be due to Pfeiffer's bacillus, but to a virus). Fleming gave a paper on 'A medium for the isolation of Pfeiffer's Bacillus' to the influential Medical Research Club in London, but it did not arouse any questions or any discussion. In the summary of his now famous paper in the *British Journal of Experimental Pathology*, all he had to say about the practical application of penicillin in disease was: 'It is suggested that it [penicillin] may be an efficient *antiseptic* for application to, or injection into, areas infected with penicillin-sensitive microbes.' (Note the use of the word antiseptic, and the absence of any suggestion for the *systemic* use of penicillin.)

Thus it was that none of the reported observations on penicillin had been put to any serious practical use until Florey began to take an interest in them. His interest started in 1929 (not at that stage derived from Fleming's paper on penicillin in that year), but he did not translate this interest into practice until after Ernst Boris Chain came from the Sir William Dunn Institute of Biochemistry in Cambridge to the Sir William Dunn School of Pathology in Oxford in 1935. Florey had engaged him because he wanted to have a biochemical section in the School of Pathology, and Chain's work on the biochemistry of the mode of action of snake venoms had interested him. But soon after his arrival, Florey asked him to undertake a different problem. Florey had been interested for some years in natural antibacterial substances, and this interest had focussed on to one in particular. Now enter Alexander Fleming for the first time in Florey's life, not in the context of penicillin — rather that of lysozyme, a bacteria-dissolving substance Fleming had discovered nine years earlier, in 1920, in his own nasal mucus. It appeared at first to dissolve only harmless germs, but later, when it turned up in all sorts of biological materials, including egg white, it was found to be active against harmful germs as well. Florey had started working on lysozyme in Sheffield in 1929, since it appears in mucus, and mucus was one of his great interests. Later he concluded that lysozyme was not essential to the animal host's defence against infection, but nevertheless he remained attached to it — what was it, and what did it do to bacteria? The first step was to get it in quantity, and in a purified form. To this end he sought the help of his near-neighbour on South Parks Road, Professor Robert Robinson in the Department of Organic Chemistry. Eventually Robinson put a young graduate, Edward Abraham, on the problem, and Abraham succeeded in purifying it (from egg white, which is a rich and easily available source), and in preparing it in crystalline form in 1937. This was notable, since lysozyme turned out soon (see immediately below) to be an enzyme, and was thus one of the first enzymes to be crystallised.

Now Florey asked Chain to find out what lysozyme was, and what it did; and Chain did that. He showed that lysozyme was an enzyme, and that the micro-organism generally used for lysozyme to work on, *Micrococcus lysodeikticus*, contained a polysaccharide (i.e. a large-molecular complex sugar) containing N-acetylglucosamine, which was split in an enzymatic fashion by lysozyme. That having been determined, there seemed thereafter to be no particular use that lysozyme could be put to in the field of medicine, since, being an enzyme, it was a protein and therefore antigenic (i.e.producing antibodies, thus causing sensitization and shock) and therefore unsuitable for systemic use in the body. While the work on lysozyme was going on, Chain also developed an interest in antimicrobial substances elaborated by micro-organsms, and he made a study of publications on them, and in so doing came upon Fleming's hitherto largely unnoticed paper in the *British Journal of Experimental Pathology* of 1929. (It had not been all that unnoticed — Raistrick at the London School of Hygiene and Tropical Medicine had tried and failed to purify penicillin in 1932; and in 1940 even I vaguely knew about it and looked it up, thinking perhaps it was something I might follow up in the war effort, but I didn't.)

In 1938, Chain and Florey discussed a project for the study of natural antimicrobial agents, and Chain drew his attention to Fleming's paper. Florey replied that Fleming's paper had interested him (he always read the *British Journal of Experimental Pathology*, and had been one of its editors when Fleming's paper was published and had discussed it with a colleague when he was Professor of Pathology in Sheffield), but that his interest had subsided when Raistrick had failed to purify penicillin in 1932. Since Raistrick was an experienced biochemist, and had spent most of his time at the London School of Hygiene and Tropical Medicine isolating the products of moulds, this was a reasonable conclusion. Nevertheless, they agreed to tackle three antimicrobial products of microbes, namely penicillin, a lytic enzyme from *Bacillus subtilis*, and pyocyanase from *Pseudomonas pyocyanea* (also mentioned by Fleming in his paper in the *British Journal of Experimental Pathology*, 1929). Chain started on pyocyanase, but found it was toxic to animals, so attention was shifted to penicillin in early 1939.

There was no need to apply to Fleming for a culture of his *Penicillium*, since such a culture had already been obtained from the National Collection of Type Cultures some years before

Florey's time. Work started on penicillin. The idea was that Chain was to produce the penicillin and purify it, and Florey do the biological testing. Chain produced some crude preparations of penicillin, and Florey assayed them for biological activity; but Chain was heavily engaged on work with lysozyme and other products, and found it difficult to grow the *penicillium* mould and carry out chemical studies at the same time. In fact, it seems to me, Chain effectively stepped out of the penicillin picture at this stage.

So now enter Norman Heatley, one of the two (or three) *real* penicillin heroes. Heatley was at the Sir William Dunn Institute of Biochemistry in Cambridge when I arrived there in the Michaelmas Term of 1934, and in September 1936 he had come to the Sir William Dunn School of Pathology at Chain's suggestion to assist in a study of the metabolism of cancer tissues. With the outbreak of war in September 1939, Florey and Chain agreed that Heatley should now take part in the penicillin work. Heatley agreed, provided he should be directly responsible to Florey (I've often wondered why!). He immediately started to make an impact on the problem. Firstly, he improved the production of active culture filtrates of the penicillium, which needed to grow in shallow layers. In the beginning, enamelled metal bedpans were used, covered with a flat lid bedded on cotton wool, the inoculation of the seed culture being effected through the side tube; later he designed a pottery vessel of roughly the same shape, but square and without an opening on top; and the story is told of Heatley going up north to the Potteries to collect them, and driving back through the heavy snow in his bull-nosed Morris two-seater groaning under the weight, to arrive back in Oxford on Christmas Eve, 1939. Secondly, and very importantly, he devised a far simpler and more accurate method of measuring penicillin activity with his 'cylinder-plate' (or 'penicillinder') method of assay of penicillin. I won't try to describe this assay, but it must be obvious that it is hardly possible to investigate a substance, especially an unknown substance, unless you know how much of it you've got. Thirdly, he greatly improved and speeded up the method of extracting the penicillin from the culture fluids with ether (later with amyl acetate) by converting it to a semi-continuous process on which I will not elaborate. Fourthly, and this is a point that baffles the remains of the organic chemist in me, he employed a method of transferring the penicillin from solution in ether back into solution in water. This was very important from the point of view of the stability of the penicillin, and the further handling of it. To transfer the slightly acidic penicillin from the watery culture fluid to the immiscible ether by shaking the two solvents together, it was necessary slightly to acidify the culture fluid; but then they found that when they tried to evaporate off the volatile ether to recover the penicillin and dissolve it in water again, the penicillin was inactivated. They were baffled. Then Heatley suggested shaking the solution with slightly alkalinized water (alkali being the opposite of acid). Chain, who was an organic chemist, said it wouldn't work, but Heatley tried it, and *of course* it worked! This is why I am so surprised at those goings-on at that time. As a lad, learning organic chemistry at the University of Stellenbosch in 1930, I learned that if you wanted to transfer an acidic substance (like penicillin) from a watery solution to an immiscible organic solvent solution, you acidified the watery solution, and shook it up with the organic solvent solution. Since acid does not like being in acid, this drove your acidic substance into the organic solvent. You separated the two solutions, and then shook up the organic solvent solution with alkalinized water, which is the opposite of acid and therefore likes it, and so pulled the acidic substance out of the organic solvent. Each time you made such a transfer you rid your substance of impurities. It is an ordinary bread-and-butter chemical routine. 'Back-extraction' it is called, and in fact it had succesfully been applied in Fleming's laboratory by his young assistant, Lewis Holt, but not pushed to its proper conclusion. Yet Raistrick, Professor of Biochemistry at the London School of Hygiene and Tropical Medicine, and essentially an organic chemist, did not try it when he made his ill-fated attempt to get at penicillin in 1932. Yet Chain, another organic chemist, pooh-poohed it. And Heatley, a man of superlative intelligence and learning, did not immediately get on to it, when you might have thought it would have been second nature to him. Herein lies the subject for an essay in the history of science.

Thereafter, Heatley was responsible for the production of *Penicillium* culture filtrate; Chain for the extraction and purification of penicillin from it; and Florey for the biological and later the clinical work. By March 1940 this procedure had provided about 100 milligrams of a crude brown powder containing about 2 Penicillin Units per milligram. Since pure penicillin has 1800 Units per milligram (as was determined when it was completely purified two years later), this means that roughly only one nine-hundredth part of that brown powder was penicillin, and 899 parts of it were rubbish. Now Chain did a strange thing. He decided to test how toxic this material was, but not having a Home Office Vivisection Licence himself, he asked a colleague, J.M.Barnes, to inject 20 milligrams of the powder into each of two mice. The mice were fine, and Chain rejoiced. I say this was strange of Chain, because it had been agreed between him and Florey that Chain should stick to the chemical work and Florey the biological. But Florey was away at the time, and Chain could not, or would not, wait. Macfarlane states: 'Florey was naturally pleased by the result, but not by the fact that Chain had done the experiment he was about to do himself'. I'm inclined to wonder what that experiment really meant. All it proved was that the rubbish in the crude penicillin was not toxic to mice, but there was hardly any penicillin in it. For all they knew at that time, pure penicillin might have been toxic. Chain stated that that experiment was the turning point (and since I have not been able to discover any other turning point that he was responsible for, I can see why). He told me about it more than once, telling me that it was the crucial experiment, and complaining that Florey gave him no credit for it, and took no notice of it.

About six weeks later Heatley's back-extraction had come into use, and a penicillin preparation that was 20 times purer (or rather, less impure) was now available for a far more important biological experiment by Florey. It was the first experiment that showed the therapeutic power of penicillin against a systemic infection. Eight mice were infected intraperitoneally with a virulent streptococcus, and an hour later four of them were given a first dose of penicillin subcutaneously. The next day the four that had been given penicillin were perfectly well, and those who had not been given it were dead. As a result, Florey went all out for the development of penicillin; and at this stage enter E.P.Abraham. Having migrated from the Department of Organic Chemistry to the Sir William Dunn School of Pathology to continue work on lysozyme, he was now to work on penicillin.

Penicillin still needed a great deal more of purification. It was good enough to put into mice, but not into people, and this is where Abraham came in. He suggested that they should try and purify the penicillin by the fairly new process of chromatography (first used to separate dyes, hence the name). This was done by: 1. dissolving the crude material in an organic solvent; 2. pouring the solution down an upright column of alumina powder (contained in a glass tube); 3. pouring more solvent down the column in order to allow the various components in the crude material to separate into different layers in the alumina column (often differentiated by small differences in colour); 4. pushing the alumina column out of the glass tube and cutting out different zones; 5. washing off the substances in these separated zones with water; 6. determining which of these washings contained the penicillin; 7. obtaining the penicillin by freeze-drying the appropriate solution. Chain pooh-poohed the idea, making it the second crucial idea that he pooh-poohed.

But Abraham carried on, and got some penicillin in a reasonably pure condition, pure enough for the first clinical trials of penicillin to be carried out in 1941. These trials were carried out with success that was limited only by the scarcity of penicillin. They could not have been carried out unless Abraham had brought his chromatographic columns into the affair.

Who should have been awarded that Nobel Prize for Physiology or Medicine in 1943? The Swedish Academy could not consult Florey, and I wonder how they happened on Chain. Perhaps because his was the first name on that first published paper on penicillin from Oxford. It was in *The Lancet* in 1940, by Chain, Florey, Gardner, Heatley, Jennings, Orr-Ewing and Sanders, since Florey made it a rule that all papers emanating from his group should list the authors in alphabetical order. If I had my say in the matter, I would nominate Florey and Heatley if there were to be only two winners.

If the Prize had been awarded a little later, say in 1945 rather than 1943, then Abraham should have qualified as well, because he went on to play a very important part in determining the precise chemical structure of the penicillin molecule. From this he went on to find other antibiotics of similar structure, but not susceptible to the break-down action of the then recently discovered penicillin-destroying enzyme, penicillinase, which is produced by several bacteria. One of these antibiotics was cephalosporin, which was patented by the newly-formed National Research and Development Council. This brought in an enormous amount of royalties, more than half the total annual income of the NRDC, and those who worked on cephalosporin received a small percentage of these royalties; but cephalosporin was, and still is, in such demand that these small sums mounted up. Abraham formed a charitable trust with his share, after waiting two years for the Inland Revenue to accept the principle of it. In the end he disbursed the money in a number of excellent academical causes, and in 1980 he was knighted.

Perhaps in the case of penicillin the Nobel Committee should have departed from tradition and have awarded the prize not to persons, but to an institution, the Sir William Dunn School of Pathology, because the whole affair was a magnificent demonstration of team work, led by Florey. Many others in the laboratory were involved besides Florey — Chain, Heatley and Abraham, as we have just seen. (And Florey's able, indefatig- able, devoted technician, Jim Kent, should not be forgotten.)

In the course of my life I have known many Nobel Prize-winners, and I've come to the conclusion it takes all sorts to win the Prize. Some Prizes in Science or Medicine are given for sheer theoretical brain-work, like Dirac's for Physics;* some go for brainwork plus experimental ingenuity, like Fred Sanger's two prizes, first for elucidating the structure of proteins, then of nucleic acids; and some, like the penicillin Prize, not so much for brain power (though brain was obviously also necessary), but for character and determination, for gumption (see the *Concise Oxford English Dictionary*: 'resource, enterprising spirit, go, ready practical sense') plus hard work, experimental and clinical, in the face of all kinds of difficulties, combined with fulfilling Alfred Nobel's stated wish that the Prize should go to those who have contributed most to the common good.

In March 1959 *The Sunday Times* published an article on Chain in its 'Portrait Gallery' which more or less made him out to be the sole hero of the penicillin affair. The next day Florey asked me to write to the paper and put them right, particularly in relation to Heatley and Abraham. I was glad to do so, and wrote that I was sure that my old and valued friend Chain would be the first to agree that there were others concerned in the development of penicillin, and in particular I wanted to stress the important parts that Heatley and Abraham had played. I did not receive any acknowledgement from the paper, but the next weekend, when we were visiting the Mileses in London, Ashley Miles said to me, 'You'll have to make your peace with Ernst Chain — *The Sunday Times* has sent him your letter [actually they had telephoned him], and he's furious with you.' I didn't see why it was up to me to write to Chain (who at that time was in Rome, as Director of the Istituto Superiore di Sanita), but I did, telling him that

*Joseph Needham told me once just after he had been for a walk with Dirac, that Dirac had kept muttering 'The fewer there are, the more they rattle.' Joseph wondered what great thoughts were passing through Dirac's mind, but it turned out he was thinking of the nearly-empty bottle of aspirins in his pocket.

I understood he was annoyed with me over my letter to the paper, and that I wondered why. Surely not because I had put in a most well-deserved good word for our mutual friend of Cambridge and Oxford days? Chain sent me a long, silly reply, saying that my letter could have caused him 'to say the least, considerable unpleasantness, if not actual harm.' I had not said a word against Chain, and I wondered at the implication of a good word for Heatley and Abraham doing Chain harm. Several more letters were exchanged, with me wondering who in the Hell did Chain think he was, because to me he was just an ordinary chap scientifically, no better than me. At length he decided to forgive me. He was coming to London, and I was invited to lunch with him in the Dorchester Hotel one Sunday. I went to the Dorchester, and there was Chain, by now looking passably like Einstein, with his hair grown long, and standing out in all directions. We went into the restaurant, with the Italian headwaiter bowing and scraping and muttering *Professore* at frequent intervals. 'Ach man, they know me here', said Chain. An enormous menu, as big as *The Times*, was handed to each of us. Chain was magnanimous — 'Have whatever you like, Kits', he said. I decided to have my ultimate revenge on him. 'Just a little omelette, please', I said without glancing at the menu.

When the Contemporary Archives Centre learned that I was clearing out my correspondence on my retirement in 1979, they asked me if I would let them have any letters relating to Lord Florey. I sent them the interchange I had had with Chain, and this now forms an appendix to the Florey collection held at the Royal Society. There they remain restricted until 1989.

In the School of Pathology in those days the senior members of the staff would gather in Florey's laboratory for coffee in the mornings, to discuss laboratory affairs, and Florey's plans for the new Australian National University that was going up in Canberra. I found this unsettling, because Florey intended to leave Oxford and go there and start an institute for experimental pathology, and he expected to take several members of his staff with him. He even asked me whether I would like to go with him and the others, I suppose more out of politeness than serious intent, and I didn't fancy the idea, because I liked it too much in Oxford. And I didn't like the idea of Florey going off to the other side of the world so soon after I had arrived in Oxford. In the end Florey didn't go there after all, but the Australian National

University was well and truly founded, and is in a healthy state today.

A far more disturbing thing was that when I told Florey of my plans to tackle the problem of a certain bacterial toxin (I can't remember which), he told me he didn't want me to work on bacterial toxins, because they were too dangerous. I was amazed. He had engaged me because he was interested in having work done on toxins; and now he was scared of them! Any professional would know how to handle them. But Florey was adamant (and Florey knew how to be adamant), so I sadly scratched around for other problems to work on. During the next four years I published half a dozen fairly trivial papers, and chivvied one student into scraping through with a thesis for a D.Phil. (that's what we call it in Oxford, not Ph.D.). This student was a Chinese, called Tai. He came to Britain while Chiang Kai-shek was still in power on the mainland, but as his power waned Tai worried about the fare for his ticket back to China, convinced that the incoming regime would not let him have the money. He solved this problem by booking a passage on a particular sailing two or three months ahead, and applying to the Chiang Kai-shek government for the money for the ticket. Once he got it, he periodically postponed his sailing and got the ticket altered. By the time he was due to go back, Chairman Mao's regime was in power, but Tai still had his ticket. In the end he presented a shaky thesis, and as he went in for his *viva voce* examination he said to me, 'If I fail, the shame will be on you, for you are my teacher.' He passed, only just, and sailed back to Shanghai on his much postponed ticket. He would write to me from China from time to time, signing off as 'Your stupid younger brother'.

Late in 1949 my interest in bacterial toxins was strongly revived by an invitation to give four public lectures on 'Bacterial Toxins' at University College, London; and on four successive weeks in November I gave them. They seemed to go down well, and this encouraged me to write a book on the subject, which was published the next year by the then fairly new Blackwell Scientific Publications in Oxford [37]. It was the first monograph on bacterial toxins for a long time, one of the last having been Armand Gautier's monograph of 1896, *Les Toxines Microbiennes et Animales*. (Gautier was carried away by the magical powers of the antiserum against tetanus toxin, one drop of which, he said, would protect 10 'trillion' men. Since a 'trillion' is a million million, that drop of antiserum would have protected 2000 times the entire human population of the world today.)

As soon as the children were settled in their respective schools, Ruthie resumed her scientific career. She started in the Anatomy Department, working for a D.Phil. with Joseph Weiner, Reader in Physical Anthropology, on the physiology and biochemistry of the adaptation of humans to hot climates. She had done enough work for a Ph.D. in Cambridge, but this work had been secret war work, and therefore not publishable, and thus not presentable as a thesis. After three years in the Anatomy Department she succesfully presented a thesis for her D.Phil., and shortly after that she changed over to Nuffield Laboratory of Ophthalmology as Research Assistant to Margaret Ogilvy's Reader in Ophthalmology, who was Antoinette Pirie, an old friend from the Cambridge days. Later she was promoted to a Senior Research Officership.

Ruthie is a most able and distinguished scientist. As well as bringing up two children, and keeping a comfortable house (with not nearly enough help from me), and doing a lot of gardening (with no help at all from me), and doing a lot of entertaining at home as wife of the Master of St Cross College from 1965 to 1979, she has become a world leader in biochemical ophthalmology. She and Antoinette Pirie wrote the authoritative textbook on the subject [27]. Some years ago she hauled me off with her to Sarasota in Florida, where she was awarded the Proctor Medal of the American Association for Vision Research and Ophthalmology. Her particular interest is the lens of the eye, and why cataracts form in it. One of her most notable contributions to the subject has been her discovery of, and further research on, the aldose reductase enzyme in the lens. In December 1984 she was invited to an international conference on research on the eye in Hawaii, as the 'Honored Guest'; and the sole honoured guest at that, for the sufficient reason that the entire proceedings of this conference were devoted to the outcome of her discoveries in the field of aldose reductose, ramifications of which are now turning out to be relevant to other diseases, such as diabetes. While she was away, I met an old friend on the street, Robert Shackleton, formerly Bodley's Librarian. 'How's Ruthie?' he asked. 'She's at a conference on the eye in Hawaii' I replied. 'But there are two i's in Hawaii' said Robert. The idea of a conference on the i in Hawaii gives one to think. Which i? When I discussed this subject with David Vaisey, also of the Bodleian Library, he told me that there actually had been a learned paper on 'The n in the Isle of Iona', the idea apparently having been that that particular n is really an inverted u, and that the Isle should be of Ioua.

I have been blessed all my life by good fortune that I have not deserved, and the greatest blessing of all has been my much-beloved Ruthie, and then our two children, and the wife and the husband they each respectively chose, and the four children that they produced in their turn. (Ruthie's mother had an amazing gene that she passed on to produce a descendant tree of tidy and logarithmic symmetry. She had first a boy and then a girl; and the boy had first a boy and then a girl; and the girl had first a boy and then a girl; and the two boys of that generation each had first a boy and then a girl; and the two girls of that generation each had first a boy and then a girl. I expect my grandchildren and grandnephews and nieces to ensure that it will go on like that for ever.)

Ruthie instinctively puts others first. She is a really *good* person, just naturally and unaffectedly good. She can't help it, it just wells up from her unselfish compassionate heart. Added to this, she has a nice sense of humour, and a sense of balance. She knows how to cook, how to shop, how to garden, how to dress, how to deal with people, and how to enjoy herself. I have had a lovely time living with her these forty-five years.

And we are blessed with two particularly nice children: Simon, born during the war, and Joanna, born just after VJ Day. I used to have a lot of fun with Simon when he was a small boy, inventing and elaborating the concept of spanking machines. I would tell him how primitive man rose from spanking his children by hand to the invention of crude machines for doing the job, powered by donkeys or water wheels. With the coming of the Industrial Revolution steam was used, and I would draw pictures of Victorian spanking machines with steam-driven paddles applied to the bottoms of children supported on oak cylinders upholstered with overstuffed and buttoned leather. Simon would wriggle with pleasure, spiced with a tiny touch of fear. With the coming of the Labour Government spanking was nationalised, and Regional Spanking Factories were set up. Simon was by now no longer taken in, but he used to like my keeping up the concept with his younger friends. Once when we were motoring between Salisbury and Winchester with one of his younger friends on board, and I was giving my lecture on the nationalization of spanking factories, we came to a big sign saying NETHER WALLOP. 'And there' I proclaimed, pointing to a large factory-like building on the horizon, 'is the Southern Region National Spanking Factory!' Now of course we have electronic spanking machines in every home, controlled by microcomputers; and you can buy spanking programmes on discs or tapes, and exchange them with other parents.

Simon had an education quite different from mine. He went to the Dragon School in Oxford, and then to Westminster School in London, being a boy who liked hard pavements and plate glass windows in his environment. From there he went to King's College, Cambridge, and his parents' old laboratory, the Sir William Dunn Institute of Biochemistry. I discovered only afterwards that Simon had achieved a pinnacle that I used to dream of as a young man in South Africa, when my first impression of Oxford (and so of Cambridge) was derived from reading Compton MacKenzie's *Sinister Street*, where I learned about the Colleges, and the lordly heroes of these colleges, the Presidents of the Junior Common Room. It turned out that Simon had been President of the King's College Junior Common Room, but in his day the undergraduates were going through a heavy socialist realist phase, and his title had been Chairman of the Amenities Committee, for goodness' sake. In the course of doing research for his Ph.D. he met, and soon married, Veronica Daniel, a fellow student of biochemistry who had fled with her family from Budapest after the failed uprising in 1958. They are both doing research in Edinburgh now, and they have two dear dark-eyed, intelligent, lively children, Paul and Eleanor.

We called our daughter Joanna because that was consonant with our Dutch surname; but I wish now we had called her Johannah. She caused us minor anguish in her early days, when she and another little girl went around the corner from our house in Keble Road to Lady Florey's house on Parks Road to beg for money. Perhaps in revolt against her mildly intellectual background, she decided to be a hairdresser's assistant, and clung to that ambition for quite a long time, but in the end she took a degree in French and Russian at St Anne's College, Oxford. Her first job was with the *Times Literary Supplement* as a Russian expert, but they decided they had enough Russian experts, and she was to be their German expert. Since she had dropped German on leaving school, she left to take a job on the French course for Linguaphone, but they gave her nothing to do. Then to my delight she decided she would like to take up architecture, and so she went to Sir Leslie Martin's department at Cambridge University, where she met her true metier; and her true love, her teacher Birkin Haward. They married, and produced two dear children in the traditional order, Bruno and Mellis (after a Suffolk village that had caught Birkin's fancy).

Now they are in an excellent architectural practice of their own.

Shortly after the publication of my little monograph on Bacterial Toxins, I wrote a chapter on Toxic Proteins for a four-volume work called *The Proteins*. I mention it because it provided us with much fun a few years later in Moscow, when we went there for an International Congress of Biochemistry. On arrival at our hotel I found a letter waiting for me from the State Publishing House for Foreign Literature, informing me that they had translated my article into Russian, and proposed now to pay me royalties (surely not the right word in that country?), which I could collect if I went to the State Publishing House for Foreign Literature — '. . . where it is [they wrote], you may find out'. I found out, and collected quite a large number of roubles, which I had to spend within four or five days, because it was not permitted to take any out of the country. It was quite a business spending that money, because we could see no consumer goods that attracted us, except perhaps a fur coat for Ruthie, but she would have none of it. We took taxis wherever we wanted to go, but taxis were very cheap, and the drivers would not take tips. In the end I shed my money by giving a series of dinner parties for our friends in *salons privés* in the best restaurants in Moscow, in one of which, when I ordered vodka and champagne, a bottle of each was provided for each of us.

I travelled. In 1950 the Brazilian microbiological authorities wrote to me, as Meetings Secretary of the Society for General Microbiology, to invite the Society to send a number of delegates to the Fifth International Congress of Microbiology, to be held in Rio de Janeiro in August 1950. They realized there would be difficulties for European delegates in travelling so far, and informed me that they hoped to transport us in a ship, the *Duc de Caxias*, which would then lie at anchor in Rio Bay and provide our accomodation during the congress. I wondered what kind of ship the *Duc de Caxias* might be, and Ashley Miles suggested I walk up the Charing Cross Road and look in book shop windows, where I might see it in a nineteenth century print. The Brazilians then offered to fly a hundred European delegates to Rio de Janeiro, of whom fifteen would be British, of whom one, Heaven knew why, was to be me. The flight on a Panair do Brasil Constellation was eventful. Halfway across the Atlantic between Dakar and Pernambuco, I noticed one of the four propellors not turning, and soon after that the Captain announced that since we were not quite at the point of no-return, we were to fly back to Dakar. For five grinding hours we flew back against headwinds, with the volatile Latin crew getting life rafts ready, looking very, very worried. As we finally came down at Dakar, the entire population was lining the runway, presumably hoping to see us crash in flames. We set off again within the hour, with the population again lining the runway to see us crash on take-off. When we reached Rio in the end we were all exhausted, but were instantly revived by small cups of delicious Brazilian coffee, and the sight of that marvellously beautiful bay. The Congress was not in Rio de Janeiro itself, but in Petropolis up in the mountains forty miles in the interior, in the Hotel Quitandinha (not long previously described in *Life* magazine as 'The Fabulous Playground of the Millionaires').

Alexander Fleming was with us, and since the Brazilians had taken with exuberant Latin enthusiasm to penicillin, with the streets of Rio lined with clinics advertising penicillin as a cure for venereal disease and impotence, they worshipped him. He was constantly being set upon by people wanting his signature; so I made a deal with him: I would sell his signature for half a gram of dried snake venom from the Snake Farm at Butandan. I was interested in snake venoms because they are proteins, like bacterial toxins, though not nearly as toxic. Fleming liked the idea, and I did a roaring business, reaping promissory notes amounting to half a kilo of venom; but nothing came of them in the end.

Shortly after the visit to South America, I went to North America for the first time after the war, in response to an invitation to attend a small conference on bacterial toxins in Chicago. In the middle of my first breakfast in the hotel I was astonished by a lovely warm feminine voice saying to me 'Shall I give you a warm-up honey?', and there stood a ravishing *café au lait* girl with a most charming and inviting expression on her face. Then it dawned on me that this was the new way of offering to refill my coffee cup, not current in my pre-war days in the United States. I sailed back from Montreal, and was seated at a dining table with an odiously boring couple. She kept telling me her husband had two doctor's degrees, until I could bear it no longer, and then I told her 'Madam, if you insist, I have *three* doctor's degrees, and these from the Universities of Oxford and Cambridge. This actually was true. I had taken a Ph.D. in Cambridge, and after some years in Oxford I put in for a Cambridge Sc.D. The idea was that if you considered yourself a recognized authority on your subject you submitted your published work, sent a cheque for £50, and applied for the establishment of a *prima facie* case to be examined. After about a year you heard from the authorities whether or not such a case had been established. It was said that the chance was less than 50:50. If the case were not established, you got your £50 back; if it were, the £50 was divided between two examiners whose names were probably the best-kept secrets in the University, since they were supposed to be world authorities on your subject, as you supposed yourself to be, therefore you were bound to know them. After another year or so, you heard again from the University, whether or not the examiners had approved your application; and again the chances were said to be less than 50:50. I had had the arrogance to put in for a Cambridge Sc.D. because I thought it was tougher than the Oxford D.Sc., but after a while I began to regret that, because with an Oxford D.Sc. I would be able at Encaenia, when the Honorary Degrees are conferred, to partake of Lord Crewe's Benefaction (of champagne and peaches) together with the Honorands and the other Doctors of the University (excluding mere D.'s Phil.), in the Hall of the College of the reigning Vice-Chancellor. The party then walks before in stately procession through Oxford from that College to Christopher Wren's glorious Sheldonian Theatre, where the Degrees are conferred; and where undergraduates read their Latin Prize Essays and their English Prize Verses; and the Public Orator delivers his Oration. So I 'incorporated' my Sc.D. Cantab. for a D.Sc. Oxon., and thus had two phoney Oxford degrees, the D.Sc. and the M.A. that I got 'By Decree' after I matriculated in 1947. In the procession, the Doctors of the University of Oxford march ahead of the Honorands, being for a short while superior to them since they are not yet Doctors of the University of Oxford. On one such procession I walked just ahead of two of the Honorands, Harold Macmillan and Arne Tiselius, the distinguished scientist from the University of Uppsala. The people lining the street clapped and applauded; and Macmillan doffed his imminently Doctoral cap and bowed in all directions. I wondered who the devil did he think he was; for all he knew they were applauding Tiselius.

Dysentery Toxin

Some time in 1952, Florey grumbled that I didn't seem to be doing much work, so I told him that was because he wouldn't let me do what I wanted to do, and what he had agreed I should do, which was to work on bacterial toxins. Florey agreed now that I should, and after studying the field, I chose to tackle dysentery toxin. There had been several papers on the subject that did not make much sense, so I thought it could do with being looked into. There are several kinds of dysentery, and two specific ones: amaebic dysentery and bacillary dysentery. There are three or four varieties of the dysentery bacillus, all known as *Shigella*, after the Japanese bacteriologist, Kiyoshi Shiga. The word dysentery is often used as a euphemism for diarrhoea. It derived from *dys-*, meaning difficult and *-enteron*, meaning intestine. The difficulties referred to in this case are diarrhoea and inflammation, the former being mainly in the small intestine, and the latter mainly in the large intestine, or colon. The dysentery organism that interested me was *Shigella dysenteriae*, known also as *Shigella shigae*. I was interested in it because it produces by far the most severe and toxic manifestations of the disease.

Gareth Gladstone had not long been in the Sir William Dunn School of Pathology as Reader in Bacteriology, and was looking for a problem, so Florey suggested that he join me on the dysentery problem, and I was glad to agree. Since he was primarily a bacteriologist, we agreed that he should grow the dysentery bacilli, and I should extract the toxin from them and then purify it. Gladstone devised an ingenious method of growing the bacteria in a continuous culture that went on day and night, with crops of bacteria being drawn off from time to time. We then persuaded the Microbiological Research Station at Porton to take this over for us on a large scale, and so quite a considerable weight of bacteria was amassed. From this mass of bacteria I was eventually able to prepare the toxin in a form that appeared to be very close to complete purity by the physico-chemical criteria available at that time. What astonished me about my preparation of the toxin was its immense toxicity. Shiga toxin (as it is often called) was known to be a 'neurotoxin', since it produces a flaccid paralysis in rabbits, that is to say, the animals are rendered limp and motionless, due to a complete relaxation of all their muscles. Since the dysentery-intoxicated animals looked as if they had been poisoned by the toxin of botulism, I presumed that the action of the toxin was on the nervous system that sent impulses to the muscles to enable them to contract. (I did not at that time stop to wonder what this had to do with the symptoms of dysentery.) The toxins of botulism and tetanus were the two most poisonous substances known at the time, and now it turned out that my purified preparation of Shiga toxin was equally toxic. These toxins are more powerful by several orders of magnitude than such poisons as strychnine, cyanide or arsenic, or the snake venoms. In theory an amount of tetanus, botulism or Shiga toxin weighing no more than the ink in the full-stop at the end of this sentence would be enough to kill thirty grown men (see next chapter).

When I gave some of my toxin to J.G.Howard of the Bruce Laboratories, he showed that Shiga toxin is not really a neurotoxin, but one that simulates the action of a neurotoxin by acting on the blood vessels in the spinal cord, causing the cord to swell within the confines of the spinal column, and thus to exert pressure on nerves, and so to bring about paralysis. Shiga toxin is so extremely toxic only in the rabbit — in other animals it is still quite toxic, but not nearly as fierce as it is in the rabbit. How it acts in the human patient suffering from Shiga dysentery was still being examined when I last heard of it several years ago. I dare say detoxified partially purified Shiga toxin might be a good preventive immunizing agent against the toxic effects of Shiga dysentery infection.

That purified preparation of Shiga toxin that I made in 1950 is still being used to good effect today in the Nobel Cancer Research Institute in Oslo by Sjur Olsnes. I was pleased to learn from him that it is a better preparation than those made by the present generation of scientists with far more sophisticated techniques than were available to me. (Cancer research workers think of destroying cancer cells by attaching protein poisons like this, e.g. ricin, to monoclonal antibodies that seek out the cancer cells in the body, and no other cells. It occurs to me now to wonder whether Sjur Olsnes has this in mind for dysentery toxin.) After the purification of the toxin, I made some studies of the bacterial physiology of toxin production by the dysentery bacillus, and published two papers on it. I found it quite interesting, but I don't think anybody else did. Perhaps somebody will come across those papers one day.

About this time Dr Jacoba van Lessen sent me another cutting from *Het Nieuwe Rotterdamsche Koerant* (see pp.2-3), this time reporting that the Burgomaster and Aldermen of Amsterdam had recommended to the City Council that I should be appointed Professor of Physiological Chemistry in the University of Amsterdam. I was amazed, because I had not applied for the post, and had not been approached by the University of Amsterdam. Of course I was flattered, but I wrote to the Registrar of the University to express my surprise, and to tell him politely that I was quite content to remain in Oxford. He sent me a good-humoured reply in his quiet Dutch way, saying that the whole thing was an embarrassment to him. The fact was that the University of Amsterdam was governed by the Amsterdam City Council, and therefore all University matters had to be approved in public by the Council before they could be taken any further. This was how my name had to come up in public before it could be considered any further.

On Coronation Day 1953 Ruthie and I and the children, and my lovely new Jowett Javelin car, sailed for Cape Town from Tilbury on the maiden voyage of the Ellerman & Bucknell cargo ship *City of Exeter*. The ship was quite big, with a displacement of about 30,000 tons, and it took 100 passengers, all in one class which was first class, if not First Class, with lots of deck space for the few people on board. I'll not forget when we docked at Cape Town. Ruthie and I were standing at the ship's rail looking down at two Black porters loading heavy goods on a trolley. They were singing and laughing, and every movement they made was just naturally a dance movement. I thought I had seldom seen a jollier sight, and turned to Ruthie to share my enjoyment. A look of distress was frozen on her dear face. She was looking at something that I didn't see because I took it so much for granted. The two merry black men were dressed in filthy rags, which consisted of little more than the double-seamed remnants of their shirts and shorts. Ruthie had occasionally seen men in rags, but never in such an advanced state of filthy raggedness, and was blinded to their merriment. Another thing that struck Ruthie were the guichets in the post offices — one for Whites, one for Blacks, and with faultless logic, one in the middle for Blacks on the Business of Whites. We motored from Cape Town all the way to the 'great grey green greasy Limpopo River, all set about with fever trees' on the border with Rhodesia. On the way I saw the last of my younger brother Peter (my sister Koekoe had died before our visit); and at the end of our visit we went to the tobacco farm in Rhodesia of my eldest sister Boudina and her husband Jack Coetzer. There I saw the last of both of them. Boudina was dying, and knew she was dying, but she was very cheerful, and I tried to be cheerful, because she had been a mother to me; but it was terribly hard to say goodbye in a nonchalant manner. We flew back to Europe from Lusaka in Northern Rhodesia (having shipped the car back from Durban). It was in a Comet, the first commercial jet, and the most beautiful aircraft ever made, and the most exciting; but we were flying on borrowed time, because a few weeks later Comets were falling out of the skies over the Mediterranean Sea. We were to visit

South Africa again thirty years later, and I will discuss that visit, and my views on Apartheid, in the last chapter.

As the mid 1950s approached, Florey seemed to grow more and more dyspeptic, at least as far as I was concerned, I never knew why. He was cold with me, and could hardly spare me the time of day. Matters came to a head when Cy Halbert came from the College of Physicians and Surgeons of New York to spend a sabbatical year with me. I took him up to introduce him to Florey, and Florey was hardly civil, and for no good reason at all made an extremely offensive remark to me in front of Halbert. As soon as I got back to my laboratory, I wrote a note to Florey, protesting at the way he had behaved to my guest, and to me, and demanding that he treat me with respect in future. Florey summoned me up to his office. 'What do you mean by this silly note?' he demanded. 'What I said', I said, quaking in my boots. 'You were as cold as a fish with Halbert, and you were offensive to me in front of him. You must treat me with respect.' 'Do you want to resign?' asked Florey. 'Of course not', I said, 'why should I?' 'I'll tear up your silly note and forget the whole matter' he said. 'O.K.' I said, and departed, quivering at the knees and hoping I looked cooler than I felt. Thereafter Florey treated me with respect. He seemed to like me better and better, and to have trust in me. In fact, he soon showed that in a convincing manner.

Shortly after I arrived at the Sir William Dunn School of Pathology in 1947, Florey had engaged a recently retired Major-General of artillery as Administrator of the Laboratory. It looked like an excellent idea, and we all thought the Laboratory would now run like clockwork. One would go to the Major-General and ask him to get something done, and he would bark, 'Got that! 't'will be done!' The trouble was, 'twas never done; and after a while the Major-General departed. He was replaced by a recently retired Group-Captain of the Royal Air Force, and again our hopes rose high. One would go to the Group-Captain and ask him to get something done, and he would say, 'Let it fester old boy, let it fester!', and that is what happened — it festered. So after a while the Group-Captain departed. By then Florey had become President of the Royal Society, with even less time to keep an eye on the day-to-day affairs of the Sir William Dunn School of Pathology, so he asked me if I would be willing to take charge of the administration. I told him I would be glad to do so, and took on the job in April 1956, expecting of course to carry on with my own research at the same time.

I started by asking Mrs Peggy Turner, the Secretary of the

Department who had been there for many years, and all through the penicillin episode, to take on a number of administrative responsibilities that I could easily see she would do far better than I could — all she needed was a free hand. Then I made some much needed changes. I gave notice to the man in charge of the Animal House that he must get his house in order. He had been the 'Beast Man' at a circus, and had a certain understanding of animals, and sympathy for them, but not the slightest conception of cleanliness. All his animals were filthy and ridden with fleas. The cats were in a particularly dreadful condition. They were kept in a completely empty room with not a stick in it, and they were given nothing but tinned cat food, which was just thrown in the room with no friendly gestures. When you opened the door they retired into a corner hissing with their backs arched. I told the beast man that all his animals must be rid of fleas within a month; and that the cat room should be cleaned out and furnished with a bench or two for the cats to jump on to and off from time to time, and that they should be given fish and other feline delicacies, and that they should be picked up from time to time and fondled. 'You've bloody well got to love those goddam cats!' I told him (though I am no great cat-lover myself). By the end of that month he had done nothing — I don't suppose he had the foggiest idea what I was talking about — so I sacked him. I replaced him with Jim Kent, Florey's technician. He had been with Florey all his working life and thoroughly understood animals. Florey had no objection, since he wasn't doing much experimental work in those days, because of all his national and international commitments. Under Kent's governance the animals flourished. Everything became spotless; the fleas and other infestations disappeared; and when you went into the cat room, the cats would jump into your arms and purr. There were two other crucial appointments to be made. Mr Bush, the instrument-maker had retired, and a replacement was needed. I took a chance with Harry Stroud, who worked for an electrical firm that had been doing a lot of work in the Laboratory. He struck me as a competent man who would soon get the hang of making instruments, doing odd jobs about the Laboratory, and looking after the electrical and other installations. He did it beautifully for the next twenty-five years. Then there was the photographer. We had had a series of professional photographers, but they were not a success because they tended to regard themselves as artists, with artistic temperaments. They didn't understand what they were supposed to photograph, and were not interested. I found another job for the current photographer with a photographic agency, and in his place I appointed a young laboratory technician, Stanley Buckingham, who of course understood the scientific side, but was a keen amateur photographer as well. I knew he would put his heart in the job. He did, and still does.

After a few years everything was running so efficiently that there was no need for an Administrator as well as a Secretary, so I suggested that our excellent secretary, Peggy Turner, assume the role and title of Administrator, which she naturally did without pausing in her stride. But I did have one tricky job before I handed over to her: somebody was stealing money left in the pockets of laboratory coats hanging in the female technicians' room. I powdered a ten-shilling note with traces of anthracene, planted it in a pocket of a coat, and left it to hang in the room. Within an hour that note was missing; so I pretended to do an experiment that needed the co-operation of the women in the laboratory. I asked them all to let me study their hands under an ultra-violet light in the darkened lecture theatre. I did it in such a way that they could not see what I could see. What I was looking for was a glowing hand, because the anthracene powder, though invisible by ordinary light in the amount I had used, shines brightly under ultra-violet light. Sure enough, a hand glowed. I said nothing at the time, but later summoned the lady in question to my office and charged her with the offence. She was an Irish cleaning lady, and could not understand the nature of my evidence. She told me she would bring her husband along and he would soon teach me not to insult a lady. He came, two yards high and a yard wide. I quaked. What did I mean, he shouted, accusing his wife like that, did I want my bloody block knocked off? I was terrrified. I took them to the darkened lecture theatre and showed him the ten-shilling note and her hand under the ultraviolet light. He cottoned on immediately, and from then on it was for her I feared.

In 1962 Florey was elected Provost of The Queen's College, Oxford, and resigned his Professorship of Pathology. The Sir William Dunn School of Pathology has never been the same again.

6
THE SARDONIC SMILE

After dysentery, Gladstone and I decided to tackle staphylococcal leucocidin, the agent that assists the invading staphylococcus by destroying the white cells (or leucocytes, or phagocytes) of the blood that would otherwise swallow up the invader and destroy it. Gladstone would grow the staphylococci and assay the leucocidin, while I would purify it. After working on the problem for some time, I concluded that it was solvable, and applied to the Medical Research Council for a grant to support somebody to take over from me. I was thus able to engage Alan Woodin on the problem. He solved it brilliantly, by isolating the leucocidin in a completely purified, crystalline, state, and by demonstrating that it consisted of two parts which were active only when put together. I believe that this was the first instance of a bacterial toxin being shown to have such a bipartite structure. I have not followed the leucocidin 'literature' (as we call it, to the scorn of literary folk), and I don't know whether this work has been further exploited. Woodin was an unhappy, moody person who kept himself to himself. He moved to Cambridge, and there the poor man committed suicide.

In the meanwhile I tackled the problem of tetanus toxin. Tetanus, or lockjaw, is an ancient and ferocious disease of wounding, described by Hippocrates twenty-four centuries ago. Any break in the skin, a superficial scratch, the puncture of a drug addict's needle, often so small as to be undetectable *post mortem*, is susceptible to infection by the tetanus bacillus, *Clostridium tetani*, the spores of which are ubiquitous, particularly in pastoral soil containing animal manure. It produces an amazingly potent toxin, which to me was the Everest of bacterial toxins; and I wanted to ascend to the heights.

The tetanus bacillus was discovered in 1884 at the University of Gottingen by a twenty-two year old medical student, Nicolaier, who concluded correctly that since the bacillus did not spread through the body, and since a tetanus patient resembled a patient suffering from strychnine poisoning, it must produce a strychnine-like poison. This poison was discovered in 1890 by Tizzone and Catani, who concluded also correctly that it was a protein that acted directly on the central nervous system, as strychnine does, and had no action on any other tissue of the body.

The lethal dose for a twenty-gram mouse is one thirty thousand millionth of a gram [38]. This means that one gram should kill 600 million kilograms of living matter. Over-estimating the average weight of people at fifty kilograms, this means that one gram should kill 12,000,000 people (on the most dubious assumption that you could line them all up and give them each a shot in the arm), or that 500 grams, say twenty ounces, should kill 6000 million people, rather more than the present population of the world. (If it were administered by mouth those twenty ounces would kill only 6000 people.) Botulinum toxin, produced by *Clostridium botulinum*, is equally toxic, producing a flaccid limp paralysis, quite the opposite of the spastic, rigid paralysis of tetanus. It is more toxic by mouth than tetanus toxin, hence the food poisoning of botulism. Much of the toxicity is lost by this route, but nevertheless it was considered as a potential lethal agent during the last war, and much study was devoted to this possibility, particularly in America. It may sound like a simple and feasible idea; and if I really believed in it, which I don't at all, and had a couple of telephones and a good staff at my disposal, I think I could turn a brewery into a botulinum toxin factory within a couple of weeks. But I would be wasting my time. I suppose the idea was to put it in water supplies, and perhaps a few people would have been killed that way. But as soon as it was suspected, the toxin could be destroyed by a touch of caustic soda in the water, and boiling it to make quite sure.

A death from tetanus or botulinum toxin would leave no signs (though a reasonably competent physician would see them before death), and the toxins would certainly not be detectable in the corpse. I presented this notion to Agatha Christie once when I was sitting beside her at an Encaenia luncheon at All Souls College, and she liked it, but I don't think she wrote any novels after that. Tetanus toxin has, to my knowledge, once unsuccesfully and allegedly once succesfully been employed with murderous intent. The unsuccesful attempt was made by a Frenchman living near Paris. He applied on fake pharmacist's note-paper to the Pasteur Institute in Paris for a strain of the tetanus bacillus, put it in his wife's soup, and waited for her to die. Of course she didn't, because he was too ignorant of bacteriology to know that he should first have incubated the bacillus in the soup for some hours to enable it to grow and produce toxin (which it might well not have, anyhow); and too ignorant of tetanus toxinology to know that it would hardly work by mouth. He was found out when he compounded his stupidity by applying to the Pasteur Institute for another culture of the bacillus. Some years ago it was reported in the British newspapers that a successful attempt had been made by somebody who would know his business — a scientist on the Continent was said to have injected tetanus toxin into his wife's tube of toothpaste and bought her a new hard-bristle toothbrush that was bound to inflict undetectable wounds in her gums. She died, but his attractive assistant was said to have broken down and given the game away. However, the court apparently found him not guilty.

Besides the unbelievable toxicity tetanus of toxin, I was attracted by the crisp and clean specificity of its action. Tetanus is a terrifying disease of spastic paralysis, resulting from opposing muscles pulling against each other. It generally starts with restlessness, muscular irritability and twitching, then with stiffness of the neck muscles and difficulty in opening the mouth. Muscular spasm quickly increases, first causing difficulty in swallowing, then spreading to the main muscles: the abdominal muscles become board-like, the back arches, the neck muscles are rigid and the jaw is locked. Convulsions then begin to take place under the slightest stimulus (a light switched on, a twitch of the bed-clothes), and the whole body is contorted in a major spasm resulting from the violent contraction of all the muscles — the spine is strongly arched, spasms of the larynx impede breathing, the jaws are tightly clenched in a fearsome rictus that the older writers used to refer to as the 'sardonic smile' (*risis sardonicus*) or the 'cynical spasm' (*spasmus cynicus*), see figure 1. The patient is fully conscious, sweating profusely, exhausted from continuous muscular activity, and in dreadful pain. When the spasm relaxes, he lies in awful apprehension of the next spasm, which will certainly come. Death is due to exhaustion, heart failure, and collapse of the lungs.

Tetanus toxin acts by suppressing what is called *synaptic inhibition* in the spinal cord, i.e. in the central nervous system. There it blocks the 'don't pull' messages to certain muscles, with the result that the opposing muscles of the body pull against each other, and so cause spasms. I have tried to show this in figure 2. The drug which is most used in the treatment of tetanus is

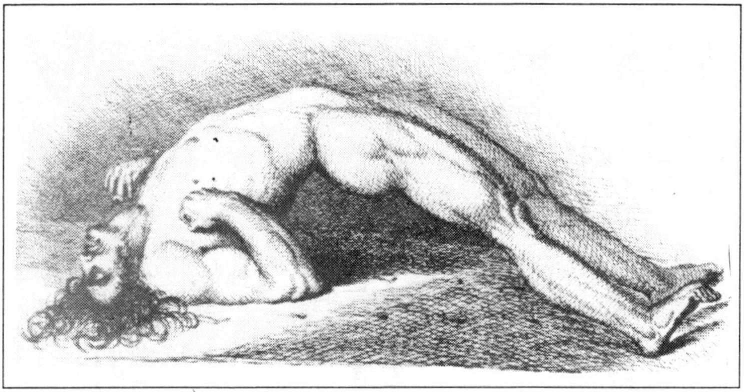

Fig. 1 British soldier in a state of 'true opisthotonus' (tetanus) as a result of wounds received at the Battle of Corunna in 1809. He was evacuated to the Royal Naval Hospital Haslar at Portsmouth, and drawn by Sir Charles Bell eight to nine days after wounding. This is the only pathological condition portrayed in the second and subsequent editions of his *Anatomy and Philosophy of Expression*, 1834.

curare, the arrow poison of the South American Indians. Like botulinum toxin, but in a different way, it acts on the peripheral nervous system, that is to say the junctions between the nerves and the muscles. It blocks the 'pull' messages and consequently the muscles remain limp, with the patient unable to move, and even to breathe, without help. In a tetanus patient this of course puts an end to the dreadful spasms, but since the patient is now unable to breathe, she must be mechanically assisted. In former times they used to be enclosed in 'iron lungs', but now more sophisticated devices are used. The treatment of tetanus patients is generally in the hands of the anaesthesiologists, who have to keep a careful balance between lethal and sustaining doses of curare; and to see that everything is done for the patient that she would otherwise do for herself without thought. I say 'she', because the second tetanus patient I saw was a woman in the Department of Anaesthetics of the Churchhill Hospital in Oxford. I will not forget her. She had sat on a tetanus-infected nail at a New Year party, and now she lay naked on a couch in a warm room, connected to a breathing machine, exuding fluid from every orifice, including her eyes, and being wiped at frequent intervals by her nurses. She was completely conscious, and aware of her situation and her surroundings; but totally incapable of movement or of speech. As I looked at her, our eyes

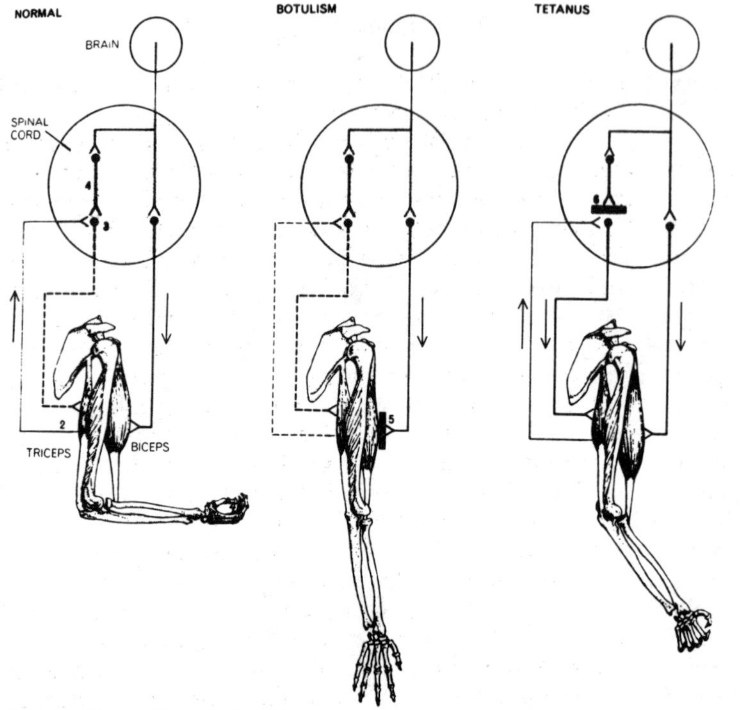

Fig. 2 From *Tetanus* by W. E. van Heyningen.

How tetanus and botulism toxins work. When you pull up the forearm a message from the brain passes down a nerve in the spinal cord to a point where the nerve branches in two. One branch goes on to an excitatory junction (or synapse, 1) in the cord, where it passes the message on to the nerve actuating the biceps, telling it to pull up the fore-arm. The pulling of the forearm stretches the triceps, causing a stretch reflex (2,3) which makes the triceps pull in the opposite direction. This is how we maintain muscular tone; otherwise we would fall over limp all the time. But if you really want to pull up the forearm, the triceps has to be told not to pull. This is done by the other branch of the nerve in the spinal cord. While the first branch goes directly to the excitatory synapse, the other goes through a synapse to a short inhibitory interneurone (4), which turns the pull-message into a don't-pull-message, and so blocks impulse 2; so the biceps pulls and the triceps does not, and the forearm comes up. Tetanus toxin blocks the don't-pull message of the inhibitory interneurone (6), so the two muscles pull against each other, with increasing tension. Finally all the muscles of the body go into a state of spasm.

Botulism toxin produces the opposite effect, by blocking all the pull-impulses at the excitatory neuro-muscular junctions (5).

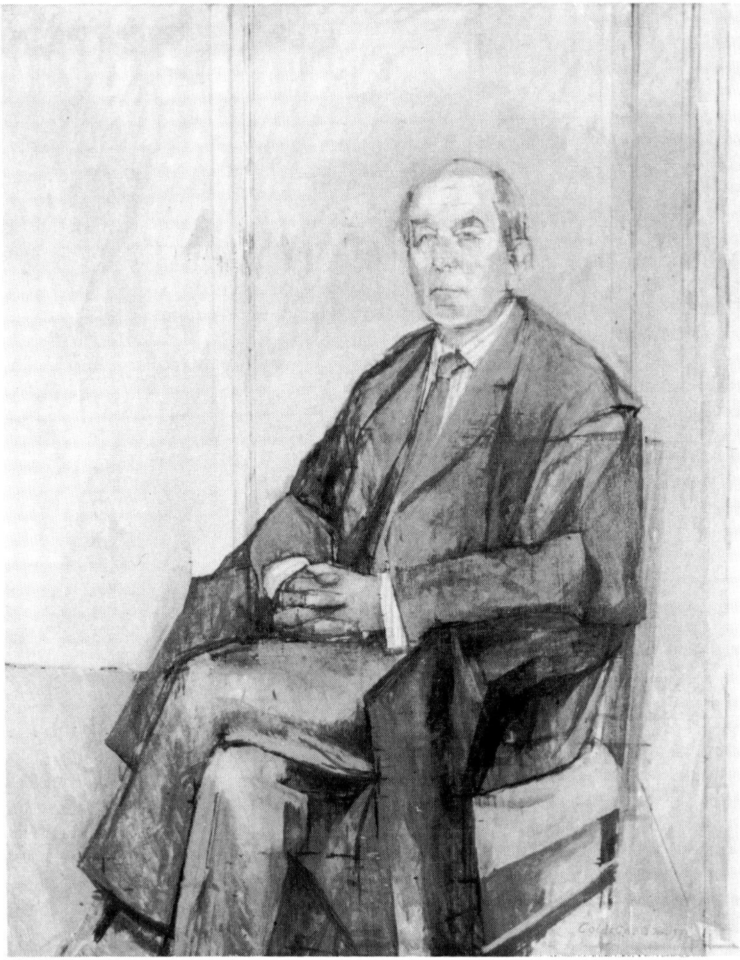

W.E. van Heyningen as Master of St Cross College, Oxford in 1972. A portrait by Sir William Coldstream.

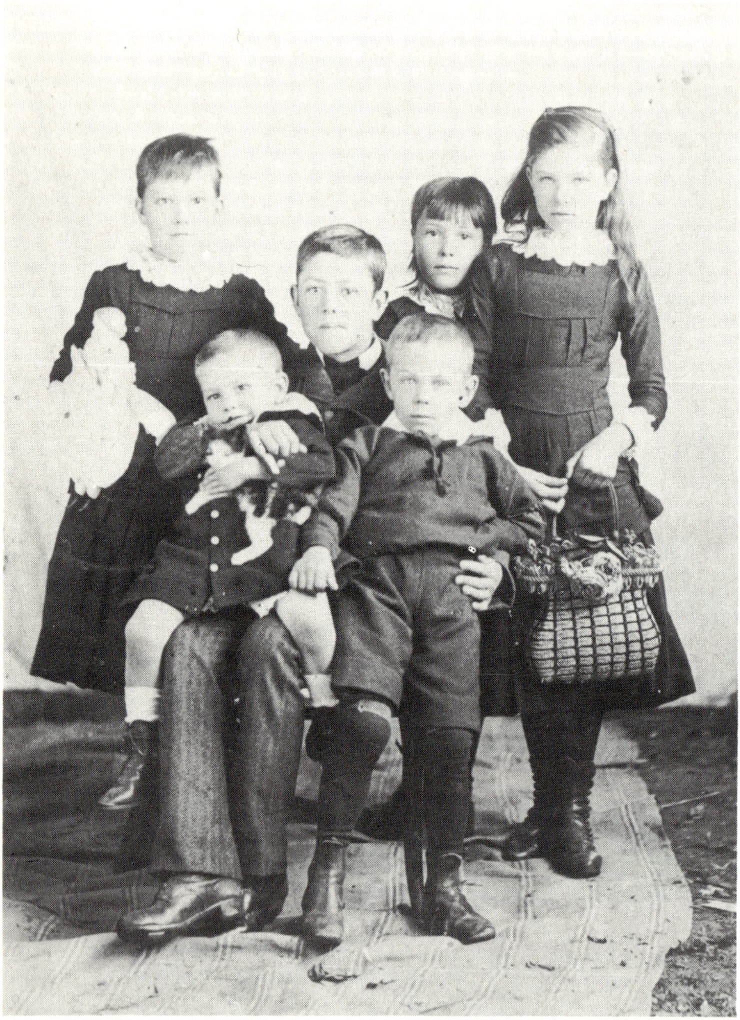

My mother, Mabel Constance Higgs (on the right), with her siblings at that time; Uncle Willie in the middle.

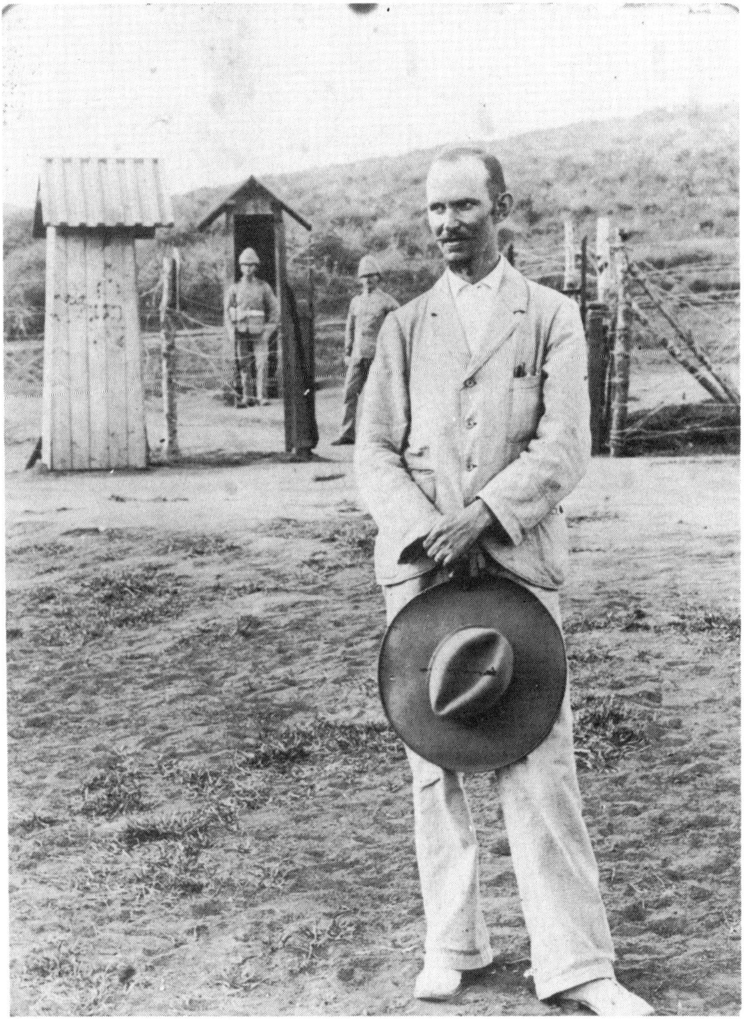

My father, George Philipus Stephanus van Heyningen, a prisoner of war of the British in the Boer War, in Ceylon.

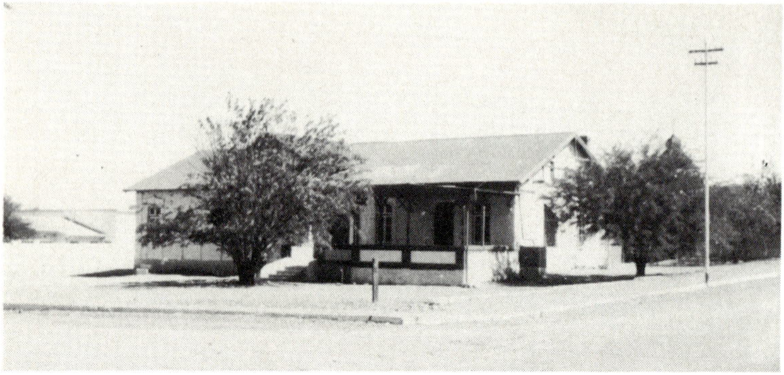

Above: the Residency at Keetmanshoop, South West Africa, with surrounding wooden paling fence removed. Below: in Cambridge, 1936, aged twenty-four years.

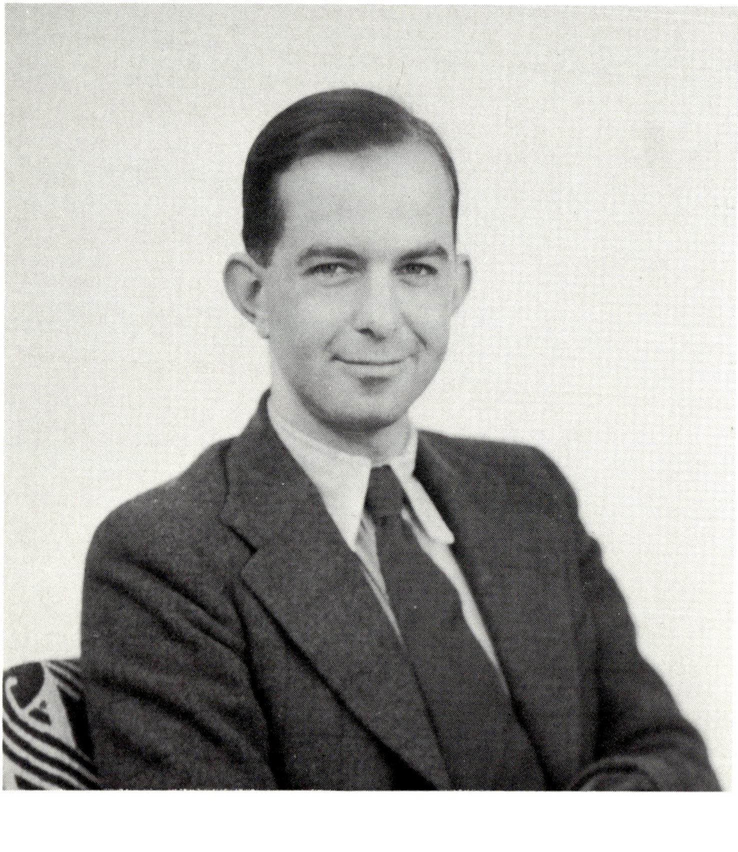

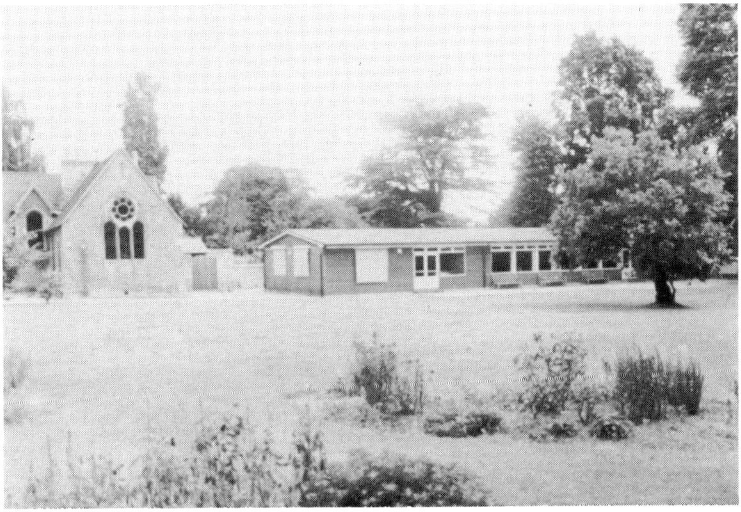

Above: the beginnings of St Cross College—the wooden hut and the old Victorian schoolroom on the St Cross site, 1965–1981. Below: a naive drawing of St Cross College—Pusey House on St Giles today.

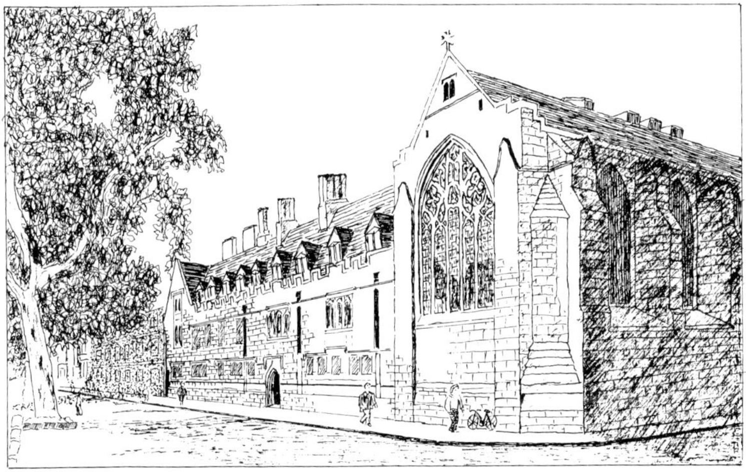

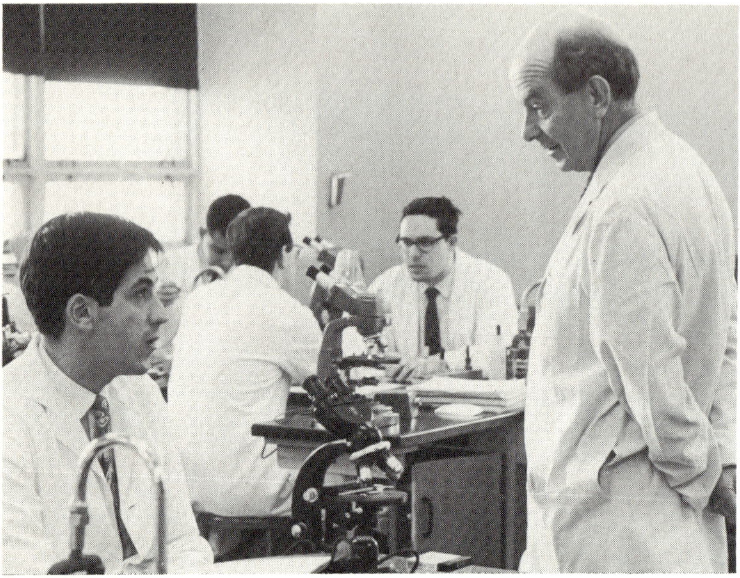

Above: conducting a practical class at Downstate Medical Center, State University of New York, Brooklyn, in 1967. Below: the dinner at the Reform Club to celebrate the completion of the portrait by Sir William Coldstream on 27 June 1972. Left to right, Ian Jenkin, Bridget Hanley, Sir William Coldstream, Kits and Ruth van Heyningen.

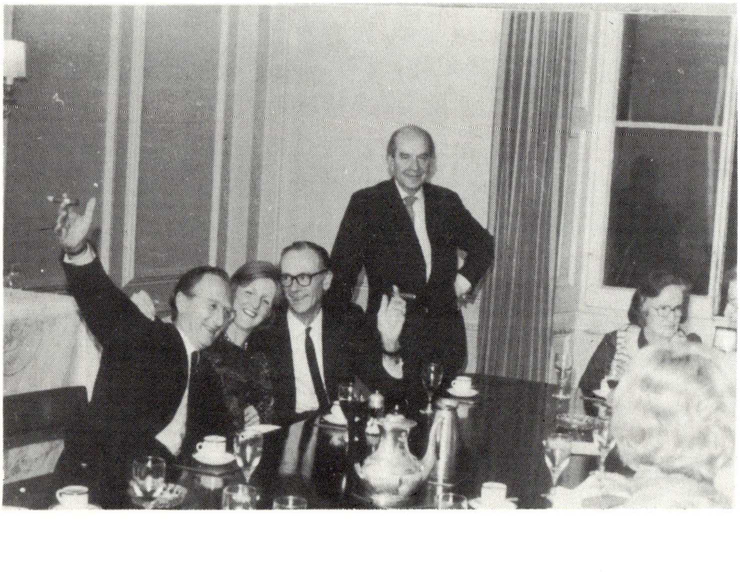

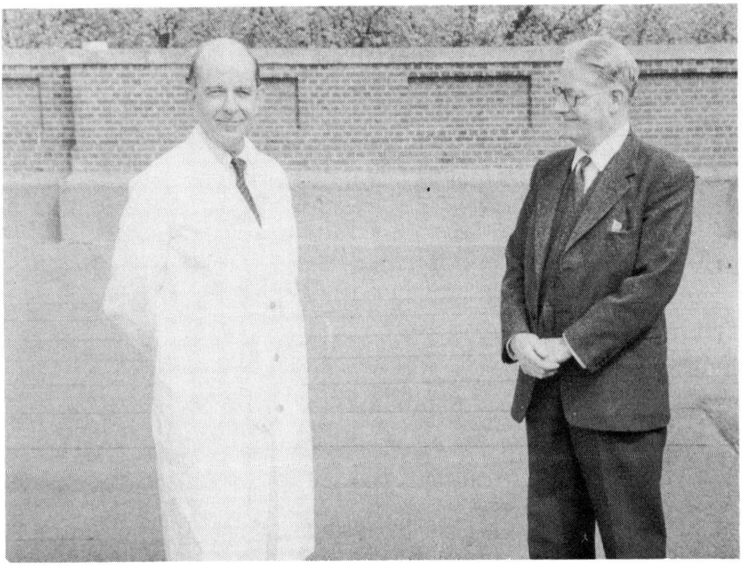

Above: with Sir Howard Florey on the roof of the Sir William Dunn School of Pathology, about 1960. Below: with S.N.De of Calcutta, who discovered cholera toxin in 1959, and Simon van Heyningen, about 1976.

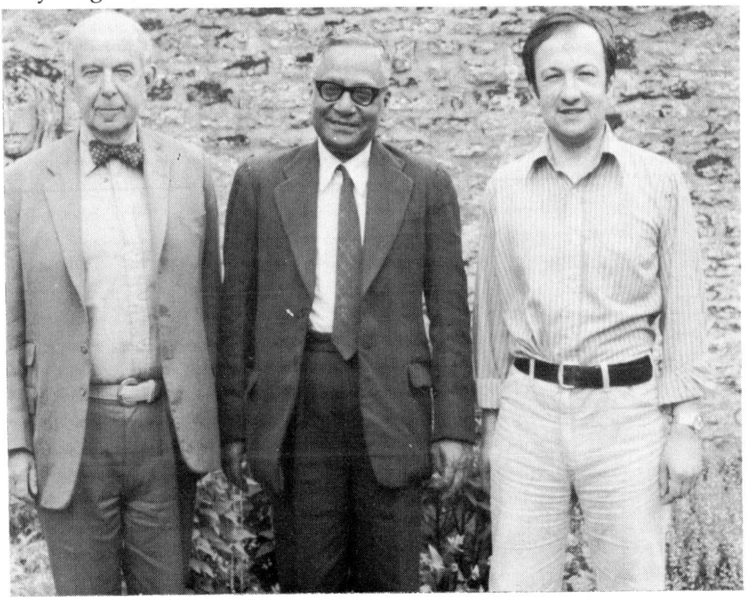

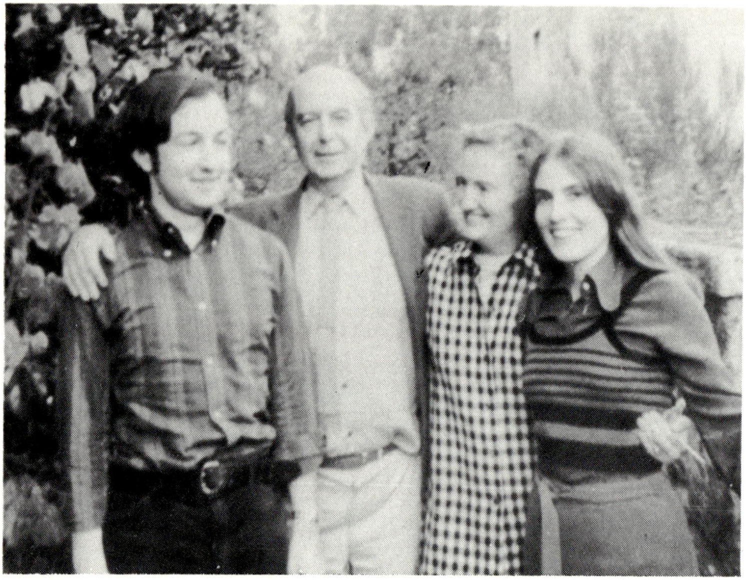

Above: with my family in 1971. Below: with Ruthie in the highlands of the Namib Desert in 1984.

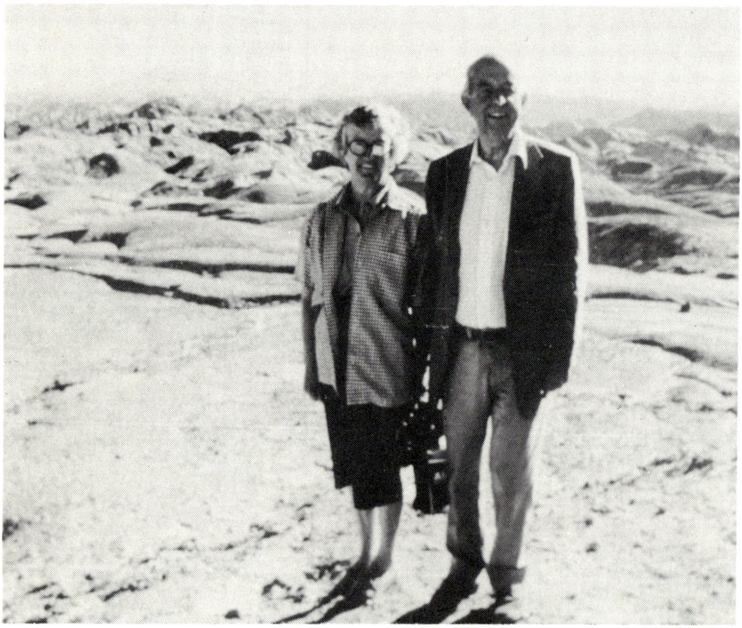

met deeply and for a long time, and it seemed to me that we communicated, I perhaps to convey to her not to fear, she would be all right; and she perhaps to convey that she understood.

I saw many tetanus patients on my (fourth) visit to Dakar in Senegal, on the western-most extremity of Africa, where I had gone for the Fourth International Conference on Tetanus in 1975. There was much tetanus in the country, as in all underdeveloped countries, due to the soil being much contaminated with tetanus bacilli abundant in the mainly pastoral economy, and due to practically everybody going about shoeless; and due to their not being actively immunized against tetanus. (It has been suggested by somebody that provision of shoes for children in underdeveloped countries would be the simplest way of reducing the death rate from tetanus.) The hospital was full of tetanus patients for whom it was not possible to provide the forced ventilation and the elaborate treatment I had seen in Oxford. All they could afford was the tranquilizer, Valium, which was some help in reducing the spasms. But it did mean that the patients were always on the edge of spasms, and could easily be sent into them. This circumstance was taken advantage of by one of our number, an American quack who made a rich living in the American Middle West by going around giving paid lectures on tetanus to the local doctors. For these lectures he wanted colour slides of tetanus patients, so he went about the wards taking flash photographs, which naturally sent many of them into spasms, thereby enhancing his pictures. Eventually I made him desist.

Immunization against tetanus is very simple, very cheap, and just about perfectly effective. Two injections of tetanus toxoid with an interval of six weeks, followed by a booster dose after six months, will ensure immunity to tetanus, probably for life, but a booster every few years would do no harm. During the last war all British and American soldiers were immunized against tetanus, but strangely enough the German and Japanese troops were apparently not immunized — I've not yet been able to determine what the Russian policy was. In the British Army in Europe and Africa there were twenty-three cases of tetanus (and something fishy about the immunization records in their pay-books) among 389,042 wounded; among the 'relatively small number' (more precise figures not known) of captured wounded Germans there were twenty-five cases of tetanus. Now practically everybody in the developed countries is immunized against tetanus.

Newborn babies in under-developed countries are particularly prone to tetanus (*tetanus neonatorum*), due to infection of the newly severed umbilical cord by tetanus bacilli, which is not helped in many of these countries by the custom of slapping a handful of cow dung on the severed cord. In the mid-nineteenth century on the Island of St Kilda, out in the Atlantic 110 miles west of the Scottish mainland, pregnant women rarely made clothes for the expected baby, because they assumed that it would die of tetanus within a few days of arrival. If the baby survived ten days, they would then make clothes for it [33].

Tetanus is a disease that is masked by the fact that it either leaves people dead, or if they recover, unmarked. If it left people maimed, as poliomyelitis does, it would be very noticeable. Its incidence is further masked by the fact that it does not occur in epidemics. It strikes individuals rather than communities or regions, and it strikes all the year round, year in year out. In many countries, including India, it is not 'notifiable', and therefore it is under-reported. When I first went to East Pakistan on cholera business, I was told there was a Goddess of Cholera, called Ghat Bomi, and a Goddess of Tetanus, called Thakuria. When a baby went into the spasms of neonatal tetanus, it would appear to be sitting up, which was miraculous. The baby had been blessed with supernatural power by Thakuria, so they would put it in a basket suspended from a tree for all to see and marvel at, and to accept the death of the baby as the inevitable payment for the blessing.

In 1973 I was invited to a meeting at the Haffkine Institute in Bombay, and was unfortunately unable to go. But they kindly invited me to send a contribution to the first issue of the new *Bulletin of the Haffkine Institute,* and I took the opportunity to make some propaganda. I sent them an article called 'Eliminate Tetanus in India', based entirely on the evidence of Indian medical authorities. They pointed out that mothers of babies with *tetanus neonatorum* did not take them to hospital for treatment because there was no point, they were doomed; so the deaths were not recorded. Moreover, when data were obtained by questioning the inhabitants of rural areas, rather than looking at the case records, the death-rate from tetanus was fourteen times higher. I came to the conclusion that perhaps 750,000 people died of tetanus in India every year, and 2.25 million world-wide. I sent an off-print of that paper to Mrs Ghandi, urging her to cut down the death-rate of new-born babies by immunizing the mothers in advance, at the cost of a rupee or two each. It is easy to prevent tetanus in a baby even before it becomes a twinkle in its mother's eye, by immunizing post-pubertal virgins, let alone pregnant women. Mrs Gandhi's Minister of Health wrote me a polite letter, telling me something would be done. I hope it will be done. But one might wonder whether it would be a good idea to stop babies dying, since the world, especially the under-developed world, is rapidly hurtling towards vast over-population, which is bound to lead to even greater numbers of premature deaths. However, there is some evidence that it might well be a good idea to prevent neonatal deaths. This evidence suggests families in which all the babies survive are smaller than families that have had infant deaths. The idea is that if babies die in infancy, more than enough babies are produced to make up for the loss. The evidence is not very good yet, and it needs more information before it can be judged properly. I do hope it turns out to be a good idea to save babies.

Tetanus toxin attracted me not only because it is so toxic, and its physiological action so clear-cut, but also because I thought I knew how to tackle its chemical mode of action. I wanted to start with the Wassermann-Takaki phenomenon of 1898. Wassermann (of the famous test for syphilis) worked in Robert Koch's Institut für Infektionskrankheiten in Berlin, and was a follower of Paul Ehrlich's doctrine of *res non agunt nisi fixata* — things won't work unless they're fixed. Working on the obvious fact that tetanus toxin acted on nervous tissue, and should therefore be fixed by nervous tissue, Wassermann and his colleague Takaki mixed tetanus toxin with ground-up brain tissue, filtered the mixture through filter paper, and found no toxin in the filtrate; it had remained fixed to the brain tissue remaining behind on the filter paper. Brain and spinal cord were the only tissues in the body that fixed tetanus toxin in this way, and the 'grey matter' of these nervous tissues was better at fixing the toxin than the 'white matter'.

This fixation phenomenon attracted a great deal of attention, since at that time it was believed that the harmful effects of all pathogenic bacteria were due to toxins. In 1906 the great Karl Landsteiner, Nobel Laureate, extracted a substance from brain which he called 'protagon', and showed that this substance had more capacity to fix tetanus toxin than any other component of brain.

But 'protagon' was not a single substance, it was a mixture; and three years later Wasserman's collaborator, Takaki, showed, or thought he showed, that the main component of protagon, a water-insoluble substance called cerebroside, was the toxin-fixer; but he was puzzled by the fact that cerebroside was far more plentiful in the white matter of brain than in the grey, whereas the grey matter was far better at fixing the toxin than the white.

There the matter was dropped for half a century, until I picked it up in 1958. I presumed that the toxin must be an enzyme, i.e. a biological catalyst, and that the receptor substance that fixed the toxin was changed in some way. In other words, this substance was the substrate of the enzymic action of the toxin, and would be changed by it. If I could identify this substrate and find out how the toxin changed it, I would have demonstrated the mode of action of the toxin at the biochemical level. We will now need to consider a little chemistry, and I beg you not to assume you won't understand it and shy away from it. You do not have to understand the chemical names.

I extracted protagon from slaughter-house beef brain by Landsteiner's method of 1906, and confirmed that it fixed tetanus toxin, and then set about trying to find what it was in the protagon mixture that really fixed the toxin. I found that a mixture of two components of protagon would fix the toxin, one of the components being insoluble in water and the other being soluble. The insoluble component was the cerebroside that Takaki had pinned his hopes on fifty years previously, but it did not by itself fix the toxin. It carried with it some water-soluble component of nervous tissue that fixed the toxin, leaving cerebroside the humbler role of merely carrying the fixer. What was this water-soluble toxin fixer?

Then I went through the 'literature' of brain chemistry to look for substances that appeared in greater concentration in grey matter than in white (since grey matter fixed tetanus toxin better than white). I could find only one such substance. It was called ganglioside. I had never heard of ganglioside, nor had nearly every other biochemist in the world. It had been discovered in 1936 by Ernst Klenk of the University of Cologne in the nerve ganglia of children suffering from Tay-Sachs disease, a disease which curiously is confined to Jews. The only other people who knew anything about ganglioside were Richard Kuhn (Nobel Prize) in Heidelberg, Gunnar Blix in Stockholm, Lars Svennerholm in Gothenberg, Erwin Chargaff in New York and Jordi Folch-Pi in Waverley, Mass. I extracted ganglioside from slaughter-house beef brain and showed that it fixed tetanus toxin; indeed it had a very great affinity for it: it fixed more than twenty times its weight of toxin. I tried a large number of other bacterial toxins, but none of them was fixed. I also tried a number of enzymes, and none of them was fixed.

I was quite overwhelmed by this discovery. It was a really serious discovery, certainly the most important I had ever made; and the fact that ganglioside was practically unknown added to its charm. That was early in 1958, and hardly had I made the discovery (and before I had published anything on it), than I received a cablegram from the Society of American Bacteriologists inviting me to give the Keynote Lecture at their Annual Meeting that was to be held in Chicago in April. 'If accepting please cable title of lecture' they said. 'Keynote, Keynote' I thought — 'THE KEY TO LOCKJAW' I cabled back. I really thought I had discovered that Key, and I still think I did, in a way. We shall see.

That April and May of 1958 was a glorious time. When the bulletin of the American Society of Bacteriologists came out with details of the forthcoming meeting, I was invited to give variants of my lecture at other places: at the Rockefeller Institute for Medical Research in New York, at the Harvard Medical School in the form of the First J. Howard Mueller Memorial Lecture, and at the University of Iowa in the form of The University Lecture.

There was the Official Dinner on my second evening in Chicago. It was my first experience of an American Official Dinner, and I'm bound to say it was a strange experience, some relic, I suppose, of the Pilgrim Fathers. I believe my American friends will agree with me if I say they are certainly not a gastronomic treat. The custom is for the big shots to sit on one side of a top table on a dais, looking over a bank of flowers towards the masses seated in circles of eight around their tables. I was at the top table, beside the notorious Mayor Daley of Chicago. At each place there was plenty to drink, already waiting for you, viz. a glass of water, a glass of milk and a cup of coffee. But no wine (no need, since everybody had already had plenty of bourbon and dry martini cocktails before dinner, and there would be more afterwards).

The Keynote Lecture was delivered to an audience of 2000 (so I was told) seated in tiers of semi-circles around the stage whence I spoke. I thought I had spoken in too great detail and at too great a length, but a large Chicago policeman who was on duty at the time reassured me: 'I couldn't figure what you were saying Doc, but you sure as Hell had 'em wowed.'

At The University Lecture in Iowa my lecture notes caught fire, but I pretended not to notice and carried phlegmatically on. The fire was due to an Anglo-American difference in paper sizes: my notes were on foolscap and the lectern was for the shorter American equivalent. Consequently the top end of my notes got overheated under the lamp at the top of the lectern. After the lecture I saw my first tetanus patient, in the University Hospital, where they have more tetanus patients than most hospitals, since it is by design the only hospital in a largely agricultural State which therefore tends towards a higher incidence of tetanus than usual. He was a young farmer, ill enough to go into occasional spasms, but not ill enough to be curarised.

During the meeting in Chicago, a very nice man called Harve Carlson approached me. He was on the staff of the Office of Naval Research of the United States Department of the Navy in Washington. The ONR did not offer Research Contracts, he told me, but he had a strong feeling that if I were to apply for one I might get it. The ONR had gained a reputation during the War for being far-sighted and innovatory in granting research contracts, and this policy had paid off. When I got back to Oxford I applied, and was awarded a most generous contract that was enough to cover all my research expenses and salaries, and to enable the modest expansion I needed. In addition, it entitled me to fly to the United States whenever I wanted, with MATS, the Military Air Transport Service, the biggest and safest airline in the world. Whenever I wanted to fly to the States, I would telephone the Navy office in the US Embassy in London, and Chief Yoeman La Prevotte would arrange it for me. On the Transportation Document of my first flight there was a section marked 'equivalent status: GS17'. I telephoned the Chief Yoeman, 'Hi Chiefie, what does this mean, GS17?' 'Man, that's *good'*, he replied, 'that means you're a Rear-Admiral in the United States Navy!'

I had a marvellous time. When I went on that first flight I had to take an Air Force bus from the US Officers' Club near Marble Arch to the US Air Force Base at Mildenhall in Cambridgeshire. When I checked in I was told there would be a three-hour delay, and as I looked for somewhere to wait I passed the Distinguished Visitors' Lounge, hoping somebody would invite me in, but nobody did. We eventually took off in a DC6 that stood on the runway with its engines running for an hour before we took off, because MATS maintained its reputation as the safest airline in the world by always making sure the engines were properly warmed up. On completing my business in the United States I reported to Maguire Air Force Base in New Jersey for the return flight, and checked in at the Navy desk, behind which stood a wonderfully beautiful girl in a Naval uniform. She gave me a heavenly smile, and said, 'Honey you don't want me, you want Protocol.' 'Is that good?' I asked. 'Honey, that's *goo-ood*!' she said, pointing to the Distinguished Visitors' Lounge. There I was looked after by two young Air Force sergeants, whose slowly-spoken Texan accents enhanced their gravely courteous manners. To my incredulous and delighted astonishment, they attached labels stamped VIP to my luggage. I still have one of them. They put me in a luxurious lounge where after a while I was joined by two Army Generals, who looked at me with wary suspicion and steered clear of me.

When it was time to board the DC6, the three of us went ahead of a long queue of Air Force and Army Colonels and Navy Commanders. On the flight back we stopped for fuel at Harmon Air Force Base in Newfoundland, where a staff car drew up at the foot of the steps down. 'I've got three VIP's on board' said our sergeant air hostess, and off we were taken in a staff car to a very luxurious Officers' Mess some distance away. As we sat at the bar, the Generals could no longer contain their curiosity about this bald-headed Limey civilian, and asked me, politely enough, what my business was. I told them I had a research contract with the Navy. Research on what? they asked. Bacterial toxins, I said. They were impressed. 'Ah! Good potential there, huh?' they said. 'Uhm, that depends' I said. They went on probing, and I continued stalling, which was easy since I had no military information to give them. This convinced them I was a good guy, doing a good job, who knew how to keep his trap shut. Thereafter they were very friendly, and we spent a convivial hour at the bar. When the Staff Officer came to take us back to our aircraft, he told us we were going to be two hours late arriving at Mildenhall because of headwinds. I expressed some dismay, because I was hoping to catch the 4.45 train back from London, and I was afraid the Air Force bus would take too long getting me back to London. 'Bus!', exclaimed one of the generals, 'You're not going in a goddam bus, you're going in a Staff Car! I'll send a message ahead.' When we landed at Mildenhall, the Station Commandant was waiting at the foot of the steps. Would I mind waiting in his office for just a few moments while I went through the customs, which he feared was obligatory? As I sat in comfort in his office drinking a cup of coffee, two British Customs officers came in. Would I be so kind as to answer just one question? 'Go ahead', I said. 'Have you anything to declare?', they asked. 'No', I said. 'Thank you, sir', they said, and they withdrew. I'll swear they backed out, but perhaps I'm imagining that. The Staff Car was waiting, and I caught my train back to Oxford. That was my last flight with MATS, because after that they changed their policy and they flew me on civil airlines. I made many such journeys to the United States, and was always made welcome when I called at the ONR offices in Washington, thus fortifying my affection for the United States of America. After some years I began to wonder whether I had made up the story of a GS17 being a Rear-Admiral. But on one of my last visits to Washington, having lunch in the mess at the Navy hospital, I asked a Naval officer if a GS17 really was a Rear-Admiral. 'Rear-Admiral?', he said, 'Hell no, it's a Vice-Admiral!'

At the time of my Chicago lecture, very little was known of the chemical structure of ganglioside, but Klenk, Kuhn, Blix and Svennerholm were working on it in Europe. Soon after my return from Chicago, I went on a tour of the Continent to call on them. My first call was on Gunnar Blix in Stockholm. He thought well of my discovery and gave me much encouragement, which I needed because I was new to ganglioside. Then I went to spend a week in Lars Svennerholm's laboratory in Gothenberg. He was not inclined to see much in my finding, but perhaps he was not interested in tetanus. However, I did learn a lot from him about separating the different gangliosides. Then I went to Cologne to see Ernst Klenk. He was pleased with me; and grateful, he said, because my discovery was the first indication of a biological role for the ganglioside that he had discovered twenty years previously. I became much attached to the Klenks, and was glad some years later to be a minor instrument in the saving of his life. He had fallen desperately ill from some intractable infection, and his wife telephoned me in desperation from Cologne to beseech me to get him some of the only antibiotic that could save him, which was cephalosporin, which Edward Abraham had recently discovered and developed, but which was not yet available to the public. I asked Abraham for help, and he, bless him, provided the cephalosporin immediately. Ernst Klenk's life was saved, but he died not long after from another cause.

When I first called on *Geheimrat Herr Professor Doktor* Richard Kuhn in the Max Planck Institüt für Medizinische Forschung in Heidelberg, he was inclined to be stiff, and I was inclined to think he was not keen to waste much time on me, but as I told him about my observation of the fixation of tetanus toxin by ganglioside he warmed to it and became enthusiastic, and in the end he gave me the rest of the day. That was the start of a friendship I was proud to enjoy, and whenever he came to London he would lunch with me in the Reform Club. Towards the end of 1960 he asked me if I would do him a favour, and of course I was glad to do so. There had been a meeting of Nobel Prize-winners that July, at which Kuhn had given a paper on gangliosides which had been published in *Angewandte Chemie. Angewandte Chemie* was going to bring out an International Edition in English, and Kuhn wanted me to translate his paper. One of the properties of gangliosides that he dealt with was that of raising body temperature (the Germans are keen on that point), and in this connection he told a story:

> One day in 1927, the great *Hofrat* Julius Wagner-Jaurreg of Vienna was sitting in a compartment of a railway carriage in Sweden, waiting for the train to take him to Stockholm, where he was to receive the Nobel Prize for Medicine in the Royal Palace. He had won the Prize for his discovery of the treatment of the insane by raising their temperatures (actually by giving them fever in the form of malaria). As he was waiting, a lady stepped into his compartment and sat opposite him. They fell into conversation, and it turned out that she too was on her way to the Royal Palace, and she too was going to receive the Nobel Prize. Hers was to be the Prize for Literature, for she was the Sardinian poet, Grazia Deledda. She had written a romance about a young man who was insane, and in his insanity stumbled about the Macedonian marshes, and so got soaked, and so got a high fever, and so was cured of his insanity.

Kuhn concluded that this showed how close the Arts and the Sciences could be. Actually my translation was never published in *Angewandte Chemie,* and I can only hope it was not my fault. But Kuhn's story did appear in English several years later. Some time in 1974 my eye happened to fall on a column by Alan Brien in *The Sunday Times,* and was caught by the name of Grazia Deledda, among a dozen other names. Brien wanted to know how many of these names his readers would recognize. I wrote and told him that I recognized Grazia Deledda's, and repeated Richard Kuhn's story. Brien printed the story, and reported that Grazia Deledda's name was the only one that had been recognized. They were all the names of Nobel Prizewinners in Literature, and the point he was making was that they were soon forgotten.

It sooned turned out that the structures of the several gangliosides were complicated. Essentially they consist of complexes of three sugary components (call them G, Gn, and L and never mind what they are) and a fatty component (call it C); and the variations among them are largely concerned with the sugary complex. These variations are due to variations in the number and positioning of sialic acid groups (call them S) attached to the G or L components (and to other S groups already present). In nervous tissue there are four main groups, viz. GGnSLC, SGGnSLC, GGnSSLC SGGnSSLC. Suffice now to say that we are interested only in gangliosides with S groups attached to L; and that in the end I was able to show that the tetanus toxin-fixer is GGnSSLC. In case I retain your interest as far as Chapter 10, please remember this.

Now that I had found that tetanus toxin was fixed by ganglioside, I confidently set about finding out what happened next. Since I assumed that the toxin was an enzyme, I expected it to bring about some change in the GGnSSLC ganglioside. But nothing happened. The ganglioside was unchanged. I was baffled. I had reached a 'So what?' situation. Tetanus toxin was fixed by ganglioside, so what? My dream of explaining the mode of action of one of the two most poisonous substances known was not going to come true. I took another tack, which led me up a maddeningly frustrating garden path.

At that time I had Jane Mellanby working with me, and a highly intelligent young research technician, Diana Messenger. We did an experiment, and please don't assume you won't understand it, and please do try to follow it. We incubated tetanus toxin with macerated brain tissue (i.e. nervous tissue) for some time, and then extracted the tissue in a certain way with certain organic solvents; and then we examined the extract by a process called 'thin layer chromatography'. At the same time we did the same thing with two variants: the first was to substitute botulinum toxin for tetanus toxin; the second was not to add any toxin. The mixture with tetanus toxin was to see whether, compared with the control without toxin, tetanus toxin brought about any change in the nervous tissue as revealed by thin layer chromatography of the extracts; the botulinum mixture was there since botulinum toxin is also a very potent neurotoxin, and perhaps we could learn something from that mixture. I must briefly explain thin layer chromatography: a flat plate of glass, about a foot square, is covered with a thin layer of silica gel; drops of the above-mentioned extracts are placed side by side on the silica gel, and the plate is then stood vertically in a glass jar with a particular organic solvent in the bottom of it, with the silica gel just dipped in it. The organic solvent slowly creeps up the silica gel, and in so doing it carries the different constituents of the extracts with it. These different constituents move at different rates according to what they are. After some hours the solvent reaches the top of the plate, by which time the various constituents of the drops have settled at different stages of the upward path. The plate is then sprayed with a dye which reveals these different spots. In this way differences in the three different mixtures are revealed.

One morning Diana Messenger came to us with a plate in her hand and a sweet smile on her intelligent face. 'I think you're going to like this' she said. I saw at once that this experiment had brought us to the very gates of Paradise. 'How beautiful the feet of the Messenger that bringeth good tidings!', I exclaimed, and I whipped out my cheque book and wrote Diana a cheque for a million pounds. 'Oh thanks', said Diana deadpan, pocketing the cheque.

The reason why I was so pleased was that we could all see at once that the plate appeared to carry two beautiful messages. The first showed the way to find out what the substance was that tetanus toxin acted on in nervous tissue, and what happened to that substance. The second was almost more exciting, and totally unexpected. It suggested that botulinum toxin acted on the same substance that tetanus toxin acted on, and in the same way. This would mean that the two neurotoxins had the same mode of action at the biochemical level; but since they acted at different situations — tetanus toxin in the central nervous system, botulinum in the peripheral, they had different physiological effects. Perhaps the fixation of tetanus toxin by ganglioside distinguished between the two toxins, steering tetanus toxin to the central nervous system.

The diagram below is an attempt to show what we saw. It represents the thin-layer chromatographic plate, turned through a right-angle to read from left to right:

	start						*finish*
Tetanus:	A	B	C	D	E		:
Nothing:		B	C	D	E	F	:
Botulinum:	A	B	C	D	E		:

The 'Nothing' line suggests that our particular extract of normal nervous tissue contained substances B, C, D, E and F. When the tissue is incubated either with tetanus toxin or with botulinum toxin, substance F is destroyed and a new substance, A, appears, suggesting that both the two toxins converted substance F into substance A. We then obtained a very small amount of substance F by preparative thin-layer chromatography of the *same extract* of nervous tissue incubated with Nothing. We incubated the tiny preparation thus obtained of F with tetanus and botulinum toxins, and showed that they both eliminated substance F. We could not find any substance A, and that was disappointing, but not surprising since we had handled only a trace of F. At least we had shown again that both tetanus toxin and botulinum toxin destroyed F, and thus appeared to have the same action.

In scientific research it is almost more interesting finding a clear way to tackle a problem than actually tackling the problem. The tackling of the problem is then no more than a mopping-up operation if you have picked on the right line of approach. What we now had to do was to find out what F and A were, and we set about this agreeable task with enthusiasm. Disaster struck us immediately. The first thing to do was to repeat the observation we had made. But we could not. The thin-layer chromatograms of the 'Nothing' tracks were exactly the same as the 'Tetanus' and 'Botulinum' tracks, with no sign of the presence of F, or of the absence of A. We tried again and failed. Over the next three months we tried two or three times a week and failed. It was maddening to get to the gates of Paradise and then to be turned away, but in the end we had to give up. Of course, if you can't repeat an observation, you can't publish it; but we did. Jane Mellanby and I were invited by the Swiss journal *Médicine et Hygiéne* to write a short review on tetanus, and at the end of it we pointed out seven similarities between tetanus and botulinum toxins. The last of them was a brief account, with an apology and photographs, of the unrepeatable experiment. We did the same in the *Proceedings of the International Conference* on Tetanus that was held in Bern in 1966. So if one day somebody demonstrates that tetanus and botulinum toxins have the same mode of action at the chemical level, I hope they will not forget that Jane and Diana and I demonstrated it first. That failure to repeat that crucial experiment was not entirely a disaster, for it led me to take a momentous decision on another front (see Chapter 9).

About this time, I received a fat letter from Antigua. I wondered who on earth would be writing to me from that remote isle. It was from an American doctor working there for an oil company. He had a tetanus problem, and wanted my advice, for he had been advised by the Commonwealth Serum Laboratory near Boston that I was the world's greatest expert on tetanus, no less. (If I were to take the trouble to deny that, somebody would think I took it seriously.) This was his problem: about six months previously he had stepped barefooted on a thumb-tack (i.e. drawing pin), shaft length *7.54* millimeters(!). Eleven days later he started feeling a tingling in the shin of that foot, which he concluded must be the onset of tetanus (!); this despite the fact that he was actively immunized against tetanus, and had had booster shots every six months (!). He gave himself a shot of tetanus antiserum (!), but the symptoms persisted; so he went to New York for advice. At the Bellevue Hospital (it has a large psychiatric division), they gave him a drug (which I knew to be a tranquiliser), and advised him to consult the Commonwealth Serum Laboratory. The Commonwealth Serum Laboratory passed him on to me. I realised it was my duty to speak to the poor man with the Voice of God, so I wrote him a letter. 'I am sure', I thundered magisterially, 'and you may be sure, Doctor Smith, that you are not suffering from tetanus.' I went on to advise him to cease and desist from taking tetanus antiserum, which would only aggravate his itches. Sure enough, he wrote back to thank me for my excellent advice, and to report that he was already on the mend, with every prospect of complete recovery.

7
UNIVERSITY AFFAIRS

Early in 1962, Florey and Professor Sir Ewart Jones (Organic Chemistry) decided to launch me on a University political career by proposing me for election by the various professors of science as a Curator of the Bodleian Library, and in May 1962 I was elected, until the first day of Michaelmas Term 1966. I remained a Curator, having been re-elected every six years thereafter, until the first day of Michaelmas Term 1985, when I really had to go. Since the idea was for me to be engaged in University politics, I shall try to give you an idea of the political structure of the University.

The Collegiate University of Oxford

The Universities of Oxford and Cambridge are entirely independent of each other, but uniquely similar; and different from any other university in the world. They may be compared (not too closely) with the United States of America in that they each consist of a federation of a number of independent, self-governing, self-perpetuating, often bloody-minded, institutions, to whit the Colleges, owing allegiance to a federal government, to whit the University. There are other universities embracing Colleges, or Houses, such as Durham in England, and Harvard and Yale in the United States, but these are subordinate parts of their universities, not independent institutions.

In Oxford there are thirty-five Colleges ranging over seven centuries in dates of foundation from 1249 for University College to 1979 for Green College: twenty-eight of these Colleges are primarily for undergraduate students reading for their first degree (which is invariably the B.A., whatever the subjects studied), but also for graduate students reading for higher degrees; six take only graduate students; one, All Souls, is composed only of Fellows and takes no students at all; one college takes men only, and three take women only. When I first came to Oxford it was different, when there were four fewer colleges, and twenty-one took men only and five took women only.

The colleges are each governed by a Governing Body of Fellows, presided over by the Head of the House, whose title may be Dean, Master, President, Principal, Provost, Rector or Warden. The Fellows are elected by the Governing Body, and in the undergraduate colleges they may act as Tutors of the students and receive their salaries from the college. Most Fellows also have University appointments, such as professorships, readerships, lecturerships (never lectureships as in all the other British universities), and keeperships in the University Library (the Bodleian) and the Ashmolean Museum. The income of the Colleges comes from the students' college fees and from endowments, which in some cases are considerable, being derived from gifts of money, property and land, much of it coming from the times centuries ago when the Heads and their Fellows, being in Holy Orders and therefore celibate and consequently childless, had no-one but their Colleges to whom to leave the fruits of their rich benefices. The University also owns valuable property, not all of it disposable; but most of its income today comes from the Government through the University Grants Committee, and from students' university fees.

As far as students are concerned, the function of the University is to grant degrees, for which purpose it sets the necessary examinations that must be passed. The University provides the libraries (the Bodleian and the Departmental and Faculty libraries); the Museums (the Ashmolean, the University Museum, and the Pitt-Rivers Museum of Ethnology and Prehistory, and others); and the many scientific laboratories. And it provides the teaching staff — the professors, readers and lecturers who give lectures and provide laboratory demonstrations and exercises. No students are obliged by the University to use any of these facilities, except for medical students, who are required by the General Medical Council to provide evidence of attendance at certain lectures and demonstrations. All the University requires of students wishing to attain degrees is that they should pass the examinations set by the University. The University having provided the objective and the means of attaining, it is the function of the Colleges in the first place to choose and accept students, and then to see, by means of tutorials, advice and periodic college examinations, that the students make proper use of the facilities provided and pass the examinations for the degree. Students in colleges are not so much taught knowledge and skills, as the where and the how to acquire them.

It has come about in time that the City of Oxford, because of the University and the Colleges, is one of the most beautiful cities in the world. The buildings of these institutions, in styles ranging over seven centuries, are, most of them, beautiful and interesting. The thirty-five Colleges, the vast Bodleian Library, the Sheldonian Theatre, the Examination Schools, the University Church, the Old Ashmolean Museum of the History of Science, the Ashmolean Museum of Art and Archaeology, are not arranged according to any plan, but are gathered together in a hugger-mugger agglomeration set on the majestically curving High Street, on the broad Broad Street, on the stately Radcliffe Square, and on innumerable narrow streets and alleys, with delightful surprises at every corner.

The Confederal Governance of the University

As far as the dons are concerned, the University of Oxford is governed by a democracy that is the envy of other universities, except Cambridge which is much the same. This government is a kind of parliament of which all dons are members. It is called Congregation, and it meets once a fortnight during Term. It is the legislative body of the University, and amongst other business it decides what proposals should be put to the Hebdomadal Council (see below) for amending, repealing or adding to the Statutes of the University; it considers general resolutions that can be put before it by Council, or by any twelve dons; it confers degrees, including honorary degrees (and sometimes decides not to, as was recently the case with Mrs Thatcher); it approves the appointment of the Vice-Chancellor every four years. The most junior member of Congregation has a vote that has as much weight as that of the most senior Regius Professor, and he has the right to speak on motions, and to propose them, if he can find eleven others who agree with him. It is a right that he uses often, and without fear.

The Hebdomadal Council meets once a week, as its name implies, during Term. It is to Congregation what the Cabinet is to Parliament (and is always called the 'inner cabinet' of the University by the *Oxford Mail*). Seven of its twenty-five members are *ex officio*; the rest are dons elected (for six years) by the dons, i.e. members of Congregation.

Under Council, the General Board of the Faculties is responsible for the academic administration of the University, i.e. teaching and research; administration of the funds available for these activities; and co-ordination of the sixteen Faculty Boards that concern themselves with the business of their respective faculties. Again, elected dons are in the great majority.

Then there are five special Boards, four of them venerable and distinguished: the Visitatorial Board that deals (rarely I think) with disciplinary matters concerning dons; the Delegates of the University Press; the Curators of the Bodleian Library; the Visitors of the Ashmolean Museum of Art and Archaeology; and the new Libraries Board, the need for which I have never quite grasped.

The Curators of the Bodleian Library

The Bodleian Library is the oldest public library in Britain, and probably the world. It is not the biggest library in the world, but it is the finest; and in Britain is second in size only to the British Library (formerly part of the British Museum) in London. It is about the same size as the libraries of Harvard and Yale Universities in the United States. It has a million maps and nearly five million books, which occupy seventy-six miles of shelving (stacked side by side, not end to end); and a further mile and a half are taken in every year. It costs about £5,000,000 a year to run. The biggest library in the world probably is the Library of Congress in Washington, with the Lenin Library in Moscow second, or *vice versa*.

Oxford's library was started in 1327 on the north side of the University Church, but in a very poor way. In the early fifteenth century it began to flourish from various benefactions, particularly those from 'the Good Duke Humphrey' of Gloucester, brother of Henry V, so much so that it was decided to build a new room for it over the new Divinity School. This room is still known as Duke Humphrey's Library, and is the most glorious of the many beautiful rooms in the Bodleian. But as a result of the political and religious upheavals between 1530 and 1550, and the poverty of the University, the library was dispersed, and for the next fifty years the University was without a library, the dons and students having to rely on their college libraries.

It was Sir Thomas Bodley who saved the library of his former University. In 1598 he retired from a diplomatic career and devoted himself to restoring the abandoned library — 'I concluded at the last, to set up my Staffe at the Librarie dore in Oxon; being throwghly perswaded, that in my solitude, and surcease from the Commonwealth affayers, I coulde not busie my selfe to better purpose, then by redusing the place (which then in every part laye ruined and wast) to the publique use of Studients' [26]. Duke Humphrey's Room was refitted and stocked with books, many of them given by Bodley. The first librarian, Thomas James, was appointed, and the Bodleian Library was opened on 8 November 1602. Within a few years Duke Humphrey's Room was extended; and then the library expanded into the top floor of the contiguous new Schools Quadrangle. This sudden increase in the size of the Bodleian was necessitated by benefactions of books from Bodley and his friends, and even more so by the agreement Bodley made with the Stationers' Company in 1610 by which the Stationers undertook to send a free copy of every book they published to the Library. This in effect made the Bodleian a copyright library 150 years before the British Museum was founded.

The reason why I assert that the Bodleian Library is the finest library in the world is because of its quality rather than its quantity. It has the finest assembly of manuscripts and printed books, and the finest *collections* of manuscripts and printed books, in the world. Many of these were bought at the most opportune time by Bodley himself, and shipped by him by barge up the River Thames to Oxford; and given by others — such as Archbishop William Laud (MSS and printed books); and Thomas Barlow (printed books); Francis Douce (MSS and printed books); Francis Junius (MSS); Richard Rawlinson (MSS and printed books); and John Selden (Oriental MSS and printed books) — in the rescue of the monastic libraries after the dispersal of the monasteries by Henry VIII.

Added to these wonderful collections, and the acquisitions since then, is the glorious fact that the Bodleian Library is housed in a most beautiful assembly of buildings, and reading rooms within them. We have the Old Schools, originally consisting of the superior faculties of Theology (the Divinity School), Medicine and Law; the Schools of the Seven Liberal Arts; the Two Tongues; and the Three Philosophies. Their names are still beautifully painted in Latin above their entrances: *Bibliotheca Bodleiana; Schola Astronomicae et Rhetoricae; Schola Geometrae et Arithmeticae; Schola Grammaticae; Schola Linguarum, Hebreciae et Grecae; Schola Logicae; Schola Metaphysicae; Schola Naturalis Philosophae; Schola Musicae; Schola Philosophae et Moralis; Schola*

Vetus Iurisprudentiae; Schola Vetus Medicinae. After nearly forty years, it still gives me pleasure to go into them. They no longer house these schools — the Divinity School houses Bodleian exhibitions, and the other Schools house a smaller exhibition room, offices, and the Curators' Room. On the two floors above the Schools are the great Upper and Lower Reading Rooms. Then we have the Radcliffe Camera, a beautiful cylinder capped by a hemisphere, built by James Gibbs between 1737 and 1749 with money bequeathed by the famous and very rich physician, John Radcliffe (I've been told his *earned* income, in the 17th century, was £20,000 a year). We also have the New Bodleian, designed by Sir Giles Gilbert Scott and finished just before the last war. It is detested by many, but I think it is not at all bad, and at least it has the merit of being much bigger than it looks. A little further out there are other establishments of the Bodleian. There is the large Radcliffe Science Library, established by the Radcliffe Trustees following instructions in his will. It is a dependent library, but distinct, and as science libraries go in Europe, it is second only to the Technical Institute Library in Hanover. Then we have the Rhodes House and Indian Institute Libraries which house everything pertaining to our former Empire; and the large new Law Library.

I don't suppose there was anybody in Oxford more ignorant of the Bodleian Library than I was when I was elected Curator. When I went to call on the Librarian, J.N.L.Myres, in his office, he seemed to me to be wondering who on earth this ignorant scientist might be. I got the impression that he, like most non-scientific dons in Oxford at that time (and like many still today), thought all scientists were ignorant of real learning; and he did not count ignorance of science as real ignorance. He started by consistently mis-spelling my name, and I believed, unfairly I'm sure, it was deliberate; so I put a stop to it by telling him one day that if he persisted in disfiguring my name, I would transpose the 'r' and the 'e' of his. That worked. Actually I admired Myres, and got to like him. He has the most impressive command of the English language (and I dare say of other languages too), and when he resigned the Librarianship some years later on a matter of principle over a disagreement with Council, the wording of his statement was pure joy to read.

At that first meeting with Bodley's Librarian, I asked him if he would give me letters of introduction to the Librarian of Congress in Washington, and to the Director of the New York Public Library, since I was about to visit those cities, and I was keen to learn more about great Libraries. The Library of Congress is probably the largest and most well-equipped of them all. Its first function is to serve Congress and Congressmen. If a Congressman wants to have some information about, say, agriculture, he doesn't go to the Department of Agriculture, he goes to the Library of Congress. The Department of Agriculture might not be disinterested, and might give him a biased slant. And besides, the assistants in the Library of Congress would do all the work for him and write a paper on the required subject. Like the Bodleian Library, the British Library in London, the Cambridge University Library, the National Libraries of Scotland and Wales, and the Library of Trinity College, Dublin, and I presume other national libraries, the Library of Congress by law gets a free Copyright copy of every book published in the country, and the fact that many more books are published in the United States than in the United Kingdom is one of the reasons why it is bigger than our immense British Library.

I went to the Library of Congress, was shown around its immensity, and then called on the Librarian of Congress, Lawrence Quincy Mumford (whose name sounds like a Bostonian in one of J.P.Marquand's novels). The great American poet, Robert Frost, was with him, and they were both very pleasant. I suppose they assumed I knew something about books and libraries, but I'm sure it would have made no difference to them if they knew the depth of my ignorance. Then I went to New York, and to the New York Public Library on Fifth Avenue at the corner of the sleazy west side of 42nd Street. As the Library of Congress has a special obligation to Congress, so the New York Public Library has a special obligation to the City of New York, and its businessmen and tradesmen, to whom it supplies all kinds of information that they require, including every edition of every telephone directory in every State. Before I called on the Director, I had a strange revelation. I went to the lavatory (should I have said powder room?), where I found that you had to put a dime in a slot to gain entry to the cubicles. Two or three of them were free of charge, but they had no doors to them, so those that used them were exposed to public gaze. I was astonished that the poor should be subjected to such indignity, especially in a country like America.

The Director was most pleasant, and after he had shown me around his Library in a general way, he gathered his senior staff in his office, and asked me if there was anything in particular that I wanted to see in the Library. I replied yes, there were three things that I would like to see: Jefferson's holograph of the Declaration of Independence; their collection of Afrikaans books; and the Manhattan Telephone Directory for 1938. I was much privileged to be allowed to see the Declaration of Independence, since it is a sacred and fragile document, very seldom exposed to light. Bronze door after bronze door clanged open and shut as we went into the sanctum where it was kept. It is just about the most noble, and the most beautifully and economically expressed document I have ever seen, and I was acutely conscious of the privilege that I was enjoying. Then we went to the Afrikaans collection, which I had heard was comprehensive. It may have been, but it was not very interesting (since then some very good novels have come out of South Africa).

Then we came to the Manhattan Telephone Directory for 1938. There is of course no room in any library for all the telephone directories ever published in all the United States, so 1938 was on microfilm, projected by a very large, gravely courteous Black man. All the senior staff were gathered around. The Black man asked me, 'Any particular letter of the alphabet that interests you, sir?' 'Yes please', I said 'C'. 'Any particular name under the Cs, sir?' 'Clarke', I said. 'Clarke with an e or Clark without an e, sir?' 'With an e', I said. 'Any particular first name, sir?' 'Margery', I said. 'Margery with a g or Marjory with a j, sir?' 'With a g', I said. 'Thank you sir', he said, 'you have been most helpful.' He flipped through his machine and found the page I wanted. The Director then said that he and his staff were most curious, and would be grateful if I would tell them why I was making this inquiry. I said the answer was simple. I was doing some experiments at the Rockefeller Institute on the East Side at 70th Street and York Avenue, and staying in the Faculty Club there. Every time I wanted to go downtown I would walk westwards to Lexington Avenue and take the downtown bus. In 1938 I used to know a girl called Margery with a g Clarke with an e, and I often used to visit her in her apartment which was on the corner of Lexington Avenue and either 62nd or 60th Street. But I couldn't remember which, and I wanted to gape sentimentally at the correct corner; which I had just now learned was at 60th Street. At this the gravely courteous Black man just about exploded with laughter.

For the first two or three years of my Curatorship I was nothing more than a passenger at our regular meetings twice a term, and on a few other occasions during the year, under the presidence of the Vice-Chancellor. I had only a dim idea of what was being discussed, but I enjoyed being part of the great institution, revelling in the idea of being the first alumnus of the Reddersburg Secondary School to play such a part, and surely the last. Perhaps my fellow curators were grateful for my silence. At any rate, I was put on the Committee for the Radcliffe Science Library within a few months, presumably because I was the only curator who was a scientist; and the next year I was elected to the Standing Committee, which meets once a week to prepare the business for the meetings of the Curators. The Chairman at the time was the distinguished Latin scholar, Sir Roger Mynors, a pleasant and courteous man who seemed to take my seldom-uttered opinions as seriously as any others. I was to remain on the Standing Committee for the next twenty years, during the course of which I gradually began to understand the scope, the working, the obligations and the needs of the Bodleian Library; and with that grew my great love for it, and its traditions. Two of these traditions are the annual Perlustration in Trinity Term, and the annual Visitation in Michaelmas Term. The Perlustration is a visit by the Curators to inspect a particular part of the Library selected by the Standing Committee. The Visitation is preceded at noon on a Saturday by the Bodleian Oration in the Convocation House, always delivered by a Student of Christ Church (which is what that College calls its Fellows). He (perhaps one day he may be she) is brought in by the Dean of Christ Church, and followed by the other Students, exuding a whiff of the Madeira they ritually consume before setting off for the Convocation House. The Oration is always delivered in Latin, on the subject of Bodley or of Hebrew studies in alternate years. After the Oration the Curators proceed to the Visitation, which takes place in the Curators' Room, and consists of counting the books in the Library. Since it is not possible to count all the five million books, we receive a list of books that are reported missing. The scientific books seem always to be missing in the greatest number, and the theological in the smallest. The theologians might believe that their readers are the most honest, but perhaps the scientific books are the most useful. Before the present austere times the Visitation was always followed by the Bodleian Luncheon, a jolly and vinous affair in one of the colleges, with many notables invited; but now we have a much more austere little affair that we have to pay for out of our own pockets.

Eventually I had to take over the chairmanship of the Standing Committee from my friend Norman Davis. He had been an excellent and witty Chairman, but was obliged to stand down on his retirement from the Merton Professorship of English Language. I had reached retirement a year before him, but because of some quirk in the rules I could go on being a Curator for another six years, and he could not. I was reluctant to take on the chairmanship because I thought that would be stretching my amateurishness too far, but I knew I had to take it on, because there was a most necessary and most difficult and painful job to be done; and after a year I succeeded in doing it. The Curators and some of the senior staff gave a little dinner for me in Nuffield College. After that, at the annual appointment (which generally amounts to a re-appointment) of the Standing Committee, I declined to continue my membership of it, since I had already been on it too long. At the end of the academic year 1984-1985 it was technically not possible for me to be re-elected Curator, and a good thing too. The Curators gave a glorious dinner for me in Christ Church in the week before Christmas 1985.

The Hebdomadal Council

In May 1963 the Warden of Merton College, Robin Harrison, and the Linacre Professor of Zoology, John Pringle, proposed me for election to the Hebdomadal Council. Pringle told me it was because I was 'without rancour'. This pleased me, because he was referring to the part I was then playing in the non-dons movement which I will come to in the next chapter. They thought that in this role I should now be involved in the higher politics of the University. This was also part of getting more scientists involved, since there were only four of them on Council, and two were about to retire. Altogether six scientists were put forward, and on 30 May two of them were elected, leaving the total number on Council unchanged. This got into the news the next day — 'Scientists fail to win more seats' in *The Times*; 'Scientists outvoted in Oxford elections' in the *Daily Telegraph*. The two scientists who were elected were Professor Sir Lindor Brown (Physiology) and me; in fact I was fourth of the seven elected, the three ahead of me being veteran Members of Council standing for re-election. I was amazed, delighted and terrified.

Well I might have been terrified, for at the very first meeting I attended I thought I was going to be blasted out of the Council chamber. I had received the minutes (always called Acts) of the previous meeting of Council and the agenda of the coming one, and various other papers, and had noted that the Department of

Experimental Psychology was apparently going to get less room in a proposed new building on South Parks Road than it had thought. I had also noted that item 7 of the rules governing the Business of Council stated that 'Papers circulated to members of Council must not be published or made the subject of public comment by members of Council, who, subject to that rule, must use their own discretion in discussing the contents privately with persons whose opinions they desire to know'. Therefore on the day before my first Council meeting I had telephoned the Professor of Experimental Psychology, Carolus Oldfield, and asked him what he thought about the proposed reduction in the amount of space to be allocated to his Department; and he was amazed and disconcerted. I reported this when the subject came up for discussion. Consternation! The Rector of Exeter (my College then), normally a very nice man, grew red in the face. 'You have been talking about Council business to a person who is not a member of Council' he thundered. The Warden of Wadham's usually red face grew redder. Glares were directed at me from every direction. I was utterly terrified and unable to utter a word. Then the Registrar, Sir Folliott Sandford, bless him, stood up and read out item 7 of the Business of Council, and I was saved, and so was the Department of Experimental Psychology.

My second meeting of Council was equally terrifying, and not at all in a dignified way. The meetings were held in those days in the Delegates' (of the University Press) Room in the Clarendon Building on Broad Street, around a huge table. The seat that had been allocated to me by the Registrar was at the end of the table furthest from the door of entrance. About halfway through the meeting I was seized suddenly by an imperious need. I had no idea what the protocol was in such a situation. Did one raise one's hand and say, 'Please Mr Vice-Chancellor Sir, may I leave the room Sir?' Then to my left I saw a door. I thought I could find my way quietly through it towards the amenity I needed. So I slipped through it: into total darkness. Immediately in front of me was another door. It was locked. I was in a space in the thickness of the wall, and the only way out of it was back into the Delegates' Room. In my panic I rattled the handle of the door through which I had just passed, but it would not open. After another hundred years I got it open and emerged into the presence of Council, slunk past them and out of the main door. When I had completed my business in the crypt of the building I slunk back to my place, wishing I had never been born.

The Hebdomadal Council Papers ruined my week-ends during Term for the next six years. A thick packet of about a hundred closely printed pages would arrive every Saturday morning and I would have to desert my family all week-end going through them in time for the Council meetings on Monday, trying with difficulty to understand them. The fact is I was not much good on Council, but it was useful to me to be on it because it gave me an understanding of how the University works that was helpful to me at the time. This was especially so since the Franks Commission of Inquiry was set up soon after I came on Council 'To inquire into and report upon the part which Oxford plays now and should play in the future in the system of higher education in the United Kingdom, having regard to its position as both a national and an international University: And *in the light of its findings on this subject* to consider in particular: '. . . ten subjects, one of which, V, was of particular interest to me for reasons that will be clear in the next chapter. This subject was 'Whether in general present relations between the autonomous colleges and the University require reconsideration. And specifically, '(a) whether the position concerning holders of university posts who do not hold college fellowships requires further consideration'; . . . (d) whether colleges might devise methods through which they could co-operate with each other in the use of their financial resources for the greater benefit of Oxford'; and '. . . (e) whether the present system of college contributions to the University is satisfactory;.' The Franks Commission worked hard, and produced its report in two thick volumes in 1966. It will come up in the next chapter.

I didn't enjoy Council as much as the other members seemed to do. I failed to understand quite a lot of what was being discussed, largely because much of what was being said was said very quickly, very elliptically, and very softly by Lucy Sutherland, Principal of Lady Margaret Hall, at the same time as Maurice Bowra, Warden of Wadham, and Bill Williams, Warden of Rhodes house, were carrying on a loud private conversation. I heard them but not her. One thing that did give me great pleasure on Council was the brilliance of the Registrar, Sir Folliott Sandford. He seemed to know 95 percent of what there was to know; but what was even more admirable was that he always knew at once where to look up the little he did not know, and had the necessary books and papers to hand. After the meetings, the members of Council would gather in twos and threes on the steps of the Clarendon Building and discuss things, but I always seemed to be walking down those steps alone. After I had served my six years I was invited to stand for a further term, but I decided no, and I've never regretted it. Besides, I had other interesting preoccupations, in addition to my research in the Sir Willliam Dunn School of Pathology. There were the Curators of the Bodleian Library, there were the Visitors of the Ashmolean Museum, and there were two new Colleges to get founded.

The Visitors of the Ashmolean Museum

In 1969 Congregation to my joy elected me a Visitor of the Ashmolean Museum for the normal period of six years. I was re-elected again in 1975, and again in 1981, which means that I can go on until the end of September 1987, if I'm not shamed into going before then. I give you these tedious details to illustrate the fact that being a Curator and a Visitor have enabled me to remain a Member of Congregation long after my rightful time. But in 1987 enough will have been enough as far as the University is concerned, and possibly even for me.

The Ashmolean Museum of Art and Archaeology is the oldest *public* museum in Europe, I dare say the world. I'm not supposed to say that, because at the tercentenary of the Ashmolean in 1983 there was an international conference on 'The Cabinet of Curiosities' in Oxford, and some obscure delegate from some obscure museum in some obscure country claimed that his was the oldest, which it is not, but out of politeness we are now obliged to say only that the Ashmolean is the oldest in Britain.

The former Bodleian Curator in me is inclined to claim that the Ashmolean Museum owes its foundation to Sir Thomas Bodley, founder of the first public library in Britain, who took the first step by providing a gallery for objects of antiquity in his Library that was opened in 1602. In it or near it were placed the ancient marbles bequeathed by another benefactor of the Library, John Selden, in 1654, and the Arundel collection of marble inscriptions given by Lord Henry Howard in 1667. The Museum was actually founded by Elias Ashmole, with the 'closet of rarities' given to him by John Tradescant the Younger, who had enlarged the collection made by his father, John Tradescant the Elder. Ashmole had offered the Tradescant collection to Oxford on condition that a suitable repository be built, and so it came about that what is now called the Old Ashmolean was built by the Oxford mason, Thomas Wood, on Broad Street, next to the Sheldonian Theatre and the Bodleian Library. It is one of the most beautiful of the many beautiful buildings in Oxford. The first Keeper of the old Ashmolean Museum was Robert Plot, who was also the first Professor of Chemistry in the University, and under him the Ashmolean 'became the principal centre for scientific research within the University', and remained so for almost two hundred years.

In 1845 the new University Galleries, built with benefactions from Francis Randolph and Roger Newdigate, were opened on Beaumont Street. It is a Greek Revival building, designed by C.R.Cockerel 'with his sculptural approach to the classical language of architecture', and it is, according to *Country Life*, 'probably the most striking and original classical design of its date in Europe'. It was intended to house the University's antique sculpture, including the Arundel collection in the Bodleian Library, in the Randolph Gallery on the ground floor; and pictures from the Bodleian on the first floor. In the meantime the Ashmolean Museum on Broad Street had acquired a number of important antiquities — Anglo-Saxon material; some of the material from Sir Arthur Evans' excavations at Knossos in Crete; and some from Sir Flinders Petrie's excavations in Egypt. The time had come for a more systematic redistribution of the University's wealth, and much of the contents of the old Ashmolean Museum was transferred elsewhere — the library and the coins to the Bodleian, natural history and ethnography to the new University Museum and the New Pitt Rivers Museum in Parks Road. On the initiative of Sir Arthur Evans, the remaining collections, including the Tradescant collection and the largely archaeological material, were moved to the University Galleries in Beaumont Street, which had been newly enlarged by C.D.E.Fortnum to house these accessions, and his own gift of bronzes and ceramics. In 1899 the name 'Ashmolean Museum' was transferred to the Beaumont Street Galleries, with Evans as Keeper, and the Broad Street building became the 'Old Ashmolean', later to house the Museum of the History of Science. The Ashmolean Museum now has four Departments: Antiquities, Western Art, the Heberden Coin Room, and Eastern Art. It is one of the leading museums in the world — just notice how many times acknowledgements are made to it when you look at programmes on the television that have to do with antiquities, Western and Eastern art or coins. No wonder I am proud to be a Visitor of such a Museum.

The Visitors of the Ashmolean do not play as active a part in the Museum's affairs as the Curators of the Bodleian play in the

Library's affairs. The reason is that most, if not all, of the Curators use the Bodleian Library for their work every day; and very few of the Visitors use the Ashmolean Museum at all. It is in a sense no more to them than it is to the man in the street or the earnest tourist. This is a fact of life, neither a disparagement of the Visitors, nor a suggestion that they are not necessary.

The Ashmolean Museum is a lovely museum. The atmosphere is not at all institutional, and when one enters it, one feels as if one were entering the noble house of some very rich friend with consummate taste and discretion. As soon as I was elected Visitor, I called on the Keeper of the Museum, who was also Keeper of Antiquities (there was not yet a Director), and on the Keeper of Western Art, Kenneth Garlick, the Keeper of the Heberden Coin Room, Humphrey Sutherland, and the Keeper of Eastern Art, Jim Harle. Again I was conscious of my ignorance, but they were kind, and none blinked an eyelid. Up to that time the Keepership of the Ashmolean had rotated among the four Departmental Keepers, but following the Brunt Report the new office of Director was created. David Piper, now Sir David, came to us, one of the nicest men I know, from the Directorship of the Fitzwilliam Museum at the University of Cambridge. Previously he had been Director of the National Portrait Gallery in London. We were fortunate in having such as him for our first Director, but he has now retired.

Not long after I became a Visitor, I was elected to the Standing Committee; and not long after that the Vice-Chancellor asked me to take on the chairmanship of it. Thus it was that I came to be Chairman of the Standing Committees of both the Bodleian Library and the Ashmolean Museum at the same time. If that was not a record for Oxford, at least it was for the Reddersburg Government Secondary School. (When Ruthie and I went to South Africa in 1984, we visited a cousin of mine, whose wife was an amateur painter. There was a mystical sort of *oeuvre* of hers on the wall, and I could see she attached great importance to it. She saw me looking at it, and asked me what I thought of it. I thought to myself that only a few weeks ago I had presided over the appointment of a new Keeper of Western Art at the Ashmolean Museum in Oxford, with Sir David Piper, Director of the Ashmolean Museum, on my right, and Sir Michael Levey, Director of the National Gallery in London, on my left; so I should be able to find the right words to say. 'It scares the Hell out of me', I said. She purred.)

Recently I took part in the appointment of the new Director of the Ashmolean Museum. It was a ticklish business, involving my making telephone calls to America, but we got the right man, Dr Christopher White, Director of Studies at the Paul Mellon Centre for Studies in British Art in London.

8
GETTING TWO COLLEGES FOUNDED IN OXFORD

The Oxford that I came to at the beginning of 1947 had just started to change from the Oxford it was before the war. In the early 1920s, the University played a small part in Oxford, amounting to not much more than a repository of books. If it had ceased to exist, the Colleges would hardly have noticed the difference, except that they would have had to rely on their own primitive laboratories, and confer their own degrees. By the late 1930s they could hardly have managed without the University laboratories. After the war, a great change took place in the function and size of the University. In the wake of a great widening of academic interests, there was a great increase in the number of members of the University, both of dons and of students, and many of these students were graduates of other universities coming to take higher degrees at Oxford. This widening of interests was particularly marked in the expansion of existing science and the introduction of new science, but there was also an introduction of new subjects in the arts. Between 1939 and 1962 there was a small decline in the number of Readers and University Lecturers in the older Faculties of Theology, Law, *Literae Humaniores* and Mediaeval History; and strong increases in Modern European Languages, Oriental Languages, Social Studies, Anthropology and Geography, and in the Physical and Biological Sciences, and in Medicine.

By the late 1950s nearly half of the University academic staff, though nominally — *and obligatorily* — attached to colleges, were not fellows of those colleges. At that time there were 560 fellows and 426 non-fellows. But of the 560 fellows, half were not on the staff of the University — they were not appointed by the faculties of the University, and not paid by the University. They were employees of the colleges, known as CUF (Common University Fund) lecturers, with the University contributing to the colleges for their salaries. If these CUF lecturers were excluded, there were 282 academic servants of the University who were Fellows, and 409 who were not.

Yet those Fellows of colleges who were not servants of the University had access to information concerning the University that was not available to academic servants of the University who were not fellows of colleges. Not only that, most of the informed discussion about University matters, and the plot-laying that went with such discussions, went on in the Senior Common Rooms of colleges. Let me quote, however improper that may be, from one of my volumes of *Hebdomadal Council Papers*, to wit an extract from a paper sent to Council by one of the colleges in this connection:

> Although we regard a college fellowship as predominantly an 'office' we feel that it has acquired 'status' and in many cases considerable amenities. These two aspects lie at the root of present difficulties and cannot be overlooked. There is an additional aspect which does not seem to have been touched upon either in the Harrison Report [I'll come to that later] or in the colleges' replies, viz. the dissemination of information about purely or mainly university matters. To put it bluntly, it is much easier to know what goes on in the University if one is a member of a governing body [of a college] than if one is not. Taking one example only, we refer to the distribution of Council documents throughout the University in the formative stages of policy. These are frequently sent to Heads of Houses with copies for each member of their governing bodies but not to members of Congregation as such. We note, for instance, that although the report of the Harrison Committee was circulated to all resident members of Congregation, the comments of the colleges on the report were not. It seems that our administrative procedures have not been brought fully into line with the growth and development of the University outside the college system.

And this was not the only way non-fellows were excluded from the affairs of the University, not by any regulation, but by custom and prejudice. They were not on any of the central bodies of the University, like the Hebdomadal Council, the General Board of the Faculties, the Curators of the Bodleian library, the Visitors of the Ashmolean Museum, the Delegates of the University Press. With the beginning of the turn in the tide, I was the first of the non-dons (as we called ourselves, or Kaffirs, as Maurice Bowra once good naturedly called us) to be on any of these bodies.

And many of the non-dons were most distinguished in their fields, and some of the scientists were Fellows of the Royal Society yet not fellows of any college. (But none of the non-scientists was a Fellow of the British Academy, which is not a reflection on the non-dons, rather a reflection of the fact that the colleges preferred non-scientists to scientists). Many non-dons (including me) had distinguished visiting scholars coming from time to time to spend sabbatical periods in Oxford working with them, and they were embarrassed by their inability to invite them to the common room of any college or to dine at any High Table. It was not that the non-dons were of lower academic status than the fellows, they were not, and several of them, for example, were Readers in the University.

On Thursday 28 September 1961 two non-dons began to move. Martyn Webb, then a University Lecturer in Geography (now in Australia), and M. Macdonald Spencer, Secretary of the Institute of Education (now Emeritus Fellow of St Cross College), began to speculate on the possibility of getting a new graduate college founded in Oxford for the purpose of absorbing non-dons as fellows, and graduates as students for higher degrees. These graduate students were a largely post-war phenomenon in Oxford, and they led a shadowy life in the colleges, which had always been superbly geared to look after undergraduate students, but had no idea of what to do with their graduates. Their supervisors were generally not fellows of the college, but outsiders appointed by the University. Webb and Spencer called a meeting of about twenty non-dons to discuss the matter, where it was decided to draw up a paper dealing with the problem of the non-dons, suggesting several solutions to the problem, including the foundation of one or two new colleges. The draft of this paper was discussed at a further meeting of non-dons, at which I was present. This led to a further meeting on 15 November, in the Geology Department. One of the non-dons was John French, a colleague in the Sir William Dunn School of Pathology. On the way to Geology he told me he had been asked to ask me if he could propose me as chairman of the meeting. I agreed, I was proposed, I accepted, and so it was that I became the spokesman for the non-dons. So I headed a committee to represent the views of the non-dons to Council (of which I was not yet a member). Council's 'Committee on the relationship between the University and the colleges' appointed a sub-committee on 10 May 1962 'to submit a report to the committee setting out the facts of the problem of closer integration of university employees into the college system (and the related problem of a revision of Statt. Tit. XXV) and suggesting some ways in which this problem might be solved'. (The Statute with the Title XXV defined the offices, the holders of which might be elected to professorial fellowships, and need not concern us.) The members of the sub-committee were Mr A.R.W.Harrison (Chairman), soon to be Warden of Merton College; Dr J.W. Linnett, Fellow of the Queen's College; and Dr E.A.O. Whiteman, Fellow of Lady Margaret Hall, representing Council; and Dr R.H.Freeborn and me representing the 'Committee of Non-Fellows'. Shortly after that, there was a large meeting of non-dons in the Taylor Institution at which I stated that if the University should fail to do anything about us we would jolly well start our own college. I then resigned my chairmanship of the non-dons because I thought that as I was about to sit on the Harrison committee (as it came to be called), I should distance myself from the non-dons for the time being. Tom Tinsley took over the chairmanship from me, and under his guidance the Oxford Collegiate Society came into being. It met from time to time over cold-table lunches in various institutions such as Halifax House or Rhodes House, acting as a peripatetic make-shift college for the non-dons. It was the fore-runner of the two new graduate colleges that came into being on the first day of Michaelmas Term, 1965.

My first instinct when Richard Freeborn and I met the other side of the Harrison Committee was that they were the enemy, but this instinct evaporated as soon as we sat together with them. Robin Harrison was the gentlest of souls, and Linnett and Anne Whiteman were entirely reasonable and sympathetic. It soon became clear to me that all three of them were on our side, but realistic about the problems to be overcome. Our report came out in November 1962. It proposed 'that all members of the graduate staff of the University ought to have some form of affiliation with some form of graduate society, that this cannot be fully achieved without the creation of new societies (and the expansion of existing ones), but that homes could and should be found for many within the existing colleges'. It went on to state 'if the University expands much further without anything being done, they [the non-fellows] will form the majority. If they do, *then Oxford will cease to be a collegiate university* [my italics] and will become instead a university with some colleges affiliated; our proposals are designed to prevent this from happening.'

The Colleges were invited by the Vice-Chancellor to comment on the Harrison Report, and their replies were referred to the 'Committee to review the relationship between the University and the colleges', which, in February 1963, set up a further committee consisting of Sir Arthur Norrington, President of

Trinity College, as Chairman; Robin Harrison; Derek Hall, Fellow of Exeter College; and Anne Whiteman; with no non-dons. The report of this committee was published in January 1964, by which time I was a member of the Hebdomadal Council. It placed the non-fellows in three categories:
(1) those like Readers (about thirty), who were especially eligible for fellowships, and should be found fellowships in existing undergraduate or graduate colleges,
(2) those whose undergraduate tutorial teaching fitted them for fellowships of undergraduate colleges (about sixty), and should be found fellowships in such colleges,
(3) those who did little or no undergraduate tutorial teaching, for whom new collegiate societies should be founded.
The report noted that the creation of about 200 fellowships would bring the proportion of fellows to students back to what it had been in 1938.

The policy proposed in this report was approved in principle by Congregation on 25 February 1964, and Council appointed a committee under Norrington to make detailed proposals for carrying out that policy. The other members of the committee were Robin Harrison; John Bamborough, Principal of what was then called Linacre House; Professor W.D.M.Paton (Pharmacology); Anne Whiteman; Derek Hall; and, representing the non-fellows, Alan Jones and me. Alan Jones was a good man to have on our side. He was a graduate of St John's College, Cambridge, where he had first taken a First Class degree in Classics, then a First Class degree in Oriental Languages, and he was now a University lecturer in Oriental Languages. He was very well-informed, being good at his homework; and he was subtle, and capable of being devious when necessary. He could be very tough and obstinate, and he knew when to be reasonable. It was a good committee, and we worked and thought hard under the tough and good-humoured guidance of Thomas Norrington, as Sir Arthur was less formally known. Our report came out in November 1964, stating that the policy approved by Congregation implied the decision 'that there ought not to be a division, among university officers of comparable standing and duties in the University, between those who hold college fellowships and those who do not'. This led to three conclusions:
'(a) There must be a clear definition of university posts which carry with them entitlement to a fellowship,
(b) There must be a statutory obligation to provide fellowships for all holders of such posts,

(c) The number of fellowships should be large enough to provide for them all.'

The concept of 'entitlement' to a college fellowship was not new. It had been in the Statutes of the University for some time, and applied to all professors; now it was to be extended to all readers, university lecturers, senior research officers, and holders of homologous offices. It is of course not an enforceable statute, because the whole point of a college in Oxford (or Cambridge) is that it is a self-governing, self-perpetuating, independent body of fellows, and nobody, not even the University, can tell it whom it may or may not elect to a fellowship. We were of course well aware of this, but pressed on. We were not drawing up a new unenforceable statute, merely expanding one that already existed. How legal the concept of entitlement to a college fellowhip is, I do not know. Even now there are still some entitled dons in Oxford for whom college fellowships have not been found, but as far as I know none of them has sued the University or a college (which college?). I expect it is in fact not enforceable by law.

The committee estimated that in order to carry out this last recommendation about 160 new fellowships would have to be found. (This figure does not match up with the figure of 409 non-fellows I mentioned earlier — this is because some of them had by then been elected to fellowships at undergraduate colleges after the publication of the Harrison report; and some of them did not hold posts which we thought were homologous with university lecturerships.) The committee expected at least fifty of the remaining 'entitled' non-fellows to be elected to fellowships in existing colleges, leaving about a hundred fellowhips to be found. For this purpose the establishment of two new colleges was recommended, for fellows and graduate students of both sexes. (The committee had been inclined to recommend only one new college, but I persuaded them that the realities demanded two of them.)

As to premises for these two new colleges, sites had been found where it was thought possible to make a start without new building, or much rebuilding of what already stood on them. These were the former Vicarage of St Cross Church with the Old School, handily situated quite near the centre of Oxford; and a handsome 18th century house quite a lot further out at Court Place in Iffley. As to finances, the University Grants Committee provided the money for the two sites, and the rest of the charity we needed began magnificently at home. A consortium of the richer colleges, led by All Souls, Christ Church, Merton and St John's — I intone their names with reverence — provided capital grants totalling £29,000, and annual grants of £18,000 (a lot in those days) for each of the colleges for ten years.

I began to think about who might be the Heads of these two new Houses. In agreement with Thomas Norrington, I went to see Isaiah Berlin in All Souls to ask if he would consider being the Head of one of them. Isaiah Berlin is a famous philosopher. He is an amusing man, and a nice man, and a man of many talents; but since I have never really been able to understand what philosophy is about, I am not competent to judge his philosophy, as so many enthusiastic journalists so warmly do. He is also very, very difficult to understand, because he talks very softly, and very quickly, and very elliptically, but I believe I got the drift of his reply, which was no, thank you; but if he were to be Head of one of the new houses, it would have to be the one at St Cross. In the event he did become Head of one of these houses, but it was not St Cross.

About this time, Florey was elected Provost of The Queen's College, and he resigned the Professorship of Pathology, to my sorrow. Shortly after that, he told me that the college intended putting up a new buiding for graduate students (which it subsequently did, not far away in St Clements — a huge strange building by James Stirling with good points and terrible points). He wanted me to be a sort of sub-provost of this institution, and a Fellow of Queen's. The temptation was terrible. Queen's is a noble college, and secretly the colonial (and possibly the snob) in me preferred the idea of a traditional, old, established, rich, college to the uncertain possibility of a poor new do-it-yourself college that was bound to be looked down upon, at least for a long time. Of course I did not accept Florey's invitation.

9
St CROSS COLLEGE, OXFORD

Getting the College started

Once the decision for the two sites had been made, the members of the Oxford Collegiate Society were free to choose which of the two colleges, provisionally called St Cross College and Iffley College, they would like to join. Somehow they divided into roughly equal groups, though I can't remember now why any of them should have chosen a site so far from the centre of things as Iffley. Of course, Ruthie and I chose St Cross.

Then, among the St Cross group, arose the question of who should be the Head of the new College. It was not within the gift of the future fellows to choose their Head, because the business of the two new colleges was for the time being in the hands of the Hebdomadal Council, since the college was not yet a self-governing institution with a charter of its own. But Alan Jones somehow, I've forgotten how, had a say on the committee that had to do the choosing, and I, being a member of Council, would eventually have to be informed of the decisions of that committee. Having done my bit over getting the affair launched, I retired to my laboratory in the Sir William Dunn School of Pathology.

There we had just made the wonderful observation I have reported in chapter 6. This was the experiment that had taken us to the very gates of Paradise, showing us exactly what step to take next in order to determine the mode of action of tetanus toxin at the chemical level; and not only that, the mode of action of botulinum toxin as well. We were now in the early stages of trying to open those Pearly Gates, that is, trying to repeat that experiment; and just beginning to lose our minds in our first failures to do so.

Alan Jones came to see me, presumably acting on behalf of the prospective St Cross fellows, to tell me that he would like to put my name forward for the Principalship, which was the title Council had in mind for the office of the Heads of the new colleges. I told him, truthfully, that if it had ever occurred to me that I might be the Head of one of the colleges, I had dismissed the idea. I did not want the job, since I was more interested in my research, and for my research I needed my laboratory, and my position in the Sir William Dunn School (which I hoped would soon be an *ad hominem* Readership, since Florey had told me that he had put me up for it). A little while later Alan Jones asked me again, and I said no, thank you.

Jane Mellanby and Diana Messenger and I continued at the rate of three attempts a week to repeat our wonderful experiment. By the end of a month we were at our collective wits' end. On one particular morning I was feeling very far out on the end of my wits, because in addition to the experimental difficulties, I was having clandestine telephone conversations with detectives in the Oxford police. One of our female technicians was getting nasty poison-pen letters that distressed her a great deal. She didn't want me to talk to the police about them, so I was doing it secretly. At this stage Alan Jones walked in with another suggestion that I change my mind about the Principalship of St Cross. 'All right dammit', I said, 'go ahead.' I told him that they must not expect me to apply for the job; and that I had to be able to keep my Senior Research Officership. At that point Jane and Diana and I decided we had had enough of our failed experiments.

Alan Jones is a man who gets his way, and I began to view the idea of becoming Principal of St Cross College as a distinct possibility. Then Alan reported to me that there were those on Council who were opposed to having me, on the grounds that I was a second-rate scientist, and I think I know who carried that idea from whom to Council. Council's people went to The Queen's College to ask Florey what he thought of me. 'If you don't appoint van Heyningen', he said, 'you'll be bigger fools than I thought.' The indefatigable Jones then went to Florey to ask him to support the proposal that I be appointed Principal, and Florey agreed to do so. I suppose that turned the balance.

A few days later Alan told me secretly that I was going to be appointed. I had told Ruthie and Alan that if I were appointed Principal I would tell the Fellows, 'Let's not be formal; don't call me Principal, just call me Prince.' Now Ruthie was away in New York. I sent her a cable 'Very secretly call me Prince', and got from her a few days later the sweetest letter I have ever had in my life. I was certain then that I was on the right tack. The next afternoon in the laboratory I received a telephone call from Sir Folliott Sandford, the Registrar. They had decided to appoint me

Principal of St Cross College, a letter would follow, would I accept the appointment? Certainly, I said. I told Jane and Diana. Jane rushed up and kissed me warmly. Diana wouldn't have dreamed of doing such a thing. The formal letter of appointment followed, and I formally accepted the appointment as Principal of St Cross College, Oxford. In all the 800 years of Oxford University's history, there had been only thirty-two Founding Heads of Colleges; now I was going to be the thirty-third.

St Cross was considered only a provisional name for the college, and I dreamed of other names. Oxford had produced many famous alumni during those 800 years, and I wondered why no college had been named after any of them (and why there was no Isaac Newton College in Cambridge). Christopher Wren, of Wadham College, was the first name that came to my mind; then those two famous scientists of University College: Robert Boyle, 'son of the Earl of Cork and Father of Modern Chemistry'; and Robert Hooke the physicist, and Curator of Experiments to the Royal Society. But then I realised that colleges could not afford the luxury of honouring the great — they needed to sell their names to the best bidders. So the very first thing I did was to write to the Queen of the Netherlands. It was a Sunday, and I had just read in the papers that the Queen had a personal fortune of £303,000,000. Surely it would make no difference to her to round that off to a neat three hundred million? On an impulse I wrote to her. I had no college writing paper, and no secretary and no typewriter, so I wrote in my own hand on a plain sheet of paper. I suggested that perhaps she might like to commemorate the years during the war when Britain was so honoured and proud to give shelter to her and her family and her entourage. I told her the name of the college was provisional, and that we would be honoured to change it, with her consent, to 'Queen Juliana College', or 'The Royal Netherlands College.' I did not mention my Netherlandish ancestry, or my great-grandfather who had been a Knight of the Order of the Netherlands Lion, leaving all that to my Netherlandish signature at the bottom of the page. On the envelope I wrote nothing but 'Her Majesty the Queen of the Netherlands.' I posted it quickly, before reason could step in and change my mind. I didn't expect a reply, but after about three months I did indeed get one, from the Ambassador of the Royal Netherlands Embassy in London. It was really friendly. He informed me that the Queen had given my letter much thought, but had reluctantly concluded that circumstances did not enable her to make a contribution to the college. He wished me well in warm terms. I believe I was very close to getting those three millions.

The University asked me to draw up plans for putting up a provisional college on the St Cross site, under the guidance of the highly talented University Surveyor, Jack Lankester. I went to look at the site. It was about an acre and a half, next to St Cross Church, otherwise known as Holywell Church, with its churchyard, which, with so many distinguished dons buried there, some of them with beautiful headstones, is a collective monument to Victorian academic Oxford. The buildings on the site consisted of a pretty stone Victorian schoolroom, with the teacher's cottage attached, a brick Victorian rectory, and another stone schoolroom, built before the first war. These buildings had in the recent past temporarily housed some University department, and were now overgrown with bushes, weeds and grass. The idea was that the buildings on the site should be refurbished and adapted to serve as the college. Jack Lankester and I studied the buildings, and he told me that just mending the roof of the rectory would use up half of the money available, which was the £29,000 that All Souls, Christ Church, Merton and St John's had provided, bless them all again. So we decided to raze the rectory and the later schoolrooom, and put up a provisional wooden hut in their place. The old Victorian schoolroom would be the library and meeting room, and the hut would consist primarily of a large Common Room with a room for the Principal, a general office, a small kitchen, a cloakroom and lavatories. Thus it was that I decided that the principal social activity of the college would be a simple lunch, carrying on the custom of lunching together that had been established by the Oxford Collegiate Society. I had only one difference with Jack Lankester. Space being short, he wanted to put one cubicle each in the men's and women's lavatories. I said to him 'Dammit Jack, I can't tell my friends in the Reform Club I'm Principal of a two-bog college in Oxford.' So we had five, three in the women's and two and a thingummy in the men's.

The hut was built, and the space previously occupied by the rectory turned into a lawn and a car park. Then I had a very pleasant time furnishing the college. I was lucky, and perhaps the college was lucky, because it was not yet formally constituted and so I had a free hand — otherwise we would have been held up interminably while the Governing Body of the college decided on matters of convenience and taste. I went to Heal's in London and to Gordon Russell in Broadway for the furniture; to Sanderson's for the wall-paper and curtains; and to Sotheby's for oriental rugs to put on the polished hardwood floors. I was determined that once you were inside the college, you would not know that you were in a wooden hut, and it worked.

I had to find a Porter. When I had first gone to inspect the site, I had been challenged by a cheeky little man with a cockney accent. He was Mr Collins, the verger of St Cross Church, living in the cottage that was an integral part of the Victorian school. I saw difficulties in throwing him out of the cottage, and I liked his cheek, so I appointed him Porter of the college.

The college buildings were not quite ready, so the first meeting of the Governing Body of St Cross College, Oxford, was held in the Mure Room of Merton College at 2.15 p.m. on Tuesday 5 October 1965. (This was the second week of Michaelmas Term — normally the University doesn't come to life until Full Term, which, curiously enough, is shorter than Term, and starts on the third Monday. Governing Body meetings are always held on Wednesdays in Full Term, when by general agreement there are no University meetings. All subsequent meetings of the St Cross governing body were held on Wednesdays.) None of us had ever been on the governing body of a college, and to this day I don't know whether our meetings were any different from those of the established colleges. Needless to say, that first meeting of ours was highly charged with triumph and expectancy. The very first decision we took was to elect Mac Spencer and Tom Tinsley as Fellows by Special Election. They were every bit as good as any of us, but owing to a technicality, the appointments they held in the University did not 'entitle' them to fellowships of the college. The next decision was to change the title of the Principal, which none of us liked, since it seemed more suited to a school or a reformatory. Some wanted President, some wanted Master. I liked Master, in the Cambridge way, and Master it was. My elation was tempered by remembrance of the story of the young man who had bought a second-hand rowing boat, then a little sailing boat, then a bigger boat that needed two to manage it, so he hired a bum on the waterfront to help him. So now he was a captain, so he bought a nautical cap emblazoned 'Captain'. He went home to his Mama in Brooklyn, and said 'Look Mam, I'm a Captain!' 'What do you mean my boy, you are a Captain?' 'I got a boat, I got a crewman, so I'm a Captain.' 'My boy', said his Mama, 'by me you are a Captain; by your sister you are a Captain; but tell me, by the Captains are you a Captain?' By the Masters was I going to be a Master?

Thereafter that term we were so busy and enthusiastic getting the college off the ground that we met every Wednesday instead of the two Wednesdays a term that were usual, not that we knew what was usual. The second meeting was also in the Mure Room, but the third, on Wednesday 27 October was on our own territory, in the library in the former school. By now I had arranged with a firm of caterers to provide our lunches, which we ate around coffee tables and some larger tables in the Common Room. It worked well, and I see in my diary that in the first two terms I had a good number of the Heads of Houses and their wives to lunch. After some time the firm of caterers began to give increasingly clear signs that they were no good, so we dismissed them. I asked Mrs Collins if she thought she could prepare our lunches, now that she knew what we needed. She thought she could, so we engaged her, and she and her husband served us well.

Almost too well as far as Mr Collins was concerned. I'm not at all sure that he was ever in London, but he put on a fine Cockney accent and, when it suited him, an unctious one. Having adopted St Cross Church as our College Chapel, we decided to have an annual service of thanksgiving in it, and I chose St Crispin's Day for it. I waited in my room while the Fellows and their spouses gathered in the church. When everything was ready, Mr Collins, garbed in his verger's cassock, came to lead me into the church. This necessitated emerging onto the street for a few yards, where some people had gathered to look on. Mr Collins took it upon himself to chant, 'Make way for the Master! Make way for the Master!' all the way from my room to the church, and there was nothing I could do about it.

After a Term or so, the Fellows of Iffley College, who never actually moved into Court Place in Iffley where they were originally intended to go (and I don't blame them), made a move. They invited Isaiah Berlin to be their Principal. Isaiah Berlin told them that he would accept their invitation if he could raise the money to get the college properly on its feet. This he did. He got a promise of £1.5 million from the Ford Foundation in America, if he could raise an equal sum from the Wolfson foundation in England; and he got a promise of £1.5 million from the Wolfson Foundation if he could raise an equal sum from the Ford foundation. He had the advantage that he was a good friend of McGeorge Bundy of the Ford Foundation, and a good friend of the Wolfsons; and he is a distinguished and famous man. It was good sense, but I was surprised that he was interested in the

Iffley proposition, even if I could see that he was in a good position to raise the money.

The only trouble was that Council had already ruled that neither of the new colleges should approach any of the big foundations without consulting Council, and bringing in the other college. Naturally I had already had my eye on these two very obvious foundations, and in my total inexperience in matters like these was trying to work out a way of approaching them; but I had no connections. Isaiah Berlin succeeded in raising his £3 million, and some people were shocked, but I was not. I was sure that if he and I had jointly approached these two foundations, we would not have got £3 million each, and not even £1.5 million each, because the foundations, like Isaiah, would think that £3 million was the minimum for founding a college. So I didn't make a fuss, and some people were surprised. When I went to the next meeting of Hebdomadal Council, Lady Ogilvy, Principal of St Anne's College, told me I was a saint, but I was merely a realist. But we didn't do too badly in our humble hut: about six months after our foundation, John Sparrow, Warden of All Souls College, wrote to me: 'I congratulate you on what I hear from all sides about the impetus you are giving St Cross. Quite as important as £3 million pounds, though I dare say that cash may seem to you a more immediately important consideration.'

When I look at St Cross College today, in one of the most beautiful buildings in Oxford, on St Giles, right in the heart of the City, and at Wolfson, in a vast concrete structure so far away from the centre that they have to run a bus, I am glad we were obliged to move slowly.

Trying to Raise the Money

It wasn't that I wanted to move slowly, far from it, but I was very ignorant of *how* to raise money. We started off badly. A good friend of ours in London, that is of Ruthie and me, was keen to help us through a friend of his who was high up in the Civil Service in London. This man thought he knew how to approach a certain very rich person in England (sorry to be so mysterious), but we had to go about it with the greatest of caution, and in the meantime I was not to approach anybody else. This lasted for six months, and nothing came of it, with no move made as far as I could see. I won't say we missed other opportunities in the meantime, I don't know, but the inaction while waiting did rather take the wind out of my sails for a while.

Then I fell naively into the clutches of a professional fund-raiser with an office — perhaps I should say an address — in Berkeley Square. This was not long after the Americans had followed Yuri Gagarin into space in Geminis III to VI, and the fund-raiser was up to date. I won't go into details, I'll just quote the opening sentence of the fund-raising brochure they suggested . It went: 'St Cross is a new concept college with all systems go!' That made me realise that I must go it alone.

I started by looking for charity at home, since that is where it is said to begin. I tried Mr Amey, the Oxford gravel millionaire. Things looked hopeful to start with, when he and his wife accepted an invitation to a dinner we gave for them in our wooden hut. He arrived saying, 'This evening's going to cost me a lot of money!', but in the end it cost him nought, for he sent his son-in-law to tell me we were not going to get anything from them.

I tried another Oxford millionaire, Robert Maxwell, and he behaved disgracefully. I had been to see him in the great mansion on Headington Hill (that he rents from the city, I've been told), and he appeared to be very forthcoming. I invited him and his wife to lunch in the college, and we fixed a date about two weeks hence. We got all worked up about that in the college, but on the day before the lunch he telephoned to say that other business had come up, so we postponed the lunch for another two weeks. The morning of the great day came, and we were all ready and expectant, when he telephoned. He had to go to a meeting of the parliamentary kitchen committee — what was it I wanted to talk to him about anyway? Oh nothing in particular, I said. A few weeks later Lady Berlin invited Ruthie and me to a luncheon party in their house. Robert Maxwell would be there, Isaiah told me, and that would be a good opportunity for me to touch him for money. That was thoughtful of the Berlins, but I asked them to seat me as far away from Maxwell as they could.

I met the Dutch director of Shell, and he, influenced perhaps by my name, introduced me to the British director, Lord Rothschild, who was most kind. He gave a dinner party for me in a Pall Mall club, I can't remember which; and he invited me to give a talk about the college to senior executives in Shell House. That was really difficult, but I felt I must do my best. I told them that, as far as I was concerned, the life of an academic was idyllic as long as you didn't mind being poorly paid. I suggested that we might consider a scheme of regular exchanges, with dons doing six months hard in industry or business, and businessmen learning and reflecting in the groves of academe (as they say). I was invited to visit the Shell laboratories at Port Sunlight, and put up in the Grosvenor Hotel in Chester, where the next morning I was amazed and embarrassed to be called back as I walked out and asked to pay the bill. I got no money from Shell, so I must suppose I was not good enough for them.

Not long after that I heard that the newspaper magnate and owner of *The Times*, Lord Thomson of Fleet, had a secret telephone number which he answered personally. That was a challenge for me to rise to, and to it I rose. I found out what that number was, and I see no reason why I should not disclose it now, since it won't bother Lord Thomson, if it bothers anybody at all. It was Temple Bar 1234. I dialled the number, and sure enough, a Scottish-Canadian voice replied. 'Is that Lord Thomson of Fleet?' I asked. 'It is, who are you?' he said. 'The Master of St Cross College, Oxford' I replied, 'and I need your help.' 'Tomorrow at three', he said, 'I'll be there' I said, not bothering to look at my diary. The next morning I drove to the station to take the train, and as I walked the platform with G. B. Richardson of the University Press and Professor Herbert Hart, the loudspeaker announced a delay in the train that meant I would not be at Lord Thomson's office on time. I was certain he would not be interested in the reason why, so I invited Richardson and Hart to join me in my car as I rushed to London. I dropped them somewhere in town and drove on to Chancery Lane, determined to leave my car on a double yellow line if necessary. On the way I passed the Middlesex Hospital, so I drove into the courtyard and asked the porter to give me a parking space. He demurred. 'Good Heaven's man', I shouted, 'there's three million pounds at stake, here's three of them!' A space appeared instantly, and so did a taxi, so I arrived at Lord Thomsons' office on the top floor with half a minute to spare. I was put in a waiting room, and there I waited for a long time. I was determined not to get irritated, assuming it was a ploy intended to have that effect on me, and so put me at a disadvantage. After an hour Lord Thomson bustled in, full of apologies. 'I'm so sorry to have kept you waiting', he said, 'I've been lunching at the House of Commons, and as it is, I had to walk out on Manny Shinwell.' He was very pleasant and courteous. I liked him. As I sat opposite him across his enormous desk, he kept stroking a large pile of golden sovereigns fused together to make a paper weight, which I found reassuringly appropriate. All the time we talked, young men would come in and hold slips of paper it front of his eyes, and he would say 'Yes', 'No', or 'Hold it'. After I said my piece, he sighed: 'I'd like to help you, but I just can't.' I made one more try. 'Lord Thomson's College, Oxford' has a fine ring to it, don't you think?' He seemed to slump in his chair, as if I had struck him a blow to the heart. 'Gee, I'd like that' he said wistfully, 'but I really can't do it, I owe my bank five million pounds.'

I decided the time had come for me to seek our fortune in the United States of America, so I wrote to the Commonwealth Fund that had enabled me to spend two years in America before the war, and told them about my need for money and my intention to seek it in America. I asked them if they could give me a grant to make one or two visits to America, and they promised me $1500, which was more than enough in those days. Then I wrote to Henry Alan Moe at 30 Wall Street in New York. He had been a Rhodes Scholar at Brasenose College in 1919, and was now, among other things, Secretary of the rather grand John Simon Guggenheimer Foundation that had sent Pauline Miller on a Fellowship from the Biological Laboratories at Harvard University to spend a sabbatical 1960 in my laboratory in the School of Pathology. I asked him if he could arrange a meeting for me with a number of people whom he thought might be willing to listen to a plea from me for money for St Cross. The dear man immediately agreed to do so, and not only that, he would invite them to a dinner party at the Harvard Club in New York. I asked him then if he would include Dr Julius Stratton among the guests. I had previously written to an old friend from my pre-war days at the College of Physicians and Surgeons in New York, called Fred Rosebury. He was a man of humble origins who had at that time been the laboratory's instrument maker (and he and I had published a paper on an instrument of our joint devising), telling him I would like to see him on my trip. He had replied that I should see Julius Stratton, Chairman of the Board of the Ford Foundation in New York, who was a good friend of his. Stratton had been Head of the Massachusetts Institute of Technology in Cambridge, Mass., and he, Fred Rosebury, had migrated from New York to be his instrument maker. He would put in a good word for me with Stratton. (And when subsequently I met Stratton, he welcomed me with open arms, such is the strength of the true democracy of the United States of America.)

Since I had so much travel money from the Commonwealth Fund, I decided to sail first class to New York on the *United States* in the hope of meeting rich people on the way. It was a ghastly, tedious voyage. The sea was very rough all the way, so all the passengers were sick except apparently me; and the wind was so strong that it was not possible to go on deck, so I was cooped up indoors with all those queezy people. On the last day but one I met one important person, Sir Michael Perrin, Chairman of the Wellcome Foundation Limited. I had prepared a paper on 'The Origins and Aims of St Cross College, Oxford', in which I preached about St Cross's intention to get away from an 'ivory tower' attitude to knowledge, and he told me he thought it was good. He thought the 'ivory tower' attitude was fairly new; and that the divinities used to have a definite article like the humanities. The divinities were God's business; the humanities used to be concerned with what humans could deal with, and this included science, applied science and technology, and applied knowledge of other kinds. He did not believe we would get any money in Britain, and thought that our only hope was in America, at least to start with.

Within a few minutes of landing and checking in at my hotel I was on the 7th Avenue Express Subway down to the Wall Street station, and in Henry Allen Moe's office at 30 Wall Street. Dear Henry Allen Moe — I believe he was as much concerned about St Cross College as I was. He had arranged a splendid dinner party, and only Julius Stratton and John M. Schiff were unable to come, but had said they would like me to call on them. It was a miracle that that dinner party in the Harvard Club was only a near-disaster and not a total one. On the fateful day New York was struck by a blizzard of such proportions that almost the entire edition of the *New York Times* was devoted to it. By 6.00 pm the snow was several feet high on the streets, and there was practically nothing moving on them. Nevertheless, the dinner party took place, but with several absentees. In fact the only people present, apart from Moe and me, were Dr Farinholt of the Sloane Foundation, Dr Mannie Piore, head of science at IBM, and Dr Bueche, head of science at General Electric in Schenectady. They were all sympathetic, and they invited me to visit them at their institutions.

Thus I moved about the Eastern States from Battle Creek, Michigan; through New York, New York; Philadelphia, Pennsylvania; Princeton, New Jersey; Schenectady, New York; to Washington, DC, to put my case to the Avalon Foundation;

the Bollinger Foundation; the Celanese Corporation; General Electric; IBM; the Kellog Foundation; the Macy Foundation; the Old Dominion Foundation; the Rockefeller Brothers Trust; the Rockefeller Foundation; the Sloane Foundation; and the Xerox Corporation. All of them asked me variants of the question 'What is the project of your school?' What could I say? How could I hope to explain to them that our project was to save the collegiate structure of the University of Oxford? I tried, but they were not convinced, because I don't think they had the foggiest idea of what I was talking about, and I don't blame them; nor do I blame myself.

But I had a few more things to do in New York. The first was to call on John M. Schiff at 40 Wall Street, to whom I had had an introduction from Sir William Hayter, Warden of New College. Schiff was the head of Kuhn, Loeb and Company, which I understood to be one of the world's greatest merchant banks. He started by asking me what I had done so far in Britain, and I told him about my visit to Lord Thomson of Fleet, and how he had told me that he couldn't help me because he owed his bank £5,000,000. 'He's damn right', said Schiff, 'he owes it to me.' But Mr Schiff was also unable to help me, in spite of my optimistic expectations.

Then I went on the first of several visits to the Ford Foundation to see Julius Stratton. He was very, very kind to me. He understood my problem perfectly, and told me he had no doubt that I would be supported to the hilt, by which he meant that $10 million should be forthcoming. He would urge it strongly, and was confident of success. I was to call again in a few days and he would report progress. I called again in a few days, and progress had been good — in a few days it would be confirmed. In those few days disaster struck. (I seem to have used this expression many times already, but that is the story of my life at that time.) Overnight, really *overnight*, the Ford Foundation had completely reversed their educational policy. They were going to put all their money into supporting the Blacks. There was nothing for St Cross. Julius Stratton was devastated, not about helping the Blacks, but about not being able to help me. There was nothing more to be done, or said. It was no use wishing I had arrived in New York just a week earlier.

I went on the first of several visits to Mr Benjamin Sonnenberg, to whom I had been given an introduction by Sir John Foster of All Souls College. Foster had told me I might find him interestingly eccentric, and perhaps dressed as a London Bobby.

Sonnenberg was the man who had invented publicity — publicity such as you don't see anymore in New York except for the Easter Parade and St Patrick's Day, with parades and bands marching down Fifth Avenue. He had a magnificent large house on Gramercy Square (or is it Park?) which it was an education and a pleasure to see, with an equally large house next door for his servants. When I was admitted by a maid, I was conducted, by design I'm sure, through a large silver pantry that looked like Aladdin's Cave, and up an elevator to his private apartment within his house. He was dressed in a sort of Edwardian manner, but not as a Bobby. He was enthusiastic about St Cross, and convinced that the money could be found, if we went about it the right way. The right way was for me to be eased into the consciousness of the right people in the United States. There should be a lunch party organized for me by the editor of *Scientific American*; there should be another lunch party for me organized by the Editor of *Time Magazine*; there should be yet another lunch party organized for me by the Editor of the *New York Times* in the editorial office on the 14th floor of the New York Times Building. He would invite the Editor of *The New Yorker* and me to lunch in his house, so that I should get written up in 'Talk of the Town'. I asked him how all these arrangements could be made, and he said he would make them. I agonized over whether he expected payment for this, since he was a professional publicity man, but anything I could pay him would be peanuts, especially compared with his obvious wealth, so I decided to assume that he did not. On my next visit to New York a couple of months later I called on him again. He didn't say anything more about those lunch parties, but he put before me a proposition that shook me rigid. It was that I should organize a visit by ocean liner to New York of the Vice-Chancellor of the University of Oxford and other notabilities, including Dorothy Hodgkin who had recently been awarded the Order of Merit and the Nobel Prize. I worried even more about her than about the Vice-Chancellor, because that sort of thing was even less her cup of tea. They would be met at the pier and led on a parade down Fifth Avenue, and then entertained by the Du Pont family in their mansion in Wilmington, Delaware. I couldn't see my distinguished colleagues agreeing to this, so with some regret I faded out of Mr Sonnenberg's engaging life.

I went to see a dear man, Gustave Stern. I had previously gone up to Boston to see my friend Pauline Miller, who had spent a sabbatical in my laboratory, and she had introduced me to two great friends, who were the nicest people in the world, John and Carol Enders. John was at Harvard Medical School, and had won the Nobel Prize for his work on the polio vaccine. He had given me an introduction to Gustave Stern, who had arrived penniless in the United States and built up an enormous chemical industry, starting from selling canary seed. He lived in a great apartment on Central Park West, and I was admitted by a maid into a large hall, the walls of which were covered cheek by jowl with enormous paintings by Chagal. I had read that morning in the paper that Chagal was due to arrive in New York by sea that day, and when Mr Stern came to greet me, I told him that. 'Ah, Marc and I are old friends', he told me shyly, 'he is coming to visit me tomorrow.' The apartment was filled with an astonishing collection of paintings. More than a dozen Chagals, a dozen Picassos, more than half a dozen Braques, a couple of Renoirs, a couple of Pissaros, several Vuillards, and a couple of Rouaults that converted me to Rouault. In the children's rooms, where other children might have posters of Spanish bullfights, there were enormous Bernard Buffets, originals of course.

Mr Stern was wonderfully courteous. He introduced his two children to me, telling them it was a great honour for them to meet the Master of an Oxford College. He told me he deplored the fact that the Master of an Oxford College should have to look for money. He had a great reverence for learning, and it didn't seem the right time for me to tell him that I was not as learned a man as he thought. John Enders had told me to expect a surprising suggestion from him, and that is what I got; and very interesting it was. He suggested that I should go to the big American Labor Unions. He mentioned in particular Mr Meany, who was head of the C.I.O./A.F.of L. Union. These unions were tremendously powerful and tremendously rich, by several orders of magnitude richer than the British Trade Unions. They did not know what to do with their money, and they might well think it would be a good idea to be patrons of a College in Oxford. I liked the idea. Mr Stern told me that he had a friend who was a professor of labor relations at the City College of New York, and he would ask him to look into this idea. He would write to me.

When I got back to Oxford I wrote to thank him for his kindness; and to put an idea in his head, which was to consider leaving some of his paintings to St Cross College, since I thought that works of art were of the greatest importance to the College. We would give him a legal undertaking not to sell any pictures he might leave to us. I never heard from him, and feared that I had put him off with my suggestion about the pictures; but when I met John Enders a few months later, he told me that Stern had indeed started inquiries into the Labor Unions; and had intended to leave some of his pictures to the College, but the dear man had died a few weeks after I saw him.

Then I met John Brooke-Little, Richmond Herald of Arms of the College of Arms in London (and now Norroy and Ulster King of Arms). Dear John, he tried long and hard to help me raise money for St Cross, and in the end his efforts led to our getting some money, but not much. I am deeply grateful to him. He introduced me to a very rich man called Lewis Kirby, whose wife was a Kirby cousin, and a granddaughter, or great-grand-daugher, of Fred Kirby, who had founded the family fortune. Fred Kirby and another young man had been assistants in a small hardware store somewhere near Wilkes Barre in Pennsylvania. One day the State Fair came to Wilkes Barre, and the owner of the store instructed the young men to take all the pots and pans that had been on the shop shelves for too long a time and sell them for whatever they could get. On the way to the fair, the young men had an idea: they put a price of five or ten cents on all the items, and sold every one of them in no time. Their boss was pleased with them. Then the young men decided to set up on their own with a shop in which nothing cost more than five (a nickel or a five) or ten cents (a dime). It prospered, so they decided each to set up a five and dime store of their own, which soon led to chains of such stores throughout the country. They agreed that Fred should take the territory south of the Mason-Dixon line, and the other the north. They both prospered and soon each had scores of stores. They decided to pool their resources, and the question now was, what to call this prospering nation-wide chain of five and dime stores? They tossed a coin, and the other man won. His name was F. W. Woolworth.

Lewis Kirby kindly invited me to visit him in his house, that is to say his immense mansion that stands in the country a few miles from the little town of Morristown, New Jersey, about twenty-five miles west of New York. The house was filled with paintings of his English ancestors (who came from the neighbourhood of Kirkby Lonsdale) and with a profusion of armorial bearings; and outside there were heraldic pennants on tall posts. There I met his wife and his two children, and after dinner I talked to them about St Cross College and its significance in the University of Oxford. I showed them a number of colour slides of Oxford, of our site, and of the projected building that had been designed by the architects Stout & Lichfield. It was a modern building, not outrageously so, but Lewis Kirby did not like it. He would have preferred something Gothic. Thereafter I saw quite a lot of him, either lunching with him in one of his many distinguished clubs in New York, such as the Knickerbocker, or in his mansion near Morristown. He was indeed very kind to me, and very formal in his manner. He worked hard in his office on Pine Street in the Wall Street area, where his life was made difficult by the fact that he seemed to do most of his business by telephone with Europe, which was five hours ahead of him, and California, which was three hours behind him. On one occasion, invited to spend the week-end at Morristown, I met him on a late Friday afternoon in his office on Pine Street, from which we took the subway to a railroad station on the west side of Manhattan (or was it on the other side of the Hudson River in Hoboken?), whence we travelled by the Lackawanna Railroad to Morristown. We travelled in a club car, that is, a carriage privately owned by a consortium of well-off businessmen. In the old days there was a barman and you could get drinks on board, but now it was no longer so, and the club car was a little run down. But it was still private. On it there was a woman, a broadcasting executive I was told, and she was pointedly being ignored and snubbed by all the men in the car. She had fought for her new-found legal right as a woman to seek membership of the club car, and this had reluctantly been granted. But they ignored her, and I felt terrible, hoping she would not think that I belonged to them. On the Monday morning I took the train back to Manhattan, leaving Lewis Kirby in Morristown, where he had things to do. He gave me a ticket to the club car, and the outcast lady was on board. After looking around carefully to see that none of Lewis' friends were on board to report me (I needed his money), I went to her, and apologised for the behaviour of my sex. She invited me to join her, and we had a hilarious time all the way to Manhattan.

During that week-end visit to the Kirby mansion, Lewis prevailed on me to apply to the College of Arms for an Achievement of Arms, which, in case you know as little about these matters as I did at the time, consists of an escutcheon, or shield, with a helm above it, and a crest on the top of the helm. Under the shield is the motto. I thought it expedient for the sake of St Cross to make the application (at my own expense) through

John Brooke Little, and you will find it described in the appendix. Lewis Kirby has his own stained-glass man, and he commisioned him to make a leaded stained glass picture of my Achievement, which he very kindly sent me. It hangs in the window of my study, and although I don't attach undue importance to it, I like it.

Lewis Kirby, hardly surprisingly, feared the communists. One evening at Morristown he pointed towards the horizon on the east. 'They're coming that way', he said. 'What do you mean?', I asked. 'The communists', he said, 'from New York.' Sure enough, a few years later he sold the Morristown mansion and moved to a mansion somewhere in Virginia which I understand is well-guarded. In the end I did not get much from him. I could see he was not going to make a sizeable contribution to a new building for the college, so I persuaded him at least to give us enough money to put the Victorian schoolroom in order, since we had decided that whatever building we should ever put up on our site, we would keep that schoolroom, because we had grown to like it; and anyway, it had a preservation order on it. To show my thanks to Lewis, I commissioned a stone carver to carve the escutcheon of his coat of arms on the wall, where you may see it today. (That schoolroom has something on it that I value more. I had got to know that great artist, John Piper, who in his all-embracing way had at that time taken up pottery. Some of the tiles on one of the tiled gables of the schoolroom were broken, and John Piper made several for us. That led to a friendship between John and Mifanwy Piper and Ruthie and me. They are marvellously friendly people, and one of the great pleasures in my life is to sit at their great kitchen table, enjoying Mifanwy's griddle-warm scones, and looking at an enormous poster proclaiming in large red letters on white: 'Death in Venice, from the novel by Thomas Mann, composed by Benjamin Britten, conducted by Stewart Bedford, libretto by Mifanwy Piper, scenery by John Piper'.)

Faithful John Brooke-Little indefatigably carried on with his efforts to help us. He introduced me to a strange character called Fred Lange, of Dallas, Texas, who was Chairman of the Dallas Community Trust, and a sort of entrepreneurial fund-raiser. He was called Doctor Lange, but the origin of his doctorate seemed obscure to me. I have to admit that Fred Lange tried quite hard in his way to raise funds for the college, but he would have to admit, were he still alive, that we did a great deal for his ego. We made him a Visiting Fellow, we arranged for him to give a lecture to the members of St Cross in All Souls College which was much publicized in Dallas, and by God I put up with a lot of crankiness from him. He got far more from us than we got from him. He invited me to come to Dallas to attend a dinner to mark the conferment on him by the Pope of some sort of medal for his charitable works. I flew to New York, where a young woman took me straight to the Braniff terminal, by-passing customs and immigration (Fred Lange had a friend on Braniff), and put me in First Class on the Dallas flight. Fred and Blanche Lange and their chauffeur were waiting for me at Dallas-Fort Worth airport at about 9 pm. and we drove to my hotel in downtown Dallas. On the way, at a word from Fred, the car stopped, and there before me, about twelve feet up, was a rotating electric sign saying WELCOME MASTER KITS OF OXFORD. It was on the top of his dry-cleaner's. The next day I met the Mayor of Dallas and was given a diploma making me an honorary citizen of the City of Dallas. Then I had to go to a businessmen's lunch and make a speech, and that was tough, because I knew I had little hope of getting the idea of an Oxford College across. The next evening there was the dinner in aid of Fred's getting his medal from the Pope. It was in a hotel on the periphery of the city and there again was that sign, even bigger, Welcoming Master Kits of Oxford. I've already described the teetotal American official dinner, and this was more so. Fred never touched a drop anyhow, but Blanche liked hers, and I mine, so she and I had several before going in to the Dinner. At the Dinner I sat at the top table behind the bank of flowers, with the Bishop of Texas on my right. He was a pleasant, good-humoured, easy man. I had been advised before I left Oxford that he would be there, and that I was supposed to make a speech, so I had looked up in my etiquette book how you addressed a Bishop. When my turn came I started 'My Lord Bishop, Mr Mayor, etc'. When I sat down, the Bishop clasped my hand and said 'Gee! I've never been called that before!'

Fred certainly had an entrée everywhere, so I met the Governor of Texas and was given a diploma declaring me to be an Honorary Citizen of the State of Texas. Please don't think I think anything of these Honorary Citizenships of Dallas and Texas, since they mean nothing and are given to everybody. Needless to say I was also given the ritual title to one square inch of Texas land. All this hullabaloo was exactly as it had been described many years previously by Sinclair Lewis in *Babbit*, which I don't suppose you've read if you're under seventy years of age. From Dallas, Fred, Blanche and I were driven by the chauffeur to Galveston on the Gulf of Texas, which I was very pleased to do, since Galveston is a handsome old town, with most of its beautiful 'Victorian' buildings lovingly restored. Fred had booked us rooms in a beautiful hotel right on a jetty built over the sea. The 'Welcome Master Kits of Oxford' sign was rotating above it, and when I got to my suite of rooms there were two handsomely encased bottles of whiskey, one of Scotch and one of Bourbon, which I love. But they were quite unnecessary, because after 6.00 p.m. all the drinks out on the deck were free anyhow.

Nothing came from this visit to Texas. Fred Lange carried on, but the time came when I couldn't take it any more. Two of the Fellows in succession took up the burden, and in the end a small sum, a few thousand pounds, was obtained, and for that Fred's name has been perpetuated in the College by my successors. The present Common Room, to my dismay, is called the Lange Room.

Not long after the College came into being, I came to know Douglas Fairbanks Junior, and later his nice wife Mary Lee, through a friend of Kenneth Knowles, at that time our Bursar. I was anxious to meet him in the first place because he was a friend of Paul Getty, and I was keen to get just a tiny fraction of the Getty millions. I had made a study of Getty, that is to say I had read his rather sad autobiography — sad because every chapter ends with a parting from his current wife, and every chapter begins with the acquisition of his new one. But I had found his description of the early days in the American oil industry very interesting. I particularly liked the 'Getty Special', which he invented for pushing aside broken-off drill bits that were blocking expensive deep bore holes and preventing further drilling. One evening, faced very deep down by such a broken-off bit, he drove past a monumental mason's establishment and had an inspiration. He aked the mason to make him a sort of gigantic granite pencil about eight feet long and eight inches diameter (I'm guessing at the dimensions), with a point at the end. It had to be ready early the next morning. The mystified mason made it, and Getty dropped it down the obstructed drill shaft. The gigantic pencil, in rushing all its weight down, pushed the drill bit sideways into the sandstone in which it was embedded. The place of the steel bit was now taken by the granite pencil. It was easy enough for Getty then to drill through the granite and save his shaft. That at least is one good point about Getty. Well, Douglas Fairbanks wrote to Getty to ask for money for St Cross, and Getty replied on the following lines: 'I despise Liberal Arts Colleges [whatever he meant by that], I despise Liberal Arts students [this was admittedly at the time when students were being at their most bloody-minded], and I despise Liberal Arts professors, but out of respect for you I have asked the American Trust Fund to forward $100 to St Cross College.' Since he got a large tax deduction through the Trust Fund, that donation probably did not cost him more than about twenty dollars. Douglas tried Getty again a few years later, but again without success. He tried many others, like Heinz of the baked beans (on my fifty-seventh birthday they had sent me a case full of their products, I suppose because I was in *Who's Who*, but there weren't fifty-seven cans, more like a score), but he never succeeded. I am very grateful to him, and I like him, and he likes the college and he seems to like me, because he always gets in touch with me when he is in London. He likes coming to Encaenia wearing his M.A. gown and hood, to which he is entitled by virtue of his fellowship of St Cross. I never ran into him when I was in America, but he gave me the use of his apartment on the top of the Blackstone Hotel on East 59th Street in New York, and I used it several times. Once in his house in The Boltons in London he was showing me some of his photograph albums, and there was a picture of Joan Crawford, his first wife. I was awed, because I used to think she was the most beautiful creature on earth. 'Jeepers creepers, Douglas,' I exclaimed, 'Joan Crawford!', but he made a moue. Later I learned that in the early days in Hollywood the only way to get into films had been to be invited to Pickfair, Douglas' parental home, and Joan Crawford, ruthlessly determined to make her career, had seized the poor innocent young fellow by the neck and married him.

I continued looking for money. On one occasion Kenneth Knowles, our Bursar, and I jointly and innocently committed an unfortunate gaffe. Kenneth had pulled various strings which resulted in our being invited to meet the Lord Mayor of London, and to have lunch with a number of very important bigwigs in the City. We travelled separately to London, having arranged to meet in the foyer of the Mansion House. I was wearing a tie that could perhaps be said to be a trifle *outrée*, it having been made for me from some flowered material by one of our scholars at St Cross. When I met Kenneth, he was wearing the same tie. We felt a ripe couple of idiots, but there was nothing we could do about it, we had to march into the Lord Mayor's parlour, and later to the lunch with the bigwigs. One *outrée* tie might have passed, but two *outrées* ties were too many. I'm sure the City gentlemen thought we were a couple of Oscar Wildes, and so it was that I may have let the College down.

One of the Fellows certainly thought I had let the College down, not over this incident which nobody knew about, but because I hadn't raised enough money for the College. The College had asked all Fellows to submit suggestions for raising money, and this Fellow, whose name out of the kindness of my heart I will not mention, suggested sacking me. He had forgotten, and perhaps many other Fellows had also forgotten, that I had played a leading part (if I may say so) on the Harrison and Norrington Committees, and on the Hebdomadal Council, not only in the idea of bringing the College into being, but also in getting the money for the enablement and continuation of that coming into being.

That money came from the richer colleges directly and through the College Contributions Fund, so I could justly claim my share in the responsibility for quite a large sum of money. By present-day figures that would amount to something near £2,000,000; not enough, but not to be sneezed at so lightly. And moreover, in trying to 'sell' the College, what had I to offer? There was a tendency among some Fellows of the College to talk about the College being a 'centre of excellence'. I detested this meaningless, smug expression, and wondered what excellence those who used it most had to offer?

When Kenneth Knowles and I presented the College with the very long list of foundations, trusts, charities, industrial and business corporations, and individuals that had been approached, my Fellows had the grace to be mollified. I did raise some other money apart from what I have already mentioned. Lewis Kirby opened an account for us in a Swiss bank and put about £5000 in it, in addition to helping to put the schoolroom right; my friend John Enders of Harvard gave us $50,000; and there were some other contributions, small sums compared with what we needed. I am glad to think that most of the money I raised, I raised where charity should begin: at home — from the richer colleges in Oxford; and from that other great Oxford institution, Blackwells, the booksellers.

Within a month or two of our settling down in our hut at St Cross, I invited Sir Basil Blackwell (the Gaffer, as he was always lovingly called) and his eldest son Richard to lunch. I spoke about our need for money, and I told the Gaffer that if they gave us enough we'd change the name of the College to St Cross & Blackwell. I think they were amused. The next week I got a courteous letter from the Gaffer, thanking me for the College's hospitality (courtesy flows naturally and abundantly in the veins of all the Blackwells), and telling me that owing to some new tax [one that was later to be replaced by VAT], Blackwells were not at the present time able to help me, but in the meantime he enclosed a cheque for £100 as a token. I took that small token very seriously. It was surely not a token of esteem, so I read it as a signal that I should be patient. Over the years I would call on Richard in his office over the shop about once a Term, and sometimes we would touch lightly on the subject of money, and sometimes we would not; but I would always come away with the feeling, almost the knowledge, that I must wait, and one day the money would come. One thing was quite clear to me — I must not push, and that suited me because pushing did not come easily to me. Optimism, patience and never giving up are more in my line.

In the meantime I was also in touch with another very important partner in Blackwells. He was Per Saugman, head of the publishers, Blackwell Scientific Publications. Blackwell Scientific Publications had published my book on *Bacterial Toxins* in 1950, but that was before Per Saugman was in charge. He was, however, in charge of the publication of a far better book, by Antoinette Pirie and Ruth van Heyningen on *Biochemistry of the Eye* in 1956, in fact I think it was one of his first books. Per and I had discussed St Cross's need for money, and he knew about my initial approach to the Gaffer and Richard. He was sympathetic and expressed a desire to be helpful, and I took the same line with him as I had taken with the Blackwells of not pushing. My way of keeping in touch with him over the matter was usually to engage in light banter about it, threatening to go to Maxwell if Blackwells would not help me, knowing that he shared my opinion of Maxwell.

In the end the money came from Blackwells, specifically from Blackwells Scientific Publications, just when we needed it imperatively. I will come to that later.

Keeping the College Going

During the first few months of the College, Ruthie's mother, Mildred Treverton, handed quite a large sum of money over to us, and asked us to handle it as trustees of a charitable benefaction. Since the College depended on charity, we asked her if the College could be the beneficiary, and she kindly consented. Ruthie and I agreed that the money should be spent on works of art for the college, to be chosen by us. We believed that the college should provide a civilized environment, and that this would be best attained with works of art. Works of art were a most important necessity, yet the last things that the College could afford. Therefore benevolent despotism was called for. When I presented the terms of the benefaction to the Governing Body of the College, they met with no enthusiasm, and hardly any thanks. It had on previous occasions decided they would not take any tainted money, and now one of the Fellows demanded to know whether the money of this benefaction had been honestly come by. I expect they were disappointed that the money was not going to be spent on something useful. Ruthie and I were disappointed in our turn, but not surprised.

We did not know what objects of art to acquire, or how to acquire them, but we did have two friends who could advise us. They were the art historians Lavinia Handley-Reed, who had been at school with Ruthie, and her husband Charles. They were both well-heeled, and they lived in a large house in Ladbroke Road, London. Charles advised us not to buy pictures, because they were too expensive. We would be better off, he said, with Victorian and Edwardian decorative arts which were at the time going at reasonable prices but were bound to rise in the future. Their house was filled from cellar to attic with such works of art. He also thought they would be refreshingly unusual in a college, and that they would make a better display than pictures. He not only knew a great deal about these objects, but he had an intimate knowledge of the market, of the dealers, and of the prices. Thereafter ensued a pleasant and educative time for Ruthie and me. Charles would telephone us from London, and tell us that he had collected a dozen Lalique glass pieces, for example, and we were to come to London and choose three or four of them. We'd go to London, Charles would open a bottle of champagne, and talk to us about the pieces. He would never choose the three or four pieces, we had to do that, but we were in clover because we knew that we couldn't go wrong. And Charles, knowing the dealers, and the dealers having a high regard for Charles, we always got those objects for a great deal less than we would have if we had been on our own. The next time it might be pots, and then silver. Thus it was that we bought a most beautiful tiazza by C.R.Ashbee of the Arts and Crafts Movement that had Shirley Bury at the Victoria and Albert tearing her hair out with jealousy. We also got a magnificent knight on a noble charger by Gilbert Bayes, with crazy little bald-headed pixies prancing about. To me it was a beautiful dream turned solid silver, but I expected my Fellows to be puzzled by it. We also bought several beautiful modern glass pieces by Sam Herman, but we were not new to them, because we had already bought two pieces for ourselves from Mrs Crossley-Holland in the Oxford Gallery. (Sam Herman was so pleased with us that he gave us one of his pieces.)

Now I come to a tricky subject. Charles Handley-Reed insisted that I have my portrait painted for the College by a reputable artist. I felt very shy about this for obvious reasons. Charles said it was not for me to consider my feelings, I had to face the fact that the colleges of Oxford and Cambridge all had portraits of all their heads, and it was particularly important to have a portrait of the founding head, so I fearfully gave in. There was only one artist to consider, said Charles, and that was Sir William Coldstream at the Slade School of Fine Art. So I went to see him at the Slade. He seemed to have a severe expression on his face, and he wore a sombre grey suit, looking more like a solicitor than an artist. He agreed to paint me, and we agreed the price of £1000. Thereafter I went to London nearly every Friday for the next year and a half, wondering whether the Fellows were wondering whether I was going to see my psychiatrist or my mistress or both.

At the first sitting Coldstream produced a canvas for a portrait that was nearly life-size. I was dismayed, and asked if we could not have something more modest, a head and shoulders half the size, but he would have none of it; it had to be from head to heels (in fact the feet were not included: they are often left out in full-length portraits). I decided to wear my black working gown rather that the full doctoral scarlet regalia which are customary. At the second or third sitting, mindful of my daughter's injunction not to let my face assume the morose expression that it normally assumes in repose, I decided I must converse with the artist. 'Sir William,' I said, 'may I tell you a joke?' 'Please do' he said, so I told him a joke: 'An exhausted man came to a psychiatrist, saying "Doctor, you've got to help me, I can't go on like this." "What's your problem?" said the doctor. "Every night I go to bed, I dream, I dream the same dream. I dream I have to drive a truck from New York to Los Angeles. That's a long way, doc, and I'm worn out, I just can't do it anymore, you've got to help me'' said the patient. ''Can you drive via Chicago next time?'' asked the doctor, scribbling on a card. ''I guess so, it doesn't make much difference,'' said the patient. The doctor gave him the card, and said ''When you get to Chicago, call this number, and I'll take over.'' A week later the man came to the doctor. ''Gee thanks doc,'' he said, ''that sure did work — anybody can drive a truck from New York to Chicago!'' A week later another exhausted man came to a psychiatrist, saying ''Doctor, you've got to help me, I can't go on like this.'' ''What's your problem?'' asked the doctor. ''Every night I go to bed, I dream, I dream the same dream. I dream a beautiful lady comes to my bed; and then another; and then another; and then another; and then another. I just can't do it any more doctor, you've got to help me!'' ''Could you, er, accommodate three ladies?'' asked the doctor, scribbling on a card. ''Sure,'' said the man, ''three ladies I can manage.'' The doctor handed him the card and said ''After the third lady, call this number and I'll come and take over.'' A week later the man came back to the doctor, more exhausted than ever. ''Gee doc, I can't go on like this. It's killing me.'' ''Didn't you call the number I gave you?'' asked the doctor. ''Sure I called the number, but a voice answered, saying 'The doctor is not available, he's driving a truck from Chicago to Los Angeles''.'

Coldstream nearly fell on his backside laughing, and after that we became, and still are, very good friends. And I also came to know the other people at the Slade, and found them all delightfully friendly and amusing.

Coldsteam is a very slow and careful painter, concerned to paint exactly what he sees, such as the exact distance from the corner of the eye to the lobe of the ear. He would look at me with a ruler balanced on his finger, then with a plumbline, and make a minute mark on the canvas. Sometimes he made an invisible mark with the point of the wooden end of his brush. I was encouraged by his matter-of-fact way and his friendliness to ask if I might bring my camera to his studio, and photograph the work after every sitting. He agreed eagerly. My photographs were not very good, but when I presented them to the Department of Western Art in the Ashmolean Museum, the Keeper, Kenneth Garlick, was delighted, and had them carefully bound in a book. He told me that he was not aware of that ever having been done to any painting. Later, when the Curators of the Bodleian Library wanted to commission a portrait of the

Librarian, Robert Shackleton, I suggested Coldstream; and proposed that the professional Bodleian photographer should take photographs of the canvas from the first sitting. Those photographs too now are bound and preserved in the Bodleian Library and the Ashmolean Museum.

Bill Coldstream finds it hard to finish a painting, so after I had sat for him for fifty-three times, Uan Uglow and his colleagues told him firmly that the portrait was now finished. I said oh no it was not, because Bill had always insisted that I wear the same shirt as I wore for the first sitting. It had alternating blue and red stripes on a white background, and Bill had painted the blue stripes but not the red. Since I had taken a lot of trouble always wearing the same shirt I insisted on my red stripes. Bill put them in. His colleagues told me the portrait was the best that Bill had done, and Ruthie and I certainly liked it, so much so that I gave a dinner party in the Reform Club for Bill and all the staff of the Slade. It was a marvellously hilarious affair, and I doubt if any of us were sober. Two or three years ago that portrait was one of a dozen in an exhibition in the Ashmolean Museum of the best Oxford portraits.

While Bill Coldstream was working on me, I had asked him if he had a painting I could buy for the college with the Mildred Treverton Benefaction. The only one he had was a large unfinished painting of a nude professional model. I bought it and hung it in the old schoolroom that served as our library and meeting room. This upset one of the Fellows, and he demanded my dismissal. I think he got upset about it because there was a wisp of pubic hair. But it was far from being an arousing picture, it was an austere academic exercise in the painting of an austere professional nude model. The mistake I made was that the painting was too big, and it was not likely that there would ever be a suitable place to hang it. So I arranged with Anthony d'Offay, Bill's agent, to swop it for a little still-life by Bill of an orange tree in a pot.

Charles and Lavinia Handley-Reed's lives ended terribly tragically, before we exhausted the funds of the Mildred Treverton Benefaction. Charles spent all his days in his office in the house preparing the catalogue of an exhibition of all their Victorian and Edwardian decorative art, and their paintings, that was to be held in the Royal Academy. Not many days before the exhibition was due to open, he committed suicide, and the reason was that he had not prepared a single entry for that catalogue. I think I can understand why he did that. There are times when one has to do a very important job that has to be done well, and it requires a strong effort of will to get started. Poor Lavinia came to Oxford to stay with us for a few days, and we knew that she had come to take her leave of us. The day after she got back to London, she locked herself in the garage and started the engine of her car.

About the time that we were assembling the Mildred Treverton collection, I had the idea of having a computer in the College. This was in 1966, in the early days of computers, and I knew next to nothing about them, except that they were going to stay, getting more and more efficient, and being used in more and more disciplines. For example, people had just begun to use them in trying to find out what Shakespeare really wrote in his plays. There were no manuscripts, only the printed first folios, in the printing of which the print of different parts was set up by different typesetters, each with their discernable idiosyncracies. For example, they liked 'eye rhymes' – if Shakespeare wrote a couplet that rhymed to the ear, they might change the words at the ends of lines so that they looked the same to the eye. People were using computers to detect these idiosyncracies. I thought the college should have a computer that should be used as much by non-scientists as by scientists. I hoped in this way they would find themselves speaking the same language, so narrowing the gulf between them.

I went to see the man who I thought would be able to give me the best advice. He was Sir Leon Bagrit, the greatest authority on computers in Britain at the time, who had recently given the then very grand annual Reith Lectures on the BBC radio. His subject had been computers, and how they were going to sweep the world. When I saw him in his office on Portland Place he was very friendly, and warmly enthusiastic about my idea of domesticating the computer in the College. But I must not make the mistake, he said, of not doing it properly. I must give the computer at least 20,000 square foot of space (which was half the size of the Sir William Dunn School of Pathology); that space must have a concrete floor at least two feet thick; it must be air-conditioned; I must provide at least thirty kilowatts of electricity (maybe it was sixty). I was amazed. I just knew, from the depths of my utter ignorance, that computers were going to get bigger and bigger on the one hand, but smaller and smaller on the other, down to the size of suitcases (little knowing that after getting bigger and bigger, big computers would get smaller again, and small computers of the capacity people were thinking of in those days would come down to something not much bigger than typewriters).

Then I heard about computer terminals about the size of a very big typewriter that could be connected by telephone lines to big central computers. So I went to see Jack Howlett, Director of the Atlas Computer at Harwell, a few miles from Oxford. Bless him, he was very kind and understanding, and the upshot of that was that we got such a terminal in the College connected to the Atlas, and we sensibly elected Jack Howlett to a fellowship of the College. This idea of the collegiate computer was quite new at the time, and it attracted quite a lot of interest in the local and the national press. Some time after that the University acquired a large computer, and other colleges began to have terminals linked to it. Now many dons, including retired ones like me, have microcomputers, generally used as word-processors. (Since the French are pleased that they did not succumb to calling a computer a *computer*, but call it an *ordinateur*, I wondered what they called a word-processor, so I telephoned the Maison Francaise here in Oxford, and they told me it was a *machine à traitement de texte*, which is a fine expression, but impossible to verbalize.)

The College prospered well enough, and I believe it earned some respect in the University. For a fine example, Nevill Coghill wrote to me:

> You really have worked a miracle. Not only in devising, decorating, financing and putting up such a building, but (far better) in making a centre of happiness and learning for Oxford, when there was a great lack before in this very respect. It is a great work to have done, and you have done it without the slightest commotion, entirely by the reasonableness and sweetness of your nature, in a University where enmities are so easily created towards new projects. But you have won universal support and good will, as I know from many conversations.

But we could not stay forever in that wooden hut that Nevill Coghill mentioned, comfortable as we were in it. In the meantime Hebdomadal Council, on which I was sitting at the time, was worrying about entitled dons who had not yet been found college fellowships. This brought up the question of the former quarters of Linacre College. It was a moderately handsome building on St Aldate's, less than 200 yards south of Christ Church and Pembroke College. It had been built in the early 1930s by the architect Worthington, who had designed several other academic buildings in Oxford, in order to house St

Catherine's Society, which had been established by the University in 1930 to replace the former Delegacy for Non-Collegiate Students that had been founded in 1868. Its Principal, Alan Bullock, had raised a vast amount of money when times were still prosperous, and tax laws less demanding, to found a new St Catherine's College, which was established in 1963 with Bullock as Master, and housed in a magnificent modern building by the Danish architect Arne Jacobsen. The senior members of St Catherine's Society became the first Fellows of the new St Catherine's College. The Worthington building had then been occupied by Linacre House (changed to College when St Cross and Iffley [now Wolfson] Colleges came into being), which had been established by the University in 1962 with the initial object of admitting graduates of other universities coming to Oxford to work for higher degrees. A few years after St Cross had come into being, Linacre, having expanded, left St Aldate's and moved to a larger building on St Cross Road.

Bullock, then Vice-Chancellor, suggested to me that if St Cross were prepared to take in the remaining non-Fellows, or at any rate a large proportion of them, the University would let us have the vacated Worthington building. I liked the idea, for two reasons. The first was that, believing strongly in our origins, I thought we should be ready to act in the spirit of the words of Emma Lazarus' sonnet, 'The New Colossus', inscribed on the pedestal of the Statue of Liberty at the entrance to New York harbour:

> Give me your tired, your poor,
> Your huddled masses yearning to be free,
> The wretched refuse of your teeming shore,
> Send these, the homeless, tempest-tossed, to me,
> I lift my lamp besides the golden door.

The still homeless non-dons may not have been considered the cream of academic sophistication, but what would that matter in ten or twenty years' time?

My second reason for liking Bullock's suggestion was that I liked the appearance of the building, backing onto Christ Church's vast meadow; and the fact that it had been more or less designed to be a graduate college. If it needed to be enlarged, there would be space enough for it.

When I put the idea to my Governing Body, they were very cool about it. I was not entirely surprised by that, but what amazed me was the predominant objection raised. This was that the building was too far away from the centre of things. After all, Christ Church, which was less than 200 yards nearer to Carfax, had got on pretty well for the last four centuries; and Pembroke, across the street from Christ Church, had managed for the last three centuries! There were many colleges much further away, including the new St Catherine's; and where did they think we were going to find a site any nearer to the centre, for Heaven's sake? I thought they were really being rather unreasonable and unrealistic.

But after much further discussion, and to-ing and fro-ing with Council, the College began to get used to the idea, and in the end the Governing Body agreed to the move to St Aldate's. Alan Jones, my able and loyal Vice-Master, the pillar of the College, who had fought by my side on the Norrington committee that brought it into being, was strongly against the idea from the beginning, on the grounds that the College should always be free to choose its Fellows, and not have to take just anybody pushed in our direction by Council. Of course that was a reasonable attitude, and perfectly understandable, but our history imposed a duty on us, at least I thought so; and besides, being beggars we couldn't be choosers.

A few hours after that crucial meeting of the Governing Body, Bullock telephoned me. Alan Jones had been to see him to object against our decision. This was unheard of treason! The College was furious. 'Burn him', they cried. I was the most furious of all at this treachery from my old comrade in arms, and of course I told him so. Alan Jones always thinks things out very very carefully, and he now claimed that since the College was not yet independent, and therefore did not have a Visitor to whom any member of the College could go in the case of a dispute, as was possible in the established colleges, he had gone to the Vice-Chancellor. This did not lessen my rage at the time, but at the bottom of my heart I knew that Alan Jones was not the rotter he seemed to be. On the contrary, being faithful to his perception of his principles in relation to the College, he did what he saw as his duty, mindless of the odium that he knew would be heaped on him. He had as much right to say that it was I who had betrayed the College by proposing that it should be a rubbish bin for dons that no other colleges wanted as I had to take my stand at the foot of the Statue of Liberty.

In the event he succeeded, because after all that fuss the College abandoned the idea of taking over the former Linacre building. His period of office as Vice-Master came to an end quite soon, and I advised him not to stand again, so Tom Tinsley, another good man, succeeded him. After some years Alan Jones was invited to accept a paid Fellowship of Pembroke College, which obviously he accepted; but I know that his loyalty to St Cross is undiminished. There is another good former St Cross Fellow now in Pembroke, for the same reason as Alan Jones, and when Alan Jones talks to him about 'the college', he means St Cross College.

It was just as well that we did not go to St Aldates, otherwise we would not have ended up on St Giles, where we are now, which nobody could complain is too far from the centre of things. And we are in one of the most beautiful buildings in Oxford. It is Pusey House, designed by the architect Temple Moore in 1911, started in 1914, and finished by his son in 1926. Most people think it is centuries old. Temple Moore was one of those architects who thought that Gothic was the perfection of architecture, and that there was therefore no point in trying to improve on it. The *Dictionary of National Biography* says of him that 'his buildings, although purely Gothic, appear to have been designed with no restraint save that of his vigilant good taste', and that applies particularly well to Pusey House.

About two years before I retired, one of the Fellows of the College had come to me to propose a thrilling possibility. He was Michael Brookes, the University Land Agent, and therefore in a good position to know about buildings in Oxford. He told me that Pusey House was financially badly pinched, and suggested that we propose a kind of marriage with them. Pusey House is a distinguished Oxford Institution, listed in the University Pocket Diary under 'OTHER INSTITUTIONS (not being part of the University but having associations with it).' Its origins lie in the Oxford Movement started in the 1830s by Edward Bouverie Pusey, Professor of Hebrew and Canon of Christ Church, John Keble, Fellow of Oriel and Professor of Poetry, and John Henry Newman, Fellow of Oriel and Vicar of the University Church of St Mary. They had become alarmed at the spread of rationalism in the Church of England, since they feared that it would detract from the holiness of religion. To counter this trend they wrote a number of tracts maintaining that 'the true doctrines of the Church of England were contained in the writings of the fathers and of Anglican divines of the 17th century.' That is how they became to be known as the 'Tractarians'. Pusey House started with the inheritance of his library and the foundation, 'Dr Pusey's Library' on St Giles Sreet in 1884, which was intended to carry on his work. It was rebuilt on the same site in present splendid form, which contains one of the largest and most beautiful of the many chapels in Oxford.

Michael Brookes suggested that we offer to buy essentially those parts of Pusey House that were not used by the three Anglican priests in it, and that we should offer Pusey Fellowships of the College to the three priests. They were known as the Librarians Residentiary, viz. the Principal Librarian and two Librarians. So I went to see Cheslyn Jones, the Principal Librarian of Pusey House. It was slightly sticky, but not nearly as sticky as I thought it would be. The upshot of that was that a lengthy series of negotiations was put in train. When I was within about a year of retiring I thought it proper for me to withdraw from those negotiations, and handed my responsibilities over to one of the Fellows. In the end, before I retired, agreement was reached that the College would buy, for £350,000, a 999-year lease of those parts of the building that were not essential to Pusey House, as well as the large piece of land at the back. I was very happy that there was now a prospect of my beloved college being housed in a beautiful building in a beautiful and advantageous situation; and although I am not a religious man, I was happy for the College instantly to acquire a distinguished religious history, and such a beautiful chapel, without which no college is a proper college, but which no college newly-built today would consider having.

In the meantime the £350,000 question was: where were we going to find the money? Clearly the time had come to shift from friendly stiff-lippedness with Richard Blackwell, and friendly banter with Per Saugman, to a direct request for a specific sum for a specific purpose. I had just nerved myself to go to Richard when I received a telephone call from Per Saugman at a strange hour of the night. This is how Per puts it in his tribute to Richard in a privately published booklet, *In Memory of Richard Blackwell DSC, MA, Hon D Litt 1918-1980*:

> Perhaps the venture that somehow gave us the greatest pleasure was our involvement with St Cross College. It was to be our last. The story is well known, but the College was looking for a considerable sum of money to improve its location, and had been doing so for twelve to fourteen years. They invited me to lunch one day, and it became quite an expensive meal, but it seemed right that Blackwell's should celebrate its centenary through its contribution to the University. Richard and I dined together that evening to discuss the suggestion and I could see him become captivated by the idea; he suddenly said "Tell the Master

he has got his college." I rang Kits van Heyningen at midnight and apologized for the late call — and gave him the news. He said he practically fell out of the bed, for his agony as a fund-raiser was over. The next morning he called on RB, and Richard said "Don't forget to remember PS." Here again his generosity came to play; this was very typical, and they have not. But the College had named its main quadrangle the Richard Blackwell Quadrangle, and we have been given a link that we could not have bettered.

Those who had invited Per to the lunch he mentions were his fellow Dane, Bent Juel-Jensen, and the Vice-Master, Tom Tinsley. After all the years that I had patiently stalked Per Saugman, it was they who brought him to his knees.

What Per Saugman means by that phrase 'and they have not' in his penultimate sentence, but is too modest to mention, is the fact that the Dining Hall of the College is named the Saugman Hall. Both Richard Blackwell and Per Saugman were particularly kind to me over this benefaction. At the College's Founders' Feast soon afterwards, Richard made a speech in which he made a point of stating that the benefaction was a benefaction to me; and he and Per have also said the same thing to Ruthie.

The benefaction was publicly announced, and made over to us, at a glorious luncheon given by Blackwell's in Merton College (of which Sir Basil was an Honorary Fellow) to celebrate their centenary on a very cold Wednesday, 3 January 1979. It was a dream come true for me; St Cross had succeeded. Sir Harold Macmillan was there at the High Table, not as Chancellor of the University, but as a fellow-publisher. Richard Blackwell presided, and I sat between Sir Basil Blackwell and the Lord Mayor of Oxford. Speeches were made, and then the time came when Per Saugman presented me with a bunch of papers that signified the gift of £350,000 for St Cross that was going to enable us to move from our wooden hut to Pusey House opposite St John's College on St Giles. It was the noblest building on that noble avenue in the heart of Oxford. I had to make a speech, in front of the finest speech-maker in Britain, Sir Harold Macmillan, but I was so exalted, I could do anything. I stood up feeling almost frigidly confident, and told them how I used to dream about Oxford in South West Africa after Christina had been there, and how she had spoken about the colleges, and about Blackwell's, with equal admiration, so that in my childish mind I thought Blackwell's was a college too. I told them my little joke about St Cross and Blackwell. I reminded the Chancellor how John Sparrow, Warden of All Souls, had once introduced me to him saying I was the Head of 'the nicest College in Oxford', and I had added 'and of the poorest', and now I felt I was Head of the richest. I sat down feeling as fine as any man could ever hope to feel.

But dreadfully sadly, Richard Blackwell did not survive long after that luncheon. Just over a year later, on 26 February 1980, he died after a long illness that he had borne calmly in the knowledge that it was fatal. His place in Blackwell's is now taken by his son Miles, a Fellow of St Cross, as his father was. Miles, like all the Blackwells, is a man of infinite courtesy, such as is seldom seen these days. All the Blackwells, and Per and Pat Saugman, who, as Richard told the *Oxford Mail*, are part of the family, have always been very warm-hearted and kind to me, and I am devoted to them all for that kindness as much as I am for their corporate generosity. When I think about my College, the source of my greatest pride and contentment is the fact that practically all the charity we have received, after all my efforts all over Great Britain and the United States of America, began at home here in Oxford: from the other Colleges, and particularly from All Souls, Christ Church, Merton and St John's; and continued at home here in Oxford, from Blackwell's.

At Encaenia that year, the Public Orator of the University in giving his Creweian Oration 'in Commemoration of the Benefactors of the University according to the intention of the Right Honourable Nathaniel, Lord Crewe, Bishop of Durham', made the customary references to benefactions received, and to those who were retiring. I was sitting in the circle with the other Heads of Houses, with Henry Chadwick, Dean of Christ Church by my side. As to benefactions the Public Orator said

> But the gift which has particularly fired our imagination during the bleak winter was that of £350,000 under covenant from Blackwell's, which has in effect secured at one beautifully timed stroke the future of St Cross College, an institution as lively as it is, academically speaking, youthful. Eventually it should also benefit Pusey House, which has long served the spiritual needs of many of our number and the memory of the great Churchman whose name it bears. One of our younger booksellers has said that Oxford has been in so many ways kind to his profession; and added 'there can be no place anywhere more agreable in which to sell books'. I know that within the walls of Blackwell's this well-conceived gift is not only intended to commemorate the centenary of that great firm, itself one of the glories of this city, but is regarded as a symbolic repayment of the very real debt which it felt to be owed to Oxford. We can be sure that it has been accepted with deep gratitude and appreciation to match the spirit in which it has been offered.

As to me, the Orator said 'Dr van Heyningen retires from the Mastership of St Cross College: he must be very happy that the benefaction for which he must have been hoping and dreaming for so long has now been translated into reality', and as he said it, the Dean of Christ Church, bless you Henry Chadwick, held my hand and squeezed it.

The College gave a glorious farewell dinner for me in Magdalen College Hall, giving me the feeling (which on rare occasions had evaded me at meetings of the Governing Body) that I was appreciated. They also gave me some beautiful teak garden furniture inscribed in abbreviated Latin in the way of the Latins: GVLIELMO EDV. KITS VAN H. PROTOMAG. SOCII COLL. SANCT. CRUC. H.C. MCMLXV-MCMLXXVIIII.

After I retired on 30 September 1979 the periodical *Oxford* (December 1979) had this to say:

> Dr W. E. van Heyningen came to Oxford in 1947 to join Lord Florey's group at the Sir William Dunn School of Pathology in order to continue that work on bacterial toxins which has been the focus of his scientific career. With previous research experience at Cambridge, Harvard, and the War Wounds Committee of the Medical Research Council, his major scientific studies at Oxford have related to the study of tetanus and cholera toxins.
>
> In 1965, the appointment of Kits van Heyningen as the first Master of St Cross College represented for him a challenge equal to any he had faced in his scientific research; and it is the measure of the man that his personal commitment to the successful development of the College has been as unwavering as his commitment to medical science. Though the establishment of the College represented, after a long and hard struggle, a victory for Kits and his fellow members of the non-Fellows movement, the subsequent task of translating this new Society into a full Oxford college has had to face and overcome numerous difficulties. It is therefore the cause of great satisfaction to his friends, within and outside the College, that at the moment of his retirement the hopes and plans of St Cross finally are becoming realities.
>
> Though grateful to its sister colleges for their generous financial support upon which it depends, the overriding aim of St Cross is the achievement of its financial independence by its own efforts. Kits has never ceased to pursue that aim with energy and determination. On more than one occasion he came so close to success that the subsequent disappointment when the desired major benefaction eluded him would have caused many to lose heart. He never did lose heart and finally, at a time when the College was in most urgent need of financial support, he had the well-deserved pleasure of welcoming the generous help from its friends at Blackwell's.
>
> Within St Cross, the first Master's most valued contribution during

those early difficult years has been the leadership and encouragement of a large, heterogeneous, and active group of impatient and independent-minded Fellows. Most of us have, on occasion, disagreed with him; and he with us. With Kits as Master, however, the sense of frustration within the Fellowship which inevitably followed disappointed hopes, never led to disillusion but to a strengthened and very real sense of corporate identity and purpose. Within that wooden hut and under the most difficult circumstances, the meaning of the word Fellowship has been demonstrated and its values created. That achievement has been assisted powerfully by the personal qualities of Kits van Heyningen: a generous nature and a lack of rancour; a sense of humour and a sense of style; and, above all, his devotion to the ideals of the society of which he was Head.

No final impression of the first Master of St Cross would be complete without reference to Ruth, his charming wife, Fellow of St Cross and distinguished scientist. To both Kits and Ruth we wish a long, busy, and happy retirement.

10
CHOLERA

In 1967 I was invited to be a Visiting Professor in Residence at the State University of New York's Downstate Medical Center in Brooklyn. The visit was not for long, about six weeks in October and November, and this suited me very well; and it suited Ruthie too, since she had a lot of reading and writing to do, and the Medical Center had an excellent and comfortable library. I had been invited by the acting chairman of the Department of Microbiology and Immunology, Dr Jack Craig, at the instigation of the Chairman, Professor Thomas P.Magill. Tom Magill, I was soon to learn, had an ear for language, considering himself a microbeologist, or one who knew about microbes; rather than a microbiologist, or a very small biologist.

The start of our visit was not as auspicious as intended by Tom Magill and Jack Craig, who met us at the New York airport and drove us to the Downstate Hall of Residence, where we had been given a thoughtfully sumptuous apartment with flowers in the vases and food in the refrigerator. We were to meet later for dinner at Gage & Tollner's, a smart and old-fashioned restaurant established in Brooklyn in 1879, but Tom and his wife, Elizabeth (Betty), arrived late. She had been mugged as she entered their Brooklyn apartment and pushed into a dark closet, expecting to be murdered any moment, this tending to be the way of life and death in Brooklyn. After some time Tom was mugged in his turn and joined her in the closet, where it took some time for it to dawn on them that they had been forgotten by their doped mugger. Strangely enough, I did not recognize Betty immediately, although I had met her a few years previously in the house of our neighbour in Oxford, and had been impressed by her, because she was a beautiful and interesting woman, and I had monopolized her. She told me in Gage & Tollner's with her tongue in her cheek that it was she who had been responsible for my being invited to Tom's department, because I had monopolized her at our neighbour's and she had modestly taken this for kindness.

In the Department of Microbiology and Immunology, Jack Craig told me about cholera toxin. I knew nothing about cholera, but thought I knew vaguely about cholera toxin, because Pierre Grabar had told me about his work on it at the Pasteur Institute in Paris. What Grabar had told me about cholera toxin, or what he mistakenly thought was cholera toxin, had been totally unconvincing and uninteresting; what Jack Craig told me about cholera and cholera toxin was thrilling. He had recently spent some time at the Pakistan-SEATO [South East Asian Treaty Organization] Cholera Research Laboratory in Dacca in East Pakistan, where he had played a large part in demonstrating the existence of cholera toxin, and the important part it played in the disease.

Cholera had been confined to India until the beginning of the last century, but in 1817 it erupted eastwards and westwards on the first of seven great pandemics (of which the last is still with us). In its travel westwards the first pandemic got no further than Tiflis in Armenia and Astrakhan in Russia. The second reached Moscow in the autumn of 1830, Hamburg and then Sunderland on Tyneside in north-east England in October 1831, and New York in June 1832, killing 23,000 people in Great Britain and perhaps two to six times as many in the United States. A second wave in 1849 killed 53,000 people in Great Britain and twice as many in the United States. The third pandemic killed 23,000 people in Great Britain in 1853-4, and none in the United States. The fourth killed 14,000 people in Great Britain 1866 and 50,000 in the United States. The fifth, in 1881, caused much less havoc in Europe than those that preceded it, but is notable for the fact that it was the one studied in the summer of 1883 by the French and German cholera commissions under Isadore Straus and Robert Koch in Egypt, and later by Koch in Calcutta. The sixth pandemic, from 1889 to 1923, caused many deaths in Mecca and Egypt, and in Russia, with only sporadic outbreaks in western Europe and none in the United States. The present seventh pandemic is due to a variety of the cholera vibrio called *Vibrio eltor*. It set out in 1961 through Indonesia to China and the Philippines, and westwards to East and West Africa where its particular characteristics and the local conditions make it likely it will stay. And of course cholera remains epidemic every year at its source on the delta of the River Ganges in Bengal, which is now divided into West Bengal in India with its capital, Calcutta; and Bangladesh, formerly East Pakistan, with its capital Dhaka, formerly called Dacca.

Cholera is a disease of the bowels filling with water, which is discharged from both ends of the alimentary tract by vomiting and diarrhoea, mainly by diarrhoea, at a rate of one and a half litres an hour, leaving the blood thick and tarry. A patient, who is being rehydrated by having salt solution pumped into his veins as fast as he loses it, can lose thirty litres a day, which in a Bengali can be not far from his entire weight. Cholera patients are mentally alert though totally exhausted and prostrated, often with an intense fear of impending death. François Magendie of the Hôtel Dieu in Paris visited Sunderland within a month of the cholera arriving there in October 1831, and wrote this to the President of the Academy of Sciences in Paris:

'. . . a person in the best of health, when he is smitten by the cholera, is in an instant transformed into a corpse! There is the same state of the eyes; the same aspect of the face; the same coldness of the limbs; the same colour of the skin, etc. Were there not the intelligence left, so to speak, intact, were there not a remnant of the voice even though almost imperceptible, one would proceed to burial at the actual moment of attack . . . to put it all in one word, the disease which is under my eyes in an instant *cadaverises* the person whom it attacks.'

Later in London he said, 'I think it is a disease which begins where others end, with death.'

As soon as cholera appeared in Europe, an understanding of its nature began to grow. In Moscow in 1830, two German expatriates in the Institute for Artificial Mineral Waters, Hermann, a chemist, and Jaenischen, a physician, recognized that all the water in the copious diarrhoeal stools of cholera patients was derived from the blood, and could not be replaced because the capacity of the small intestine to absorb ingested water was totally blocked. They suggested intravenous rehydration, but only one abortive attempt was made. When the cholera came to Sunderland two years later, William Brooke O'Shaughnessy, a twenty-two-year old physician qualified only in the previous year, saw straight into the heart of the matter. He analysed the blood and stools of cholera patients and concluded that they had lost not only the water from their blood, but also its neutral salts and the alkaline sodium bicarbonate. He suggested intravenous rehydration, remineralization and re-alkalinization with a solution of salt and bicarbonate of soda that was then successfully applied in the rescue of a terminal case by Thomas Latta. But in the end the patient was lost, because nobody realised at that time that the process had to be continued until the infecting germ had been eliminated in the natural course of events. That was understandable, because Pasteur was not to pronounce the germ theory of disease for another twenty-nine years. But the germ theory of cholera did come to the surface unofficially with the next pandemic, that started in 1852. John Snow, Queen Victoria's anaesthetist, showed that the cholera 'poison' consisted of particles that were carried from one person to another by being swallowed, and then multiplied in the alimentary tract. By studying the incidence of cholera in contiguous houses supplied either by the Southwark and Vauxhall or by the Lambeth Water Companies, he proved with marvellous precision that these particles were carried only by the water from the Southwark and Vauxhall Company, which was contaminated with sewage. He was thus able to suggest appropriate counter measures. He also stopped the cholera in Soho by removing the handle from the [then] Broad Street water pump, which event is commemorated to this day by 'The John Snow' public house on [the now] Broadwick Street. At the same time his Italian contemporary, Filippo Pacini, observed myriads of curved organisms swarming in the intestinal contents of cholera patients, and (anticipating the germ theory of disease) ascribed the cause of the disease to them, giving them the name *Vibrio cholerae*. So by the time Koch set off to Egypt in 1883 to study the cholera, everything he was going to learn there was already known, and published.

Koch reported and discussed the findings of his commission at the two sittings of *Die Conferenz zur Erörterung der Cholerafrage* on 26 and 29 July 1884 in the *Kaiserlichen Deutschen Gesundheitsamt* in Berlin; and at the *Zweite Serie der Conferenzen zur Erörterung der Cholerafrage* on 4 May 1885. Although he was 'by common consent the greatest pure bacteriologist', Koch made a mess of the cholera problem from beginning to end, even if I am probably the first and only one to say so. Not only did he fail to use the sound knowledge that Snow and Pacini had gained thirty years previously, but his own evidence implicating the *vibrio cholerae* (which he called the comma, or *Virgul Bazillus*) was involved and shaky. He used two curious cart-before-the-horse arguments (which I won't repeat now), and failed to fulfil his own postulate that the disease should be reproduced by inoculating a pure culture of the bacillus in experimental animals, back-tracking by asserting that cholera was no more a disease of animals than rinderpest was a disease of people. But never mind that — there was no real doubt about what caused cholera; where Koch did real damage was quite unnecessarily — almost wilfully — to delay the discovery of cholera exotoxin for two thirds of a century; and since cholera is an exotoxinosis, like tetanus and diphtheria, that was a serious matter. I should explain that an exotoxin is a simple protein toxin of high and well-defined activity secreted into the culture medium by a bacterium during its growth; whereas an endotoxin (which we are about to come to) is a complex of protein, sugar and fat within the bacterium that appears in solution only when the bacterial culture is old and broken down. Compared with exotoxins, the toxicity of endotoxins is ill-defined and very low.

At the first conference in Berlin, Koch ignored the outstanding symptom of cholera that had been so glaringly obvious to his predecessors, namely the profuse and unremitting diarrhoea. He asserted that the symptoms of cholera were in reality due to a poison acting systemically (that is generally, on the body as a whole) to exert a 'paralytic cardiovascular' effect on the circulatory system of the blood. At the second conference, in 1885, Koch restated his paralytic systemic poison hypothesis, and suggested that the poison belonged to the group of so-called ptomaines that had recently been postulated by Brieger, but which in reality do not exist (even if they do still occasionally strike terror in the hearts of laymen). It was this suggestion of a systemically acting poison that diverted the search for a proper animal model for testing the action of cholera toxin, which is a local action confined to the surface cells of the small intestine. When fresh culture filtrates of the cholera vibrio were injected intravenously into animals by various workers, no effects were observed; but when filtrates of older cultures were injected, various ill-defined toxic effects were observed. For reasons that are not worth discussing now, this led to the discovery by Cantani of bacterial endotoxins in 1886, and these totally boring and irrelevant substances were then pursued for the next seven decades with apparently no-one being concerned about the fact that none of the toxic symptoms observed bore the slightest resemblance to the diarrhoeal symptoms of cholera. It was this fatuous endotoxin that Pierre Grabar had been working on in the Pasteur Institute many years ago, and put me off cholera.

At last, in 1959, realism broke through, and it is not surprising that this happened in Calcutta, where the nature of cholera was understood. S.N.De, at the Nilratan Sircar Medical College, injected cholera culture filtrate into short tied-off lengths (or 'loops') of rabbit small intestine, and observed that after a few hours these loops swelled up with a rice-watery fluid characteristic of cholera stools. His short letter to *Nature* in 1959 on 'Enterotoxicity of bacteria-free culture filtrate of *Vibrio cholerae*' is a classic of medical and biochemical history. In the end it led to the currently held view of how cholera toxin turns on the process in the gut that leads to the diarrhoea of cholera.

To return to Jack Craig in the Downstate Medical Center: he had developed another method for testing the activity of cholera toxin which was much simpler than injecting the toxin into tied-off loops of the rabbit intestine. The tied-off loop technique was not at all accurate, could not produce many results at a time, and involved surgery that was beyond the likes of me. It was fine for demonstrating the action of cholera toxin, but not for measuring it; and if you want to do biochemical research on a toxin you must be able to measure how much you're dealing with. What Jack Craig was doing was injecting minute amounts of toxin into the shaved skin on the backs of rabbits. The toxin induces an extrusion of fluid from the cells in the skin tissue (by the same biochemical mechanism as it induces an extrusion of fluid from the blood into the gut in real cholera), and this shows as a bleb on the surface of the skin — the bigger the bleb, the more toxin. It was a comparatively simple matter to make 100 to 150 injections of toxin into the back of a rabbit, so Craig had made a most useful contribution to the study of cholera toxin at a crucial time.

I was enthralled by the cholera problem as soon as I learned about it from Jack Craig, and soon after that I had lunch in New York with an old toxinological friend who had been much involved in the setting up of the Pakistan-SEATO Cholera Research Laboratory in Dacca, and was now in the higher direction of it. He was Colin MacLeod, Deputy Director of the White House Office of Science and Technology. We discussed the cholera problem, and evidently he could see that I was interested, because soon after we returned to Oxford I received a letter from Dr Robert A. Phillips, Director of the Pakistan-SEATO Cholera Research Laboratory in Dacca (PSCRL from now on), inviting me to visit the Laboratory as a consultant. Travel to Dacca would be by Pan American Airlines (First Class). I accepted the invitation avidly. I was thrilled about the cholera problem, I was thrilled about India, by which I mean the Indian sub-continent embracing India and Pakistan as it then was. I have always been thrilled by India, as most British are, and I don't think it is just the idea of the wicked old British Imperial India. There seems to be an affinity between the British and the

Indians. Ruthie and I had briefly visited Delhi a few years previously on the way back from an international biochemical congress in Tokyo, and I had found India exactly as I had expected to find it. I have since been to India and East Pakistan many times, and the strong feeling of affinity is always there. Dacca is one of the ugliest, filthiest cities I have ever been to, and yet every time I go there I feel I have come home. I can't explain it, but I don't believe I am the only Britisher who feels like that. It's the land and the people. Once in Narayanganj, the port on the River Meghna, I took a photograph of a street scene for the sole and sufficient reason that everybody in the teeming street was smiling.

The PSCRL consisted of the Laboratory and a cholera ward at Dacca, and a field surveillance station where forward medical care could be provided at Matlab Bazaar, a market community on the banks of a creek flowing into the Meghna River opposite the point where it joins the Padma River about forty miles southeast of Dacca. (The holy River Ganges suffers two indignities near the end of its long journey from its source in an ice cave at the foot of a Himalayan snow-bed to its steaming delta on the Bay of Bengal: first, when it is joined by the mighty Brahmaputra [or Jamuna] River and becomes the Padma as it flows by Dacca; then, when in this guise it is joined soon after by the Meghna and yields its name once more to that short if voluminous tributary. Nevertheless, the delta is still known as 'the many mouths of the Ganges.')

During the cholera season the PSCRL has midwives (*dhaks*) who visit every house in every village every morning to find out if there have been any manifestations of cholera. They make mental notes (being illiterate) of all cases and then telephone to summon the PSCRL's fleet of fast motor launches to take patients to the cholera wards at Matlab Bazaar or Dacca. It was at Matlab Bazaar that I saw my first cholera patient, a young woman who was too weak to stand on the scales on admission, and so was weighed in the arms of a pre-weighed orderly standing on the scales. The pupils of her eyes were rolled back, and only the whites were visible. She was placed on a cholera bed and given an intravenous drip of salt water and sodium bicarbonate; and as I looked at her, I could see her coming to life, and in an hour or two she was smiling contentedly.

I think I saw that first cholera patient of mine before I had really discussed the cholera problem in the PSCRL. Although the PSCRL was in East Pakistan, and was a SEATO affair, practically all the senior staff were competent and devoted Americans. I took to the biochemical, physiological and immunological aspects of the cholera problem like a duck to water. It became clearer than ever to me that cholera was a toxinosis, and I was probably the first experienced toxinologist to look at the disease. All the problems seemed understandable, and there seemed to be all kinds of advice I could give them. Phillips seemed to be pleased. He sent a message to Dr John R. Seal, Chairman of the Cholera Advisory Committee at the National Institute of Allergy and Infectious Disease of the National Institutes of Health at Bethesda near Washington, who was in effect in charge of the operation of the PSCRL, saying (so Seal told me later) that I was 'the best consultant they had ever had'. Phillips asked me to send a report on my visit to Seal, and to counter any suggestion that research on the cholera problem in Dacca should be confined to practical problems, leaving basic research to be done in the United States. I did so, and got a frosty reply from Seal (whom I'd never met), which drew a frosty reply from me. That led, after we had met eyeball to eyeball, to a great friendship between us that lasted until I helped to bury him in the Arlington National Cemetery in Washington in 1984.

The PSCRL was administered officially by a body comprised of representatives of the SEATO countries who met once a year at Dacca, and this body took advice from a Technical Committee that was reinforced by consultants that were selected by Bob Phillips and by the Cholera Advisory Committee of the National Institutes of Health at Bethesda. So it came about that I was invited to be a consultant, and travelled many times to Dacca, and many more times to the United States, with the ticket usually paid by the United States, but occasionally by H.M.Government.

On my several visits to Dacca I always took the opportunity on the way back to visit India and other parts of the world, like Istanbul. On a visit that H.M.Government kindly paid for, I visited Kathmandhu in Nepal. I was on my way to Delhi, but could not go there directly from Dacca because India and Pakistan were on bad terms, so I had to go through a neutral country, and Kathmandhu was fortunately almost on a straight line between Dacca and Delhi. When I reached passport control at Kathmandhu the Ghurka officer in charge got excited and directed me to a very properly dressed Englishman. He was from the British Embassy and had brought me an invitation to dinner from Lady Kellas, the Ambassador's wife. A pair of red-sashed Sepoy NCOs came that evening to take me from my hotel to the

Embassy, and when I entered Lady Kellas' drawing room I was delighted by her beauty, and by the warmth of her and His Excellency's welcome. Apparently H.M. Government thought enough of Heads of Colleges in Oxford to have advised them of my visit. Thereafter a series of the most beautiful women came in, accompanied by distinguished men, for example Madame and Monsieur France [really], the French Ambassador. Then finally there breezed in a very confident and handsome lady in a beautiful bejewelled blue gown, with flowing golden hair, obviously on close terms with the other ladies. I was in a state of undiluted bliss. At the dinner I sat beside Madame France, and she told me how she baked the croissants herself for breakfast every morning in the Embassy, because everything had to be French. After the ladies had withdrawn, the gentlemen drew to the Ambassador's end of the table; and later, as we went to join the ladies, I saw a seating plan, so I asked him to tell me who was who. Pointing to the name of the lady in blue who had blown in with such *éclat*, he said, 'And that is Miss Patricia Adams, the Mistress of the Crown Prince.' This seemed to me to be a formal statement, not just tittle-tattle; and when the Crown Prince got married a few months later, and there was such a fuss about it because so much money had been spent on the wedding, and it was on television in England, I looked for her, because I was sure she must have some official position, perhaps giving the bridegroom away.

On another visit to India on the way back from East Pakistan, I had introductions to the Maharajah of Jaipur and to the Maharanah of Udaipur. When I checked in at the Rambagh Palace Hotel in Jaipur, which was a former palace of the Maharajah, and was still owned by him, I asked hopefully if there was a message for me, but there was none, and I was told the Maharajah was playing polo in Calcutta. After a few days I went down to Udaipur and checked in at the marvellously beautiful Lake Palace Hotel that floats on its own reflection in the middle of the lake. Again there was no message for me, but as I was having a bath the telephone rang, and a sweet female Indian sing-song voice informed me that she was the Kanwaranee Nanendra Singh, and she had come to take me to the City Palace on the lake shore to be received by the Maharanah. I dressed as quickly as possible and rushed to Reception. There was a ravishing black-haired pale *café au lait*-skinned Indian lady, the Kanwaranee. She explained that she was the wife of the Kanwaranah, the Crown Prince, and that in Udaipur they speak not of Maharajahs but of Maharanahs. We were to wait for her friend, who, she whispered, pointing to the back of another Indian lady, was 'the number two wife of the Maharanah'. Soon this lady came to us, and she was equally ravishing in a pale-skinned way. We then were taken in a kind of ceremonial barge to the lake shore, where we climbed into a howdah on the back of a great elephant, for Heaven's sake. As we went up the slope towards the City Palace, with the moon shining on the howdah, I was quite overcome; I couldn't believe it really was me riding on a howdah on the back of an elephant with two beautiful princesses, going to be received by a Maharanah in a great palace. I made a remark on the beautiful English the princesses spoke, and the Kanwaranee said, 'I should hope so, I'm an English girl from Guildford', and the Number Two Wife said 'And I'm a British girl from Belfast.' In my unconsciously racist way I had assumed that the more royal you were, the paler was your skin. When we got to the City Palace, with scarlet-sashed Sepoys smartly saluting, we were received by an adjutant, and the two ladies skittered silently away. I was taken to an enormous Durbar Room where I was received by the Kanwaranah and given the most dilute gin-and-tonic I ever drank. The poor man was dead bored, and I got away as soon as I decently could.

At the first meeting I attended of the Technical Committee in Dacca, I was fortunately able to make a useful suggestion. Before Jack Craig had started testing what he assumed to be cholera toxin in the skins of rabbits, Richard Finkelstein of Dallas, Texas, had devised a test for cholera toxin which laboriously involved dosing the material to infant rabbits and inducing diarrhoea in them. Finkelstein's test was undoubtedly a test for cholera toxin, but it was not one that could be used on any practical scale. Craig's test could very easily be carried out on a large scale, but was it a test for the diarrhoea-inducing cholera toxin? Were they both testing the same substance? I proposed an immunological way of settling this matter that I had learned at the Wellcome Laboratories during the war; and it was agreed, since the question was important, that tests should be carried out on a large scale at the PSCRL. By the time of the next meeting of the Technical Committee, the tests had been carried out, showing that there was no doubt that they were both testing cholera toxin. That was a really useful practical advance, because the Craig test was quick, easy, and accurate enough for anybody to use who wanted to work on cholera toxin. I think the Technical Committee was pleased.

The Committee then settled down to devising a large-scale field trial in the Matlab *thana* (district) of the efficacy of cholera vaccine. This was a vaccine made of killed cholera bacilli, and was therefore an antibacterial vaccine rather than an antitoxic vaccine, and I was dismayed. Diphtheria and tetanus were toxic diseases that were completely and easily preventable by immunization with their toxoids against their toxins — surely we should be doing the same with cholera, which was just as much a toxinosis as diphtheria and tetanus? Seated by my side was Sir James Howie, an impressive figure, Head of the Public Health Laboratory Service in Britain, and a member of the Technical Committee. I gave him a scribbled note: 'If they won't test cholera toxoid, let's get the Wellcome Laboratories to make some, and we'll test it in Bombay.' 'Agreed!', scribbled Sir James, but I don't know what either of us thought we were talking about. Who would do the testing in Bombay? And there wasn't nearly as much cholera in Bombay as in East Pakistan!

In the end, a massive, comprehensive and carefully controlled field trial of cholera bacterial vaccine was carried out by the PSCRL in East Pakistan in 1968-9, only to yield the conclusion that the vaccine was ineffective. So then at last began a great effort in America, and at the Wellcome Laboratories in Britain, to make a toxoid from cholera toxin. We had endless discussions in Washington about it, trying to balance harmlessness of the toxoid against immunological efficacy. The Americans were fearful of injecting anything into Pakistanis that might produce even a slightly painful reaction, so they were anxious to get the toxin completely purified, and then completely detoxified. I was fearful that too much purification, and then too much detoxification, would produce a toxoid so neutered as to be ineffective. When after all that effort the toxoid was finally produced in the United States and tested in East Pakistan, it turned out to be no good. But I don't think now that that failure was due only to neutering the toxoid — I think it was due to the nature of the disease.

What really protects an immunized person is what is beautifully called the 'anamnestic response', the 'not-forgetting' response. Take diphtheria. Once you have had two injections of diphtheria toxoid separated by an interval of six weeks, and then a third injection after six months, you are probably immune to diphtheria for the rest of your life, though it might be a good idea to have a booster injection of toxoid once in a while. What protects you is not the antitoxin in you at the time of infection — that will have gone down to an almost unmeasurable level — but the fact that the antitoxin-making cells in your body's immunological system never forget; and as soon as they encounter any fresh toxin from a new infection, they immediately respond by making more antitoxin. It takes them about three days to produce an protective level of antitoxin, which is fine in the cases of diphtheria or tetanus, because these diseases have incubation periods of more than three days, that is, the germs take more than three days to grow and produce toxin. But cholera is a very quick disease, with an incubation period measured in hours rather than days. A cholera patient may be woken by a loose stool at dawn, and be dead by noon. That is why I now think that it will never be possible seriously to immunize against cholera.

But if cholera is not preventable by immunization, at least it is now very easily cured. So far I have touched from time to time on the treatment of cholera by intravenous rehydration, that is, dripping a solution of neutral and alkaline salts in water into a vein, to make up for the loss of water and salts from the blood as a result of the diarrhoea. It is not possible to replace the water and the salts simply by giving it to the patient to drink, because the cholera toxin has affected the internal surface of the gut in such a way that it not only provokes the pouring of water and salts from the blood into the gut, but it also prevents the absorption of water and salts from the gut back to the blood. While Bob Phillips was in charge of U.S.Naval Medical Research Unit Number 2 in Taiwan, before he came to Dacca to be Director of the PSCRL, he tried to find a way of making the cholera-poisoned gut absorb water and salts, and in the end he succeeded with marvellous simplicity. All that needs to be done is to add a little sugar, preferably in the form of glucose, to the fluid. The sugar opens a channel, so to speak, for the water and salts to pass from the cholera-poisoned gut to the blood. The technique is so simple that at first Phillips was most reluctant to put any trust in it, but it was further developed at the PSCRL and elsewhere, and in the end it came to be adopted. It is now the standard way of rehydrating people suffering from the dehydration of cholera, and of other dehydrating diseases that children in under-developed countries all over the world are especially prone to. It is a great, hardly-sung, blessing brought about by science; far more life-saving, really, than a cure for cancer would be.

I usually stayed in the Intercontinental Hotel in Dacca, and emerging one day from the lift onto the ground floor, I was amazed to be met by a large group of expectant-looking

Pakistanis, who seemed clearly pleased to see me. I asked the man at the reception desk what it was about me that interested them, and he told me, 'They think you are Zulfikar Ali Bhutto.' I suppose Bhutto and I did have some appearances in common – we were both bald, of the same height, of the same complexion (he pale-skinned for a Pakistani, I sun-tanned), and with vaguely similar facial features.

While I went to East Pakistan twice a year on cholera business, I went to America half-a-dozen or more times a year, as a consultant to the Cholera Advisory Committee of the National Institutes of Health. Naturally I was very pleased to do this, but do not let the word 'consultant' mislead you into thinking that I was drawing enormous fees. Other kinds of consultants may draw such fees, but not medical-scientific academics advising the U.S.Government. All I got was my economy-class tickets across the Atlantic (but first-class to Pakistan), hotel bedrooms (if I was not staying with the Seals), taxis in moderation and a tip of a hundred dollars or so; but of course I was glad to do this work. Most of the meetings were at the National Institutes of Health at Bethesda, or nearby at the Johns Hopkins University Medical School in Baltimore. Every other year there was a meeting at some beauty spot, like the Grand Canyon of the Colorado River in Utah, or Williamsburg in Virginia. These were the meetings of the Cholera Panel of the U.S.-Japan Co-operative Medical Science Program, which were held every year, alternately in the U.S. or Japan, and I went to those in America. They were the brain-child of my friend Colin MacLeod when he was Deputy Director of the White House Office of Science and Technology. In January 1965 President Lyndon B. Johnson and Prime Minister Eisaku Sato of Japan had met in order to attempt to solve the problem of the industrious Japanese exporting too much and importing too little. Nothing came of the meeting, and in order to find some way of saving face the President had incarcerated Colin MacLeod all night in the White House with instructions to come up by breakfast-time with a scheme for mutual co-operation. Colin had come up with a scheme for a US-Japan Co-operative Medical Science Program. It would be fair to say that the Japanese gained more from this than the Americans gained from the Japanese, so President Johnson could at last claim to be exporting something to Japan.

At these meetings in America, exciting developments in the cholera field were being reported, mainly in connection with the mode of action of the toxin at the molecular level. I won't go into this in any more detail for the moment than to say that an entity glamorously called 'The Second Messenger' (or 'cyclic AMP') was involved. The Second Messenger is 'turned on' by the hormones, or First Messengers, and transmits messages to the organs that are affected by the hormones. (Earl Sutherland was awarded the Nobel Prize for the Second Messenger in 1971, at the time when humourless students were apt to be concerned about whether academic research had any practical applications to the betterment of man's material lot. When Sutherland was asked whether the information he had gained would have any such practical application, he replied 'There is one kind of information that I am reasonably sure cannot be applied. And that is the information we do not have.') Now it seemed that the Second Messenger was also 'turned on' by cholera toxin.

All these interesting biochemical advances gave me pause. Here I was, talking and advising about cholera on three continents, without actually working on the problem myself in my own laboratory. It was practically an open scandal. Wasn't it time I wet my own hands on the problem? So I went to work in my laboratory, and had a marvellous time. As the young lady said after her honeymoon, 'I never knew you could have so much fun without laughing.'

I set out in the same way as I had started with tetanus toxin, to find out what it was that fixed the toxin. What was its receptor in the host's tissues? In the case of tetanus I had looked for it in nervous tissue; in the case of cholera I decided again to look for it in the tissue that the toxin worked on, that is, the epithelial cells lining the small intestine. It was very easy to obtain these by turning rabbit intestine inside-out and scraping off the tissue. I tested suspensions of the tissue in buffer solution, and found that they avidly fixed cholera toxin. I tried suspensions of all other kinds of tissue, from the liver, the kidneys, the lungs, and the heart muscle, and none of these fixed cholera toxin. I was overjoyed. It was going to be a comparatively easy matter now to find out what it was in the gut scrapings that fixed the toxin. It turned out to be even easier than I thought it was going to be. My then technician, Sylvia Main, suggested we ought also to test the cholera-fixing capacity of brain tissue. I thought she was daft. What on earth could nervous tissue have to do with a diarrhoea-inducing toxin? But I thought I must humour Sylvia, so we tried brain tissue, and to my amazement, and to the accompaniment of a smug smile from her, brain tissue fixed cholera toxin even better than the scrapings from the small intestine. Far, far better.

No matter how we diluted down the suspension from brain tissue, it fixed the toxin, even when we seemed to be working with a clear buffer solution. Obviously and amazingly, the cholera toxin receptor must also be ganglioside, and when we tested it, it was.

I had been assaying the activity of cholera toxin by Jack Craig's useful test in rabbit skin. Clearly it was now necessary to test the fixation of cholera toxin by ganglioside by other techniques of assay of the toxin, particularly the technique of inducing accumulation of fluid in the gut of experimental animals. I was not enough of a surgeon to carry out these tests, so I went to the place where they were the most skilled at them, the Department of Medicine at the Johns Hopkins University School of Medicine in Baltimore, Maryland. I went to Baltimore, carrying with me a large supply of mixed ganglioside that I had isolated from slaughter-house brain. There Chuck Carpenter, Nate Pierce, Bucky Greenough and I confirmed by all the available tests that minute concentrations of ganglioside fixed cholera toxin. Those three distinguished and experienced colleagues of mine were considerably impressed by this phenomenon. I left the large supply of ganglioside that I had brought with me with them; which was a pity, because it was unscrupulously to be used by a colleague of theirs, called Pedro Cuatracasas, whom I had met and told in detail about my discovery.

My Johns Hopkins colleagues and I wrote a paper on the fixation of cholera toxin by ganglioside and sent it to the distiguished British weekly *Nature* for publication. They turned it down (it was the first and only paper of mine ever to be turned down by a scientific journal), so we sent our paper to *The Journal of Infectious Diseases,* which published it in October 1971. This delay was most unfortunate, because it gave the opportunity to Cuatracasas to publish a pretentious paper in *Biochemistry* claiming the discovery of the fixation of cholera toxin by ganglioside, which was based on experiments which he did with the ganglioside that I had left at Johns Hopkins. He was the first of the jackals who preyed on my work.

When I got back to Oxford, I started to find out which of the several gangliosides fixed cholera toxin. Having already touched on the chemistry of the complex ganglioside molecules in connection with the tetanus toxin receptor in Chapter 6, I won't go into them now, except to remind you that there are several of them, all of them being big complex molecules, consisting essentially of a sugary component (GGnL) joined to a fatty component (C). To the sugary component there may be joined from one to four sialic acid components (S), attached either to the G or the L component or to both. I had already shown that tetanus toxin was fixed by GGnSSLC; now my colleague Carolyn King and I found that cholera toxin was fixed by GGnSLC, that one S component making the difference between the receptors of these two entirely different toxins (and it may be significant that the cholera vibrio produces a sialidase, an enzyme that splits sialic acid from gangliosides containing more than one S, turning them into the toxin-fixing GGnSLC). We determined this quite soon, but unfortunately Caroline was a bit tiresome about the publication of our results, which were consequently delayed for many months. In that time another scavenging jackal, a Swede called Holmgren, tried to steal a march on me. He was a colleague of Lars Svennerholm in Gothenberg, from whom (you may possibly remember) I had learned some ganglioside chemistry soon after I discovered the fixation of tetanus toxin by ganglioside. Svennerholm had spent most of his life isolating the different gangliosides, so it was a simple matter for Holmgren, having read our paper in the *Journal of Infectious Diseases*, to pick the different gangliosides off Svennerholm's shelf and test them one by one on cholera toxin — a trained monkey could have done that. I minded, but not too much, secure in the belief that by the captains in the tetanus and cholera worlds I was a captain.

I had started out with the cholera toxin receptor as I had with the tetanus toxin receptor, thinking that if I could determine its chemical nature I would be on the verge of knowing the chemistry of the action of the toxin — all I would have to do next was to find out what changes the toxin brought about in the receptor. But tetanus toxin did not bring about any change in its ganglioside receptor, GGnSSLC; and soon it was clear that cholera toxin did not bring about any change in its receptor, GGnSLC.

With so many people working on it, cholera toxin was by now moving fast. A flood of information was coming in about its structure, and about its mode of action at the chemical level. Let us consider the structure first. It became apparent that some of the biologically active proteins were composed of two quite easily separable parts; one part being concerned with fixing the toxin to the susceptible cells in the body, so facilitating the entry of the other part, which was the active part, into the cell, where it could do the damage. This had been shown to be the case with diphtheria toxin, and with the poisonous proteins from plants, abrin and ricin (by means of which, on the sharpened end of an umbrella, a diplomat was murdered not long ago on the streets of London). Finkelstein, who was the first to purify cholera toxin, showed that it consisted of an inactive part (which he called choleragenoid), and a smaller part which was presumably active. All this had been brilliantly foreseen long ago, in 1900, by the great German scientist, Paul Ehrlich, when he gave the Croonian Lecture before the Royal Society of London. He had proclaimed, in Latin as was his wont, that *Corpora non agunt nisi fixata,* — things won't act unless they're fixed. He postulated that toxins consisted of an active component, which he called the 'toxophore', and a binding component, which he called the 'haptophore', that fixed the toxin to its receptor on the susceptible cell and so enabled the toxophore to express its activity. Ehrlich apparently arrived at this conclusion by the light of pure reason, or by instinct, since he never, as far as can be judged, made any attempt to test his hypothesis by experiment. Yet the progress made on the toxic bacterial and plant proteins in the 1970s proved him right. And I don't suppose that any of the clever young people in the 1970s had ever heard of Paul Ehrlich's dictum — why should they have?

One of the clever young people was our son Simon, who to my great satisfaction had decided to turn his knowledge of proteins to bacterial toxins. He had been working on the structure of an active protein, a proteolytic enzyme, in the Department of Biochemistry in Oxford, but had decided to switch to more interesting proteins, and so had chosen cholera toxin. The structure of proteins is a difficult subject, well beyond my capability, but not Simon's. He borrowed some ganglioside from me, made it insoluble by a particular technique, and fixed cholera toxin to it, then treated the mixture with a solution of urea. The choleragenoid part of the toxin remained fixed to the ganglioside, and a smaller part was washed off. This smaller part was the active part of the toxin. There is nothing new under the sun — the active part was the toxophore; and the ganglioside-receiving part, choleragenoid, was the haptophore.

This work of Simon's, together with that of others, showed that the fixation of cholera toxin by ganglioside GGnSLC was preliminary to its actual action, which was performed by the component that was not fixed by ganglioside. The toxin could not be toxic unless it were first fixed by its inactive binding component to the ganglioside of the susceptible cell, and by this means enabled to introduce the active component into the interior of the cell where it could wreak its damage.

As to the active component of cholera toxin, it is another example of the unity of nature. Perhaps I should say the thriftyness of nature, that applies a few ideas in many different situations. Michael Gill determined the mode of action of the active component on a short visit to my laboratory, by showing that it is a particular enzyme, an 'ADP-ribosylase', exactly like the active component of diphtheria toxin that he and Alwyn Papenheimer had unravelled at Harvard. It is the ADP-ribosylase that turns on the Second Messenger in the case of cholera (but not of diphtheria).

With the mode of action of cholera toxin all so neatly tied up, and with the mode of action of tetanus toxin still a total mystery, I continue to wonder about the role of receptor substances, and in particular about the tetanus and cholera toxin-fixing gangliosides, in the normal economy of the healthy living body. Let us go back to what Paul Ehrlich had to say about the normal function of toxin receptors when he gave his Croonian Lecture to the Royal Society in 1900:

> That these are in function specially designed to seize on toxines [*sic*] cannot for one moment be entertained. It would not be reasonable to suppose that there were present in the organism many hundreds of atomic groupings destined to unite with toxines, when the latter appeared, but in function really playing no part in the processes of normal life, and only arbitrarily brought into relation with them by the will of the investigator . . . . One may therefore rightly assume that these toxophile protoplasmic groups in reality serve normal functions in the animal organism, and that they only incidentally and by pure chance possess the capacity to anchor themselves to this or that toxine.

What are the 'normal functions in the animal organism' of the gangliosides (that may still have been lost in obscurity if I had not determined their role in tetanus in 1958)? It has been suggested that they may form part of the cell membrane system that normally transmits information from the outside of the cell to the interior. Perhaps they are receptors for hormones, since there are several of them (and they also seem to have active and binding components) that appear to be bound by gangliosides in cell membranes. And there has been speculation that gangliosides may play a part in the regulation of cell growth, since cancer cells have been shown to have altered patterns of glycolipids, which include gangliosides.

Cholera Prevention at Home?

As soon as I discovered that minute amounts of brain tissue inactivated cholera toxin, I thought about the possibility of using mushed-up slaughter-house brain as a cholera preventative. I had visions of Bengali mothers slaughtering a goat from time to time during the cholera season, making a gruel from the brain, and giving spoonsful of it to the family twice a day. For all I know, that may be a good idea, but it has never been tested. Not for want of trying on my part. I even patented the idea.

Florey and his penicillin group had been too busy, too high-minded, too innocent, to patent penicillin during the war; and other people got rich instead. But at least the lesson was learned, and the National Research and Development Corporation came into being, with the object of patenting academic discoveries. Cephalosporin was the first substance to be patented by the Corporation, and that is how Edward Abraham got so rich (see Chapter 5). It seemed to me that the only way to get brain tested in cholera was to have it tested under the auspices of the Cholera Advisory Committee at the National Institutes of Health at Bethesda. They were supporting research by the University of Maryland on cholera in human volunteers in the Maryland House of Correction (which is a nice name for a jail), and I discussed the possibility with John Seal of getting brain powder tested at this facility, and he agreed to try to arrange it. First it was necessary to get the brain powder put up in gelatin-coated capsules so that measured amounts could easily be swallowed by the volunteers. That is where the NRDC came in. I didn't think I would ever get rich out of a patent for brain powder as a short-term cholera preventative, but I knew that the NRDC would at least pay for getting the capsules made and filled with brain powder.

In the end I took a supply of brain capsules to John Seal, and he promised to do his best to get them tested at the Maryland House of Correction, but he was doubtful whether he would succeed. He was right to be doubtful, because the capsules were defeated by bureaucracy. It was bureaucracy I could understand. The United States and Great Britain have laws that you cannot administer medicaments to people without specifying all the ingredients, and the concentrations of those ingredients. How could we specify all the ingredients of brain powder? I made a mistake putting the brain powder in medical capsules — what I should have done was to get the volunteers fed brain gruel, which would not have had to comply with any pharmaceutical regulations; but that was not possible for me to arrange at a distance.

The Passing of John Seal

John Seal was a romantic soul though he didn't look it, always thrilled by the drama of the events around us. Quite early on he told me that he would like to see a book written about the effort that was being made over cholera. He suggested that I might write such a book, but I was far too busy; and the idea did not appeal to me anyhow. In East Hampton I had met Berton Roueché, who wrote about medical science in *The New Yorker*, so with John's agreement I asked him if he would be prepared to undertake a commission to write such a book. But to my surprise Roueché seemed to find it hard to understand what I was getting at; and now, when I think back on it I can see that it was not really his cup of tea. In 1979, when I was near retirement, and all the tumult and the shouting over cholera was beginning to die down, it occurred to me that the time had come for John Seal's book to be written, and that I might write it. I put that idea to him, and he was pleased. I was pleased too, because the idea of writing the book now seemed very attractive, and I felt I knew how to write it. Besides, it would mean many visits to the United States, and I was keen to make them.

John Seal was very enthusiastic. He came to see me in Oxford, and he planned a trip right round the world for me to interview people concerned with cholera. I was first to go to Cairo to talk to the people at the U.S. Naval Medical Research Unit Number 3 (NAMRU-3, of which John Seal had been Director in his time), where in 1947 Captain Robert A. Phillips had first started working on cholera when it came to Egypt. Then I was to proceed to the International Centre for Diarrhoeal Disease Research in Dhaka in Bangladesh, which used to be the Pakistan-SEATO Cholera Research Laboratory in Dacca in East Pakistan; then to the Chulalongkorn University Medical School in Bangkok in Thailand; then to NAMRU-2 at Taipei in Taiwan; then to California, Arizona, Texas, South Dakota, Ohio and Maryland and on to Washington. Everything had been arranged, when the United States offended Taiwan for some reason which I can't remember, and this caused NAMRU-2 to be thrown out of Taipei, and since that was to be the most important of my visits, my circumnavigation of the globe was cancelled. However, I did travel over a great many of the United States, talking to cholera people as far west as Arizona and South Dakota. And I went many times to Washington to talk to John Seal and other people at the National Institutes of Health at Bethesda. I always stayed with John and Frances Seal, and the strong friendship between us grew stronger. John Seal was the United States' most devoted civil servant. His devotion to his work as Deputy Director of the National Institute of Allergy and Infectious Diseases was absolute, and his knowledge and grasp of the problems of infectious diseases was total, from the broadest principle down to the minutest detail. He could have been Director of the Institute, but it suited his temperament always to work behind the scenes as Deputy.

In the end I wrote the book, in a handsome room that had been set aside for me by the kind Keeper of Scientific Books in the Radcliffe Science Library of the Bodleian library. It is called *Cholera: The American Scientific Experience, 1947-1980* [39], by van Heyningen and Seal. It simply had to be a good book, and the many reviewers seem to think that it is.

By the time the book was written, John Seal was a very sick man, with two angelic nurses looking after him at home day and night. Dick Krause, Director of the NIAID, gave a magnificent party in his house on the NIH campus for the launching of the book. We got John to that party, and we all had a beautiful time and got a little drunk, including John.

In the end I had a telephone call from NIAID telling me that John had died, and asking me to come to Washington for his funeral. Since he had been a Captain in the U.S. Navy, and had been on the point of being promoted to Rear-Admiral when he left the Navy for the National Institutes in order to preside over the Cholera Advisory Committee, he was given full naval honours, with a service in the Fort Meyer Military Chapel and a burial in the Arlington National Cemetery. I was an Honorary Pall Bearer, which meant that I stood with the other Honorary Pall Bearers, with our right hands on our hearts, while the sailors carried the coffin into the chapel, and we then followed it in. Dick Krause read the address, referring to John's and my friendship and our work together. Then the coffin was placed on a caisson drawn by eight white horses, followed by a naval band and a detachment of armed sailors, and we proceeded from the Fort Meyer Chapel at a walking pace with the naval band playing the long way, a mile or more, through the Arlington National Cemetery with the tourists in their all-glass buses looking on. At the burial place, the bugler sounded the Last Post, the armed detachment fired several salvos, and then there took place a ceremony that I did not know of: at a barked command, eight sailors, four on each side, whipped off the Stars and Stripes covering the coffin and held it aloft in a rigid flat rectangle. Then at another command they folded it lengthwise in three or four machine-like movements until it was a foot wide; and at another command until it was a foot square, with the Stars on top. Then the commanding officer folded that square of Stars into a triangle, and handed the flag to Frances to take home and keep; and then my friend John Seal was buried.

The Magic Letters

All British scientists dream of being elected Fellow of the Royal Society of London, and thus of being able to put the letters F.R.S. after their names. The Royal Society has so much prestige that although I would love to have those Magic Letters after my name, I don't think I am good enough for them — I am inclined like W.C.Fields in another context to state that I would not like to belong to a Royal Society that would have me as a Fellow. Florey put me up for a Fellowship, but I was not elected. He put me up again, but I was still not elected. I don't object to that; but what I do object to is the large number of people who have been elected who are no better than me. I'd love to name them.

East Hampton, Long Island

That first dinner with the Magills at Gage and Tollner's in Brooklyn in 1967 was the beginning of a long friendship. Towards the end of our stay at the Downstate Medical Center, which is at the western end of Long Island, they took us for the week-end to their house in East Hampton, 120 miles out on the other end of Long Island, a little short of its eastern extremity at Montauk. It is one of the oldest towns in America, having been founded (first as Maidstone) by Kentish immigrants on 29 April 1648. I always spent some time there on my many subsequent visits to the United States.

The start of my second visit to East Hampton was mildly adventurous. I had been to see Jack Craig at Downstate Medical Center, and then asked how to get to East Hampton. 'Take the Long Island Railroad to Babylon', they told me, 'then the bus.' Babylon! Babylon! How gloriously romantic! But how horribly unromantic it turned out to be when I got there. From there I travelled in the bus, and as night began to fall, I began to hope we would soon stop somewhere where I could assuage a mundane need. Eventually we stopped outside the Armory Bar & Grill at Westhampton, and the driver shouted 'Coffee folks!' He and his passengers dashed into the Bar & Grill, and I into the other place, for only a few moments. By the time I came out the bus was gone, with all my luggage. (They had not gone in to *drink* coffee, but to *fetch* it in waxed cartons to take on the bus.) It was getting on for 11 pm and there was no-one in sight. What would I have done in England? I would have got in touch with the police. So I went into the Bar & Grill and telephoned the local police. A police car arrived in minutes, and took me to the police station, where they told me that there was no further public conveyance to East Hampton that night. But they would alert East Hampton, and would get me there in the end. They could take me in their patrol car only to the limit of their precinct, where they arranged to be met by a patrol car of the next precinct, which would hand me over to the precinct after that, and so on, until I was safely in the East Hampton precinct. Thus it was that I was handed on like a baton in a relay race from one amiable pair of policemen to another through about five precincts, finally to be met not too long after midnight by Betty Magill outside their house at 140 Main Street in East Hampton. I could not have arrived there in a more agreeable fashion.

East Hampton is a very pretty town (officially it is a 'village', because 'town' means the county embracing the village), with the Atlantic Ocean breaking on the adjoining miles of glorious beaches, and with its beautiful, wide, tree-lined Main Street, where the Magills live. It is one of the fashionable places, to which you will find frequent references in *The New Yorker*. Many of the citizens of East Hampton are rich, with apartments on Park Avenue in New York as well as their sumptuous houses in East Hampton. One of the rich people, with an immense house on the beach, was a Mr Trip, head of one of the great airlines, and since he bore the same name as an aunt of my father's, I was frequently tempted to knock on his door and beg for money for St Cross, but I could never summon up the nerve.

The Magills are not rich, but their handsome and agreeable house on Main Street is of great antiquity, with a garden planned with awesome erudition by Betty, who is one of the *Grandes Dames* of the Garden Club of America. Their many pleasant friends are always kind to me on my visits, in that marvellous friendly way that Americans are so good at, and which I sometimes get very home-sick for in England. But in spite of their open-ness, Americans are strangely shy about certain things, like, for a trivial instance, lavatories (already a euphemism), which even most of the most worldly and sophisticated of them call bathrooms. And once I was amazed by the young curate of the East Hampton Episcopalian church. It is a handsome stone church, built perhaps a hundred years ago in the English style; but the church bells are by no means in the English style — they are an electrically operated carillon playing tapes of music. One day at a church fête I suggested to the young curate that it might be a nice idea to replace the carillon with real bells, which I was sure his parishioners would be glad to ring. There was a keen band of bell-ringers at St Cross College who would be glad to come over and teach them (and all the other Hamptons) how to do it. I really thought, and still think, that it was a good idea, but it didn't catch on with the curate. He did not understand what I was saying. Then it dawned on me that the reason he hadn't the faintest idea of what I was talking about, was because he had simply never heard of church bells being rung by hand.

11
FRANCE

I have been drawn to France ever since I set foot on the dock at Marseilles in September 1934. But that was a short visit that ended the next morning, when I flew from Le Bourget to Croydon in Imperial Airways' *Hengist*. I did not see France again until after the war, when I went to Paris in November 1946, and then to Dole and Arbois in the Jura, for the *Cinquantenaire de la Mort de Pasteur*. During that memorable visit I became enamoured of France, even though I could not understand or speak a word of its glorious language. It is a language that is so ravishing to hear, especially from the lips of a stylish French woman; and in print it is so elegantly *éclatant*, with those accents acute and grave, those caps and diaereses, those frequent apostrophes sparkling *au-dessus*, and those seductive cedillas sibilating sinuously *en dessous*.

Not long after the war we had a seaside holiday at Le Val-André on the north Brittany coast. The sun shone all day and we had a lovely time; but we continued after that to have holidays on the British seaside, and it always rained. To the South African in me the idea of bathing under dripping grey skies was masochism, and finally at a place called Sea Palling which must have been a misprint for A-palling, I revolted. I told my loved ones I was never, never again going to take a seaside holiday in Britain. Ruthie gathered the two children under her wing, and the three of them gazed at me with surprise and pity — it was a fact of nature that it rained during British seaside holidays, what on earth was I going on about? But I stuck to my guns, and the next holiday was a perfect one at Menton, then at Roquebrune-Cap-Martin, on the French Riviera, which was not as crowded then as it is now. But I was not yet so totally smitten by France as I was going to be, and anyway we wanted to explore the holiday resorts of Europe, so for our next holiday we put the car on the brand new *autocouchette* that took us from Boulogne to Lyon, which was as far as it went in those days. From there we drove through Provence to Spain, to stay at San Feliu de Guixols on the coast of Catalonia. It was a very pleasant holiday, but what stands out for me was the day we spent in Barcelona, for it was an important day in my life. We passed a strange structure that looked for all the world like four immense straightened-out brownstone bananas. It was the funniest thing I ever saw, but as I turned to Ruthie, the grin froze on my lips, for I realised that I was looking at one of the most beautiful things I had ever seen. It was Antonio Gaudi's uncompleted Templo Expiatorio de la Sagrada Familia, the Expiatory Chapel of the Holy Family, begun in 1884, unfinished at the time of his death in 1926, and still very slowly being worked on. The objects of my unseemly mirth were the towers supporting and enhancing the main entrance of the chapel. They rose curvilinearly in brown stone up into the air, carved near their tops with the repeated proclamation *Hosanna Hosanna Hosanna,* and finally burst into brightly coloured, strangely shaped finials whose brightness and colour were derived from surfaces covered with brightly coloured fragments of broken pottery. If I were a religious man, that is how I would proclaim my God.

The various parts of the building were of the strangest shapes, covered with a rich profusion of carvings of animals and vegetation. Somewhere high up over the entrance there were two angels blowing trumpets. 'Observe the angels', said the English-language pamphlet, 'with their filmy garments clinging their sexy forms.' Many years later Ruthie and I paid another visit to Barcelona for the purpose of looking at and photographing every one of Gaudi's strange and beautiful buildings and edifices.

Driving back to Lyon to rejoin the *autocouchette* home, my left forearm began to ache from an infected slight injury, and this rapidly got so bad that I was unable to move the gear lever with it; but Ruthie and I were so well co-ordinated that she handled the gear lever without prompting while I footed the clutch pedal. The ache became intolerable, and I decided I must take myself to a hospital in Lyon. Lyon is a big city, and I had never been to it before, except for the station on the way down, and the drive southwards from it directly out of town; and the hospital was not on that route. But somehow I knew where it was, and when we entered the city from the west I drove straight to it without hesitation and without asking the way. A mention of Oxford and Florey ensured that I got all the attention that I needed. The point of this is not my arm-ache, but the fact that I just *knew* for certain, without any doubt or hesitation, where that hospital was. I had no idea how or why I knew. It gave me pause. If I had been a Believer I suppose I would have known.

Then we went to Greece, having decided before we went that while we were there we might perhaps look for a little holiday house to buy for a small sum on some Greek island. We even spoke to a house agent in Greece, but decided against it because Greece was too far; and much as we liked the nice Greeks, we did not like their bread or their wine; and we saw no possibility of learning their language.

So then we thought of the South of France; and Jane Mellanby and her husband, Oliver Impey, who had spent their honeymoon at Gassin near St Tropez, advised us to look for a house in La Garde-Freinet, an ancient *village perché* on a *col* up on the Maures *Massif*. It was an abandoned village, said Oliver, and we'd get a house for about £600. Oliver's mother told us that Carol Martin, Nevill Coghill's daughter (we knew him but not her), lived there, and that she was sure to help us find a house. Another Oxford friend was about to tour the South of France, so we asked him to call at La Garde-Freinet and find us a house agent.

After a few weeks we took an overnight train from Paris to Les Arcs, where the house agent met us and took us to Ste Maxime where we rented a car, and then we drove up the steep winding road to La Garde-Freinet. Already on that journey we were overcome with enchantment at the beauty of the Provençal countryside in the autumn, and of the forest of chestnut trees as we got near the top. La Garde-Freinet was everything we could have hoped for. There were many near-abandoned houses, and several less abandoned for sale. We chose the second house of the three the agent showed us in the village. The price was closer to £6000 than £600, but we were not altogether surprised. Then it was a matter of having to deal in our non-existent French with a lawyer, so we called on Carol Martin, bless her heart, who turned out to be very, very nice and very, very kind. She went with us and the house agent to the little town of Cogolin where the *notaire* was. There it turned out that the French, being dedicated and adroit evaders of taxes, had at that time their own way of selling and buying houses (it has been reformed since then). The sum that appeared on the legal document, and upon which tax was paid, was more than half of the sum agreed with the house agent, but not much more; the rest had to be paid on a later occasion to the house agent *sous la table*. The practice was universal in France, and there was simply no other, legal, way of buying a house at that time (there were articles in British Sunday newspapers explaining how to deal with this aspect of buying French property). That made it difficult for us, because although the Bank of England would let us have the French currency specified on the legal document, it would not allow us any more. So I arranged to borrow the money from my friend André Lwoff of the Pasteur Institute; went to Paris to collect it; and the next morning I met the house agent in a café-bar near the Hotel Oxford et Cambridge where I had spent the night. After we had talked for a few minutes, which was difficult with my severely fractured French, he asked me to pass him the money *sous la table*, yes, that was what he actually said; so, feeling like a fool, *sous la table* I passed it to him.

I loved La Garde-Freinet and our house in it. The local Provençaux were friendly, but our regrettable inability to talk French readily did not make for much social intercourse. However, there were several British people for us to fraternize with. Dear Carol Martin lived there permanently; her nice mother Elspeth Schubert, who had been married to Nevill Coghill and was now married to a Swedish gentleman, lived half the time in her own house in La Garde-Freinet and half the time in Sweden; the aristocratic Lady Jane Heaton, daughter of the Marquess of Ormond, lived in a magnificent converted chapel next door to the Mairie; Oswald Savage, a retired rheumatologist from London, and his wife, Kitty, lived in a beautiful house a little down the road to St Tropez; Nicolas Kaldor, the brilliant Cambridge economist, had a house in the village; Jane Jack, an English don at St Anne's College, Oxford, had a house in the village; and there was a Nuffield College don who had a house just outside the village, but we never got to know him.

There were many interesting and some glamorous towns to visit, like St Tropez twelve miles away; with Ste Maxime, St Raphael, Cannes, Antibes, Nice and Menton to the east; and Toulon and Marseille to the west; and Grasse and Aix-en-Provence in the hinterland. In our early days, St Tropez was still very pleasant, and we would enjoy sitting in the sun at Senequier's looking at all the beautiful people going by against the background of expensive yachts. And the bathing was beautiful. There was one part of the beach where they bathed bare, and there seemed to be a unwritten understanding that only the beautiful girls went bare. And a few hundred yards from this delectable beach there was a glorious restaurant — no more than a large canvas open-sided marquee with sea sand as a floor.

Ruthie and I would go there for a beautiful lunch of at least four delicious courses and a litre of ice-cold red Provençal wine, all for nine francs.

According to the Michelin Guides, Provence starts just west of Nîmes and Aigues-Mortes and stretches eastwards just beyond Aix-en-Provence, thirty-one kilometres north and a touch east of Marseilles; but to most people, including me, Provence goes all the way east, embracing the Côte d'Azur, or French Riviera, and beyond Nice to the Italian border. It is the hinterland that appeals to me even more than the coast, delightful and fashionable as it is (or used to be). I love the higher, more hilly and mountainous country with its limestone outcrops; the *garrigue* with its great stretches of bare rock and its aromatic thyme, its lavender and its rosemary, and its thistles, its gorse and its scrub oaks; the less arid parts with their umbrella pines, their cypresses, their chestnut trees and and their cork oaks, especially when their ochre trunks are exposed after the stripping of the cork bark; and the valley floors and slopes with their olive trees and their vineyards.

All this glorious country has been described lovingly, and with beautiful dry humour by Marcel Pagnol in the three volumes of his *Souvenirs d'Enfance — La Gloire de mon Père, Le Château de ma Mère*, and *Le Temps des Secrets*. He has also described it in the only novel he ever wrote — *l'Eau des Collines*, which appears in two parts — *Jean de Florette* and *Manon des Sources*. I so loved its beautiful evocation of Provence, and its tenderness and gentle dry humour, that I translated both volumes; just for the fun of it, and not with any intention of publication. But Richard Blackwell insisted that it should be published, and he was kind enough to send it to a number of publishers. I saw the letter from one of their readers (signed Graham Greene, but I don't think *the* Graham Greene), which said 'van Heyningen's translation is perfectly adequate'. That struck me as being a completely satisfactory comment on a translation — anything more than adequacy in a translation would be impertinent interference. The publishers apparently were leery of another translation of Pagnol, since the translation of *Souvenirs d'Enfance* had not sold well. But my translation is still hopefully going the rounds.

A friend of mine at the Pasteur Institute, André Turpin, was a friend of Pagnol's widow, and he told her about my translation, and as a result I was made a member of the Societé des Amies de Marcel Pagnol, and every year I get a bulletin (addressed to 'Sir William') from the Secretary in Marseilles.

But in 1976, after twelve years, we pulled out of La Garde-Freinet. There were several reasons. It was a long way to drive from Le Havre. So many people in so many cars started coming to that part of the world that it took over four hours to drive the twelve miles into St Tropez, or to the beaches. Ugly people took the place of the beautiful people in St Tropez; and on the crowded beaches fat old women took to pulling their over- and under-garments down to their waists. In La Garde-Freinet the honest little shops were taken over by trendy young people selling expensive and useless trinkets, no doubt capitalized by their parents. A great big *Village de Vacances* was being built on the slope behind us for holidays for old folk. Of course one could only rejoice for the old folk, but it added to the disenchantment.

I think Ruthie in her heart of kind hearts would have preferred us entirely to give up the idea of a holiday house in France, though she never said so, bless her, because she knew that I loved having a French foothold. So we looked for another region to seek a house, nearer to England; and we chose Burgundy, since it was within an easy day's drive by car from Le Havre, and at least it had the glamour of its noble vineyards. After some searching, we decided on the little town of Nolay, twelve miles south-west of Beaune, in the Haute (or Arrière) Côte de Beaune of the Côte d'Or, up in the higher country above the Côte de Beaune. There was much to be said for it. It is a pretty little town with a mediaeval centre, mentioned with favour in the guide books to Burgundy; three miles away is the beautiful Château de la Rochepot; the surrounding country is a quite beautiful mixture of vineyards, farmlands with white Charollais cattle, and charming little villages, some of which have interesting names, like Dezize-les-Marranges (in fortunate juxtaposition with Paris-l'Hôpital); others have given their names to famous wines, like Meursault, Pommard, and Volnay; and others have taken their names from famous vineyards, like Puligny- and Chassagne-Montrachet. And not far from Nolay there are many famous and beautiful towns, like Beaune, Dijon, Saulieu, Autun, Nevers[1].

We found a house within a day of arriving in Nolay, in the centre of the town. It was a large house, indeed the largest house I have ever lived in, handsome outside but horrible inside. We knew that our architect daughter Joanna and her architect husband Birkin Haward would be able to make something of it, and indeed they did. We ended up with a most comfortable

[1] See Table on facing page for a selection of Burgundian place names.

Amazey	Nicey
Billy	Poncey
Bondilly	Publey
Borgy	Les Quatre Oeufs
Bouze-les-Beaune	St Boil
Changey	St Forget
Fangey	Ste Opportune
Fussy (le Grand et le Petit)	St Privé
Jambles	St Usage
Joncy	Songey
Maligny	le Trembly

Table: Some Burgundian Place-names

house, with practically the whole ground floor turned into one enormous sitting room, with the kitchen conveniently part of it yet ingeniously separated from it. The messy and confused back yard was converted into a sunny, gravelled, ivy-clad courtyard. The enormous loft, with its beautiful tiled floor, was an additional handsome sitting room, but we never really used it.

For a year or two we were quite happy in this new neighbourhood, exploring the beautiful Burgundian countryside. And we found some new English friends in the neighbouring village of Change. In the early days, when we were settling in, our doorbell rang, and in came a man and a woman. 'We wouldn't have dared to knock on your door if we hadn't had a couple of pastis' said the woman, 'I am Jeanne Hubbard, and this Professor Freddie Fielden, Secretary of the Royal Fine Art Commission.' 'Oh is he?' I said, 'well, I am Doctor Kits van Heyningen, Master of St Cross College, Oxford.' Freddie Fielden and Jeanne Hubbard had adjoining halves of a pretty cottage in Change, where they were joined within a few days by Freddie's dear wife Maggie, who had gone off to Prague on an impulse. That was the beginning of a friendship that continues today, although both families have left Burgundy.

We did not see much of the Fieldens in Nolay, because our visits seldom coincided. That was a pity, because they were the only friends we had in Nolay. The Nolaytois were friendly enough, but social intercourse was sticky because of our lack of easy conversational French, and because they must have found us as dull as we found them. The reason why we had all the social intercourse we needed in La Garde-Freinet was that practically all our friends there had been fellow Britons. In addition to the lack of social intercourse, there was a lack of decent restaurants in Nolay. None of the three in town was any good, and we were no better off in Beaune, because the restaurants there (leaving aside very expensive ones like the Hotel de la Poste, which is very good) were not much better. And it was no fun driving back after dinner having perforce had less Burgundy than I was wont. So we sold the house in Nolay, and now I feel bereft not having a foothold in France. I don't feel as much as I did that I belong to France, and France to me.

This year, nine years after we left La Garde-Freinet, we returned to it to spend a fortnight in Elspeth Schubert's dear little house that she lent us. It had been newly-built in the same size and shape as the tiny decayed *Usine à Gaz* that stood there before, on the Place de la Vieille Fontaine. Being retired, we could go there in September, when the South of France was not crowded. The charm of the village, the beauty of the glorious mountainous countryside, and the nearness of the Mediterranean Sea bordered with enchanting towns like St Tropez, St Raphael, Cannes, Antibes, overwhelmed me again as much as it had when I first came there. And with my French far better than it was when we were last there, I particularly enjoyed the way the Provençaux speak, pronouncing vowels that other Frenchmen do not pronounce, and so making it easier for me to understand them, and they me. My joy at being back again in Provence was nearly submerged by my sorrow that we had ever left this Paradise.

Jane Jack, the St Anne's don, was there, and she came for two drives with us up in the mountains, then down along the coast. Near the *cap* on the end of the Antibes peninsula we passed the Eden Roc on the way to the old town, and on the way back across the foot of the peninsula we were surprised to pass Eden Roc again. We missed our way like this several times, so I wrote a little story about it:

EDENROC.DOC[1]

He and she went to Provence for a fortnight, and never came back.

They had crossed from Folkestone to Boulogne, and thence to Avignon on the car sleeper. On the way to La Garde-Freinet they had stopped for a few hours in Aix-en-Provence, where they had

[1]The computer filename of this document (whoever processed it).

been pleased to find the old core of the city thoughtfully pedestrianised, so that they could walk about peacefully without mechanized harassment.

La Garde-Freinet is an ancient *village perché* up on a col on the Maures *Massif* between the valley of the Argens on the north and the bay of St Tropez twenty kilometres to the south. In the 9th century the invading Saracens had carved a fort out of the hard metamorphic rock dominating the col; and in the following century, with the restoration of the Western Empire as the Holy Roman Empire, a village had been perched just below it like an eagle's nest, as a protection against Germanic invasions, and attacks by Moorish pirates and mercenaries of the Middle Ages and the Renaissance.

There was quite a large foreign element in the village, much of it British, most of them coming there for holidays, a few of them living there permanently. He and she had had a house there for some years in the 1970's, but had given it up. Now they had come to spend a fortnight in a house a British friend had lent them. They were again quite overwhelmed by the charm of the village, the friendliness of the Provençaux, and the beauty of the mountainous Provençal landscape; and inclined to regret their ever having given up their house in the village. Perhaps this was where they first went wrong.

They visited St Tropez several times, pleased to find that a drink at Senequier was still the agreeable experience it always had been, that the lunch at La Fraiche Grotte was still good, and that at the small, glorious, Musée Municipal de l'Annonciade, with its delightful Bonnards and Vuillards, the ground floor was given over to an exhibition of van Dongen's paintings. They bathed with friends at the beaches of La Moutte and of Gigaro.

One morning they drove westwards from near the Saracen fort, along the beautiful, high, slightly perilous *route forestière*, by the Cros-de-Mouton to the Col de Fourche, where they turned south towards Collobrières, still high up in the mountains. From Collobrières they drove eastwards along the extraordinarily rough road to the remains of the Cistercian Chartreuse de la Verne, where the austere, silent, life of the monks evidently had had its luxuries, since each of them had had his own set of rooms, together with his own private ambulatory.

From the Chartreuse they turned back westwards again through Collobrières and then southwards through the Col de Babaou and the Col de Gratteloup, after which they descended steeply through Bormes-les-Mimosas to the Mediterranean Sea at Le Lavandou. From Le Lavandou they travelled eastwards through the string of sparkling seaside towns to the big cross-roads round-about at La Foux, then northwards through Grimaud and up the mountain road back to La Garde-Freinet. They decided that the next day they would continue eastwards along the coast road from La Foux and travel as far as Cap d'Antibes.

The next morning the mountain sky above La Garde-Freinet was dark and ominous. They were inclined to abandon the drive along the coast, but decided, since they had nothing better to do, to risk the bad weather and go. That was a pity — they should have heeded that warning.

As they descended through Grimaud, the weather began rapidly to lighten; and by the time they reached the sea, it was clear and bright. The coastal road ran flatly along the beaches through Beauvallon as far as St Raphael. They paused there for coffee. Thereafter the coast road was cut into the the red porphyric rock of the Esterel *Massif* that rose almost vertically from the sea. The road was high up, and down below the sea by the *Côte* really was brilliantly *d'Azur*. As they drove along through Agay, Mont Vinaigre came into distant view, and nearer-by the massive, beautiful red escarpments, with the slopes below them cloaked with dark green verdure, filled him with nostalgia for the days when he had been a geologist.

They drove through le Trayas and Théoule, then descended steeply, down to la Napoule-Plage at the western end of the long beach of Cannes. They drove down the palm-lined Boulevard de la Croisette by the sea-front of a Cannes that still retained some of the glories peculiar to the Côte d'Azur of days gone by. Beyond the Pointe de la Croisette they reached the Boulevard Guillamont that ran along the beaches of Golfe-Juan and Juan-les-Pins. Suddenly all the charm of the Côte d'Azur was gone. The road was quite horrible, jammed with people, moving cars and parked cars, and it seemed hardly worthwhile continuing on the journey. But they had to go forward because there was no way of turning back.

Then just as suddenly, as they turned off the main road from Juan-les-Pins to Antibes in order to follow the road around the Antibes peninsula to the *cap*, everything became calm and beautiful again. The traffic fell away to almost nothing, and all was quiet and peaceful. It was time for lunch, and they were hungry. They parked the car and walked up the practically empty Boulevard Baudoin. Within a hundred yards they came upon an hotel on their right, on the water's edge. It looked rich in an understated way, and well it might have, for it was the Belles Rives. They decided to be extravagant, and walked in and asked for lunch. They were conducted through the hotel and down the steps beyond to the waterside, the truly *belles rives*. They sat under a blue sunshade at a table on the edge of the water. From where they sat everything was incomparably bright and beautiful. The Mediterranean sparkled in the bright sunlight. It was as if they were in a bygone pre-war age. They ate a small delightful lunch; they drank a half-bottle of a very expensive Provençal rosé[1] (and he heard, or thought he could hear, a distant voice softly singing 'gather ye rosebuds while ye may'; and felt a momentary twinge of fear, of terror).

They tarried quite a long while, then returned to the car and continued along the almost empty Avenue Mai Juin on the seaward edge of the promontory, towards the tiny *cap* at the end of it. Just before they reached it, they passed the Pavillon Eden Roc on the edge of the sea. They continued around the promontory, by the Pointe Bacon, through the old town of Antibes, around by the *vieux port* and the Anse de la Salis to the old Fort Carré.

They had seen all they wanted of Antibes, and were ready to go home along the same coastal route as they had taken out. Having negotiated a complicated one-way system, they got on to the N 98, which should cut across the promontory and lead them back to the crowded Boulevard Guillaumont by means of which they had struggled in the opposite direction through Golfe Juan and Juan-les-Pins some hours previously.

Just as they had braced themselves for the horrors of Guillaumont, they found themselves passing the Eden Roc, and a little later, the Belles Rives. Obviously they had missed a turning, and must retrace their steps. They retraced their steps, and soon found themselves passing Eden Roc again. They tried again, and again they passed Eden Roc. He had prided himself on his ability to find his way by car through strange towns and cities, and now he felt foolish making the same mistake again and again. They tried again. They passed Eden Roc again.

His eyes fell on the clock on the car dashboard. It said three, yet they must have spent at least two or three hours trying to find the way back, and it must be about six. He looked at his wristwatch

---

[1] That of Monsieur Ott.

— it said three, and the sun was still high. He felt again that tingle of fear. He looked at her. Clearly she had felt it too. They tried again and again, but always they passed Eden Roc. They came to a particular bend in the road. He realised that this was where they has been going wrong, and that they should turn right, not left, but he found that his hands were not turning the steering wheel; it was the wheel turning his hands, left. He lifted his hands from the wheel. The car continued its course. He kept his hands off the steering wheel, and soon they passed Eden Roc. They caught each other's eyes. He dropped his hands to his sides. They both knew now they were doomed for eternity to roll around the promontory past Eden Roc.

*

My scientific connections with France continued, largely through the Pasteur Institute in Paris, but there was one near-connection with the University of Montpellier that it fair broke my heart to sacrifice. A Professor Roux of the Medical Faculty had published a paper in a French scientific journal reporting the lethal action of tetanus toxin on amoebae, small organisms just visible to the naked eye, and easily grown in test tubes. This was most important, because it promised to provide a test-tube method of assaying the activity of the toxin that would be much quicker, easier and more accurate than the usual method of assay, which involved determining the lethal dose for mice. I was naturally very pleased about this, and studied the paper more closely. At the end of the paper, Professor Roux stated that he had confirmed his observation with all but one of the several samples of tetanus toxin supplied to him by different workers. That one sample that did not show the effect was the one that had been sent to him by André Turpin of the Pasteur Institute. I knew that Turpin was the only one of them who was really capable of purifying tetanus toxin, and that his sample was most likely to consist of nothing but tetanus toxin. The effects observed with all the other samples of toxin were obviously due to impurities that had nothing to do with the toxin. Hardly had I come to that conclusion than I received a letter from Professor Roux, telling me about his marvellous observation, and inviting me to come to Montpellier and spend a month or two in his laboratory exploiting his great discovery. I would have liked nothing better. I had always wanted to visit Montpellier, and had a great respect for its ancient university, but what could I do? There was only one thing for me to do. I wrote to poor Professor

Roux, breaking the news as gently as I could, that in effect he had discovered nothing at all. He sent me a courteous reply, which I was glad to have, because I had feared I would get no reply at all.

I had good friends and colleagues in the Pasteur Institute in Paris, and visited them many times on scientific business. In June 1959 I had been invited to lecture on my newly discovered fixation of tetanus toxin by ganglioside. Knowing my ignorance of French, they kindly told me I could give my lecture in English. But largely with the help of a friend I translated it into French, and then I got a young Frenchwoman who taught French at the Wychwood school to teach me how to pronounce it in passable French. At the Pasteur Institute the Chairman of the meeting announced that I would be giving my lecture in English, but when I got up I gave it in French, and they seemed to understand what I was saying. At least they cheered loudly, and asked many questions afterwards.

I then began to teach myself French by means of Linguaphone, supplemented by other courses on records and tapes, and found that my ease with Afrikaans was a help with French pronunciation; particularly with their Rs and their 'u' as in rue, which of course must not be pronounced 'roo', but 'r(ee)', where the brackets signify pursed lips as one breathes out the 'ee'. The difficulty for most would-be French speakers is not only pursing the lips, but pursing and unpursing them in rapid succession.

In June 1974, I was invited again to lecture at the Pasteur Institute. This was to be a grand lecture, the Louis Rapkine Memorial Lecture, and I was told I was to give it in French. The librarian of the Maison Française in Oxford translated it for me, and I read it over and over to my dear friends, Professor (of French Literature) and Madame Jean Seznec, until they were satisfied. The great day came, André Lwoff introduced me with the words I have quoted on the first page, and I gave my lecture. I had wanted to call it 'Les Delices de l'Ignorance', because all my life I have been more ignorant than people realised, but somehow I had managed to struggle on. But it seemed arrogant to expect people to come to a lecture without knowing what it was to be about, so I called it 'Les récepteurs des Membranes Cellulaires pour les Toxines Tétanique et Cholérique, ou les Délices de l'Ignorance'. They gave me a medal, and there was a great reception afterwards. There the Baronne Rothschild startled me by exclaiming 'Mais vous étiez si passionnant!' It was only later that I learned that 'passionnant' means not what it seems to mean, but 'exciting, absorbing'.

This chapter has a very happy ending for me. In August 1980 I received a letter from the French Embassy in London informing me that I was to receive a French decoration. This was followed by a reception in the Maison Française in Oxford at which the French Scientific Counsellor addressed me thus:

C'est un grand plaisir pour moi, et aussi une vive satisfaction, d'être ici pour honorer le Dr William van Heyningen.

J'ai pour vous, cher ami, une grande estime à laquelle se joint une profonde admiration. Je suis heureux que, par mon intermédiaire, le gouvernement français vous témoigne cette marque de distinction.

En tant que scientifique, je suis, en outre, fort honoré d'avoir à vous remettre cette décoration.

Vos principales contributions scientifiques se situent dans le champ des toxines bactériennes et vos premiers travaux ont porté sur les toxines de Clostridium welchii et plus particulièrement sur les toxines alpha et kappa que vous avez purifiées. Ces travaux, effectués d'abord à Cambridge avec Marjory Stephenson, puis à Beckenham avec Oakley, furent les premiers du genre. De même, vous fûtes le premier à purifier la toxine de la dysenterie at à mettre en évidence son extrême toxicité contrairement à ce que l'on pensait à l'époque, et également le premier à montrer que la production de cette toxine avait un lien avec la concentration en fer et en cytochrome.

Tous ces travaux effectués à Oxford avec Florey (l'un des prix Nobel de la pénicilline) vous ont conduit à écrire un excellent ouvrage scientifique sur les toxines, qui fut à l'époque un document de travail d'une haute valeur scientifique.

Vers 1956, vous avez entrepris des études sur le tétanos qui vous ont amené à montrer que les gangliosides agissaient comme récepteur dans le tissu nerveux pour la toxine du tétanos.

Aprés le tétanos, vous vous êtes intéressé au choléra; là encore, vous avez été un précurseur, montrant que les gangliosides étaient des récepteurs pour la toxine du choléra.

En dehors de vos travaux purement scientifiques, vous avez consacré une partie de votre temps à des tâches diverses; c'est ainsi que vous avez été secrétaire de la Sociétée Générale de Microbiologie; en outre, vous avez également enseigné et administré.

Jusqu'à un passé recent, vous avez été Reader en Chimie bactérienne à la 'Sir William Dunn School' à Oxford, dont la réputation est mondiale, et Master de St Cross College à Oxford. Dans ces dernières fonctions, vous avez accompli une tâche difficile dans laquelle vous avez particulièrement bien réussi.

A titre personnel, j'ajouterai que j'ai une autre raison de me réjouir de la distinction qui vous est offerte aujourd'hui. Vous avez commencé votre vie en Afrique du Sud, vous vivez aujourd'hui en Grande-Bretagne aprés avoir séjourné aux Etats-Unis, et vous trouvez le temps de venir en France où vous avez un domicile, et vous avez traduit en anglais deux livres de Marcel Pagnol. Vous avez en outre beaucoup voyagé. En d'autres termes, vous avez une large vision du monde et, mieux que d'autres, vous êtes en mesure d'y saisir les différences mais aussi les complémentarités existant entre les diverses communautés des pays occidentaux. Votre grande expérience scientifique et humaine est particulièrement bénéfique pour le développement de la coopération entre nos deux pays, la Grande-Bretagne at la France.

Dr van Heyningen, au nom du Président de la République et des pouvoirs qui me sont conférés, je vous nomme Chevalier de l'Ordre National du Mérite.

[It is a great pleasure and a profound satisfaction for me to be here to honour Dr William van Heyningen.

I have a great regard for you, dear friend, and a profound admiration. I am happy that the French Government bestows this mark of distinction on you through me.

Your principal scientific contributions lie in the field of bacterial toxins, and your first works were on the toxins of Clostridium welchii, particularly on the alpha and kappa toxins which you purified. These researches, done first at Cambridge with Marjory Stephenson, then at Beckenham with Oakley, were the first of their kind. Similarly, you were the first to purify dysentery toxin and to demonstrate its extreme toxicity, contrary to what was thought at the time, and also the first to show that the production of this toxin was connected with the concentration of iron and cytochrome.

All this work, done at Oxford with Florey (of the Nobel Prize for penicillin), lead you to write an excellent scientific book on toxins, which at that time was of high scientific value.

Towards 1956, you undertook studies on tetanus that lead you to demonstrate that gangliosides acted as receptors for tetanus toxin in nervous tissue.

After tetanus you interested yourself in cholera; there again you were a forerunner, showing that gangliosides were receptors for cholera toxin.

Besides your purely scientific works you have devoted part of your time to diverse tasks; thus you were secretary of the Society for General Microbiology; in addition, you have also taught and administered.

Until recently you were Reader in Bacterial Chemistry in the Sir William Dunn School at Oxford, with its world-wide reputation, and Master of St Cross College, Oxford. In these latter capacities you have accomplished a difficult task in which you have succeeded particularly well.

On the personal side, I would add that I have another reason to rejoice at the distinction that is offered to you today. You started your life in South Africa, you live today in England after having spent some time in the United States, and you find the time to come to France, where you have a house, and you have translated two of Marcel Pagnol's books into English. Besides that, you have travelled a great deal. In other words, you have a large vision of the world, and, more than others, you are in a position to understand the differences and the similarities among the diverse communities of the western world. Your great scientific and humane experience is particularly beneficial for the development of the cooperation between our two countries, Great Britain and France.

Dr van Heyningen, in the name of the President of the Republic and under the powers conferred on me, I name you Knight of the National Order of Merit.]

With that he pinned the medal of the Order of Merit on me, and gave me a little blue ribbon to wear on my lapel. The next time I went to France, I thought all the *gendarmes* would salute me, but nobody paid any attention. I don't suppose they noticed, or they thought it some British decoration. The only time it was ever noticed was in New York, twice, on the same day.

12

SOUTH AFRICA, 1984

Ruthie and I spent the months of March and April 1984 in the four provinces of the Republic of South Africa, and in South West Africa. We flew by South African Airways to Cape Town, where Customs were not as friendly as they might have been. They imposed a punishing duty on some little silver-plated picture frames with inscriptions on them, intended as thank-you presents for the relations we were going to stay with, and when I protested that they had no commercial value since they had personal inscriptions on them, I was brushed aside in a manner that gave me the uneasy feeling we were entering a police state. And we were to have a relieved feeling that we were leaving a police state when we flew back from Johannesburg, and were spoken to again in the same uncouth way by uniformed officials. But between those two mildly nasty moments we had a marvellous time, and I came away thinking that there was just a chance of hope for South Africa, provided the rest of the world allowed them to work out their own salvation, that is, the salvation of both the Blacks and the Whites. This is not to say they don't need some stimulation to get on with it. Since I have touched on the subject, I might as well grasp the nettle now, and state what I think about the situation in South Africa.

But first, over-simplifying history, I must remind the British that it can be said that it was they who were largely responsible for the present position of the Blacks. It was a matter of British goodness before the Boer War being frustrated at the end of that war, at the Treaty of Vereeniging in May 1902, by the British greed that had brought about that war. British rule over the Cape Colony (and I suppose the Natal colony) before the war had been good in that there had been equal franchise for Blacks and Whites. At Vereeniging, the delegates from the Natal and Cape Colonies argued for equal franchise in the new Union of South Africa whose constitution they were drawing up. The delegates from what was now called the Orange River Colony, who had always been drawn to the Cape (see Chapter 1), would have voted with them, but having been unwillingly drawn by the 1897 treaty of mutual defence on to the side of the Transvaal Republic during the Boer War, they voted reluctantly with the Transvaal against equal franchise; and thus it was defeated.

I am against apart-hate (spelt *apartheid*), and the Bishop of the Indian Ocean is no holier than me in this respect. Therefore I was glad to see that things had changed since I was last in South Africa in 1953 — not enough, but I think significantly. After we were met by my brother, the genuine Kits (and from then on I was Willie), and his daughter Elizabeth at the airport, we went to lunch in our hotel; and as we walked into the restaurant, I was astonished to be preceded by a Black family, and by the sight of many other Blacks already seated in the restaurant. This was something I would never remotely have dreamed of in my day in South Africa, nor yet in 1953. Again in the very grand Carlton Hotel in Johannesburg there were perhaps more Blacks than Whites in the big lobby (and more Whites than Blacks in the restaurants); and in South West Africa the relationship between Blacks and Whites seemed to be even easier. Those in Britain and elsewhere who are unwilling to be informed and are unshakable in their righteousness maintain that all this is nothing more than a meaningless veneer. But I believe that now that this liberalisation has started, it can't be stopped. It is bound to go on of its own momentum, and as it goes on, it will accelerate; and as it proceeds, both the Whites and the Blacks will adapt to the changing situation. I am not suggesting that the change should be left to its own volition. It needs constant forceful nudging; but the worst thing that could happen would be a violent push.

If Black majority rule were to be imposed overnight, as the Bishop of the Indian Ocean would like, it would be as much a disaster for the Blacks as for the Whites. If I were a Black in Africa today I would be unfortunate, but for my own safety and material comfort I would rather be in South Africa than in any of the Black states of Africa. I have not yet heard the comments of the Bishop of the Indian Ocean on the unfortunate state of the people in these Black states. Perhaps he has not made any, and I would not blame him under his circumstances. The Black slums in South Africa are of course perfectly terrible, but have you seen how the Blacks live in other parts of Africa? The reason why I have my knife in the Bishop of the Indian Ocean, otherwise known as Trevor Huddlestone, is that I saw and heard him not long ago on Peter Sissons' news broadcast on Channel 4 of the television. Sissons was interviewing the South African

Ambassador, and Huddlestone about the position of the Blacks in South Africa, and the Ambassador was putting his unpopular case. He did so with as much reason and good sense as the circumstances in South Africa permitted, and even if I was by no means in complete agreement with him, it was obvious that he had to be heard. But Huddlestone wouldn't let him be heard, and kept shouting interruptions. I thought his unshakable self-righteousness and intolerance were odious and lacking in my non-Christian perception of the Christian spirit.

Of course there are still far too many South African Whites, English and Afrikaans, who don't like the changes that have already taken place in South Africa, and would like to stave off any further changes forever; but they are doomed, because those changes are going to take place. Even the South African Government is beginning to recognize that change must take place, but the pace they are moving at is too slow, and I expect their objectives are too limited. It would be a disaster if a change were made as suddenly as the self-righteous in Britain and America (not forgetting would-be President Edward Kennedy) would like, because it would precipitate violence and dreadful misery that would not help the Blacks at all. Radical changes must certainly be made, neither too quickly, nor too slowly. What would be neither too quick nor too slow? A time must be put on it in advance, with agreed defined stages; and my guess is ten years.

My brother Kits belongs to a political party called the Progressive Federal Party (and so, I believe, does my friend Danie Craven, the great rugby hero of South Africa). The PFP believes in equality for all in South Africa. They would like to see a National Convention bringing about a Federal Government (as in the United States of America) of a Federation of as many self-governing States as necessary to represent all the different groups of peoples in South Africa (with any individual having the right to belong to any State of his choosing). This Federal Government would not be run on the winner-take-all principle, and all points of view would have a say. No general policy would be adopted unless it were agreed by the majority of States, any one of which would have the right of veto; on the other hand, no policy that was close to general agreement could be frustrated by the veto by a minority less than ten to twenty percent. Unfortunately the PFP is not a very powerful party, which is a pity, because I believe its policies could be the saving of South Africa.

It is important for South Africa to be saved, for the sake of the rest of Africa as well as its own. All Africa is in a poor state, but with South Africa in a good state, with its high proportion of educated people (for the present almost exclusively White), it could be an example and a help to the other states. I hope it is not too late.

To return to our tour of South Africa: I was terribly disappointed by Cape Town, which, with its perfect setting between the Table Bay and Table Mountain, and its beautiful old Cape Dutch buildings and streets, I had always regarded as one of the finest cities of the world. But now it is dotted about with a number of wide skyscrapers of seemingly deliberate gracelessness. I don't object to the principle of skyscrapers — but they must be lean like those in New York, and subject to the Principle of Categorical Propinquity as formulated in Chapter 3.

Kits was staying with his daughter Elizabeth, who is Lecturer in the History faculty of the University of Cape Town, in Rondebosch, a suburb of Cape Town, and he kindly lent us his car, which enabled Ruthie and me to drive all around the Cape Peninsula — 'the fairest cape of them all', as Drake so rightly said to Queen Elizabeth I. It is a mixture of California and the French Riviera, and were I not perfectly content with Oxford and Europe (and not scared of living in South Africa), I would gladly live there. From Cape Town Ruthie and I drove thirty miles to spend a week in Stellenbosch, which, with its fine old Cape Dutch buildings on its oak-lined streets, was as beautiful as ever; and so was the glorious, vineyard-clad and mountainous countryside around it. I was invited to call on the Rector of my old University; and when the Registrar asked me if there was anybody else I wanted to see, I said yes, my old friend Danie Craven, who is regarded as being very close to God in rugby-mad South Africa. He is a sort of Emeritus Professor of Rugby at the University, besides being the Head of the South African Rugby Board. When Danie and I were first-year men at Stellenbosch, he was going to be a *tokkelok*, or theology student, believing with immovable conviction that the earth was flat. None of my scientific protestations had any effect — he simply countered them with the statement that the Bible said the world was flat (at any rate, the Bible refers to the four corners of the earth). As soon as I was ushered into the great man's presence, I started hurling abuse to him in Afrikaans. Was he still so *dom* as to think the world was flat? *Ag nee, man* he replied. But he had told me the Bible said the world was flat, I said. *Ag man, die Bybel lieg,* said Danie, and the Registrar nearly fainted.

Kits drove us all around South Africa, which was fine, and

convenient, for me as well as Ruthie, who is very fond of him. We visited many Higgs relations and some van Heyningen relations, but I will not impose an account of those visits on you.

One of the places we visited was Brandfort, where I was last in 1920, aged eight years. It was a moving and pleasant experience for me, because all the buildings that I must have known those many years ago, but could not remember, were still there in a good state, two of them being used for the same purpose as they had been in my time; and my brother Kits knew where they all were. There was the school we went to, a really handsome building that I am proud of; there was my father's Magistrate's Court, which was even more handsome; there was the house that we first lived in, and where my mother died, while the *Drosdy* (the Magistrate's official residence, pronounced dross-day) was being renovated for us; and there was that *Drosdy*, now no longer a *Drosdy*.

We also visited the little town of Fauresmith, where my father had been Public Prosecutor Assistant Magistrate; and where he and my mother had set up their first home; and whence he had been taken Prisoner of War by the British on 15 October 1900, and transported for two years to Ceylon. The town still had a very old-fashioned air, and I don't believe it was much different from the town that my parents knew. From Fauresmith we drove via nearby Jagersfontein (in the diamond mine of which my father had spent his first night of imprisonment), to have a look at Reddersburg, that horrible hell-hole where we lived after my father died. I wasn't able to find the house we had lived in, and although the town had changed and grown somewhat, it still looked like a hell-hole.

We drove the forty miles on to Bloemfontein, whence the next day we flew to Keetmanshoop in South West Africa. As our aircraft flew low to touch down at Keetmanshoop, my first feeling was one of disappointment. Instead of the fiercely arid desert countryside I had loved so much sixty years ago, the land was carpeted with green, and ablaze with beautiful yellow flowers. The triennial, or quadrennial, or quinquennial, miracle had happened — the rain had fallen, and the land was covered with spreading green thorn bushes and their yellow flowers. But if I was disappointed, Ruthie was delighted. There was another surprise for us when we landed, and it was entirely delightful for both of us. A pleasant couple approached us and asked if we were the van Heyningens. They were Hans and Shirley Botma, and they had been asked by the Control Magistrate of

Keetmanshoop to meet us. He was Mr Truter, to whom I had written previously to ask if I could call on him when I got to Keetmanshoop. Hans Botma was a South African-born lawyer and Shirley was an English woman who had by now been many years in Keetmanshoop. They were marvellously kind to us, showing us the town, inviting their friends to meet us in their house, driving us about the countryside, even lending us their car so that we could do our own driving as well. They made a great difference to our visit. The Control Magistrate was equally kind when we met him in his office, and he was very interested in my father's having been the first British magistrate of Keetmanshoop.

Keetmanshoop had changed so much that it was no longer recognizable. The Residency that we had lived in was gone, and so were most of the old German buildings that I had known. They were replaced by nondescript buildings of no charm or interest. The streets were all tarred, and no longer six inches deep in sand. There were no more Herero women in their long dresses, their leg-of-mutton sleeves and their tall turbans. There were no Bushmen, but we did at least meet two small wagons on the outskirts of town, each with a Hottentot family on board. I asked the leader of one of them if they were *Bondelswarts*, and he said no, *Veldskoendraers*; I asked the other if they were *Veldskoendraers* and he said no, *Bondelswarts*.

We drove in Hans Botma's car far out westwards, past Seeheim, into completely empty country, hoping to see some really arid country, and at last we did find some that was passably arid. But we couldn't find the sand dunes that I used to play in, and still remembered so vividly. I asked the Botmas about them, but they were mystified. They were not aware of any big stretches of sand dunes, and had never heard of them. Nor had Mr Truter, nor any other of their friends. But I know there were sand dunes in the 1920s, and I wish some physiographer would look into them for me.

Then we flew to Windhoek, the capital of South West Africa, which also but hardly surprisingly was entirely different from the Windhoek I remembered as a keen Boy Scout in the 1920s. It was full of demi-skyscrapers; and little was left of the old German town, except a small row of preserved old buildings on the main street, a fine Rhenish church, and the would-be Rhine *Schlossen* on the surrounding hills, but they were fewer, smaller and far less interesting than I remembered, and hardly visible in a smother of suburbia. In Windhoek there were some Herero women, but they were a travesty of the Herero women I knew. I suppose they must have been in the employ of the Windhoek Tourist Board. Their dresses were still long, but no longer with the tight bodices and the leg-of-mutton sleeves; and their turbans, instead of taughtly curving 18 inches up, were flat-topped and flopped out sideways. They were to be found sitting on the floor in the lobbies of hotels, selling little models of themselves. All their dignity was gone.

From Windhoek we travelled in an excellent coach, with a good crew and pleasant company, to the Etosha Game Reserve in the north, close to the border with Angola. We started westwards through the Namib Desert to Walvis Bay, and at last my desire for aridity and fierce heat was satisfied. First we went through the highlands of the desert, and it was really mean country, with nothing to adorn it but black rocks and an occasional thorn bush. I loved it. Then we came to the lowlands, which were even meaner, with no vegetation at all except the occasional *Welwichia*, a cactus-like plant said to be over 2000 years old. When we reached Walvis Bay, it had become a seaside holiday place with colonies of small, quite good-looking holiday houses. I was pleased to see Swakopmund again, since it did not seem to have changed. All the handsome old German buildings were still there, and I understand that they are to be preserved. Then we went to the game reserve, which we liked, but I don't intend to give an account of that, except to report that I came away with a photograph of a couple of copulating camelopards looking like a couple of aberrant Eiffel Towers.

Our visit to South Africa came to its end in Johannesburg, where we met several of my van Heyningen relations, including my cousin Margarieta van Rooyen, daughter of my father's sister Boudina, who had died of typhoid in the dreadful Bloemfontein concentration camp during the Boer War, leaving the baby Margarieta and her baby sister and brother to be looked after by strangers, since their father was in another concentration camp in South Africa, but nobody knew where. Apart from my splendid relations, Ruthie and I did not really much enjoy our stay in Johannesburg, largely because we were scared to move anywhere. We had been warned several times that our hotel was in a dangerous part, and the possibility of being mugged had seriously to be considered; and the rest of Johannesburg, they said, was not much safer. You were liable to be attacked by three villians moving about separately, but closing in on you from different directions when the time was right. So we crept about somewhat fearfully and warily, and, having seen all we wanted to see, and having met all whom we wanted to meet, we were relieved to fly home.

I have lived a charmed life, surrounded by a loved and loving family at home and abroad, blessed with good friends, fortunate in everything I've undertaken. I thought I might call this autobiography 'The Autobiography of a Contented Man', but Joanna made a scornful moue and said, 'Why don't you call it *The Key to Lockjaw*.'

APPENDIX

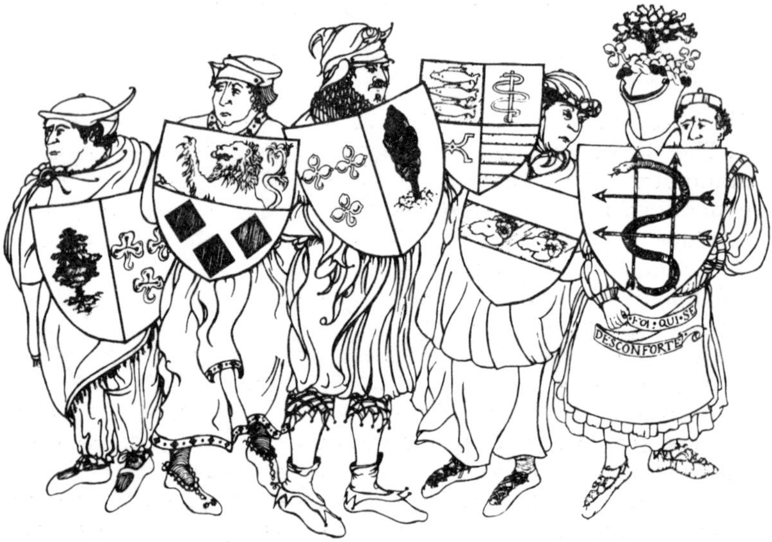

Fig. 3. Escutcheons. From left to right: (a) Hendrik van Heyningen (—Kits); (b) Hendrik van Heyningen; (c) George Philips Kits van Heyningen; (d) van Hoei Schildhouder, with the Velse arms, and below, those of Tulleken; (e) William Edward van Heyningen.

DIVERS ORIGINS

The Dutch

The *Nederland's Patriciaat* in the Centraal Bureau voor Genealogie in The Hague gives the six generations preceding my paternal grandfather. This has been possible, obviously, because each generation has had at least one male child who has survived to produce a male child. I could just as well have been more interested in tracing the female line, but things being what they are, that has not been possible. What follows is of interest only to my family and close friends.

My earliest traceable van Heyningen ancestor was Mees Claeszoon (i.e. son of Claes) van Heyningen, of Uithoorn near Amsterdam, who married Grietje Gerrits in the early 1670s. This was just about the time that Dom Pérignon invented champagne, hardly in time for the wedding. The dates of birth of Mees Claeszoon and of his first-born son are not known because the christening records of that period are missing. Since Mees was married in the 1670s, I suppose he was born about 1650. He was the atavism of my grandfather Petrus Arnoldus Conradus, who emigrated to South Africa in 1858. (I had always thought that 'atavism' had generally to do with remote ancestry, but recently I found that its Latin origin is 'a great-grandfather's grandfather', and that is the meaning I will use.)

This was the time when Rembrandt was still living; and before Robert Boyle wrote *The Sceptical Chemist*, or Isaac Newton wrote *Optics*, or Milton wrote *Paradise Lost*; or Christopher Wren began the rebuilding of St Paul's Cathedral, or von Leibnitz invented differential and integral calculus. Holland was in its Golden Age of commerce, with the Dutch merchant fleet numerically exceeding the combined fleets of England, France, Spain, Russia and Germany; and Amsterdam was the world's banking capital. It was also the Golden Age of Dutch art, when painters like Pieter de Hooch and Jan Vermeer (which unfortunately to an *Afrikaner* means John Vomit) changed the course of art by showing the world as it was, with ordinary people rather than virgins, saints or nymphs; and still lifes of ordinary things. But it was also a troubled age, with frequent wars and changes of alliance with Spain, France, Germany, Sweden and England. In 1652 Holland was for the first time at war with England, where Cromwell was at the zenith of his power. The Dutch Admiral de Ruyter was defeated by Blake, but revenged by van Tromp, who took a number of English ships off Dungeness and led them up the Channel with a broom lashed to his masthead. Peace with England was signed in 1653, but war broke out again in 1665. In June 1667 the Dutch fleet under de Ruyter practically destroyed English naval power when he sailed up the Medway, raided Chatham Docks, and made off with the Royal Barge, the Royal Charles. In the following month the Peace of Breda was signed by England with Holland and France. By the next year England, Holland and Sweden signed an alliance against France, but in 1670 England deserted Holland, and joined France and Germany two years later. William of Orange rose, and in 1673 the Dutch captured New York, and in the next year the English withdrew from Holland. In 1677 William married Princess Mary of England, and twelve years later became King of England.

This was the time too when the origins of the Boer nation were being laid down in South Africa. The Dutch East India Company, in its trade with the East Indies, needed to establish a halfway house — a refreshment station — on its new route around the Cape of Good Hope. In 1652 Jan van Riebeeck landed on the Cape Peninsula for this purpose and founded Cape Town. (I learned this fact in my tender years at school in South Africa, and it puzzled me, for in my mind refreshments were lemonade and cakes, and I could not understand how John Company could be so frivolous as to have so important a need for them, nor where in such an untamed country they could be found.)

The atavism of my father, Jacob Meeszoon van Heyningen, was born 'presumably before 1675'. The presumption is necessitated by the absence of Uithoorn birth records, and is based on the fact that the birth of his father's next child was recorded in Nieuwendam in 1675. On 14 May 1702 he married a girl with a name that is unpronouncable in English, Trijntje Outgers Out, and they had five children, three of whom died young. The first of the five, born at Oostzaan on 28 February 1703, was Claas, my atavism. Claas married Grietje Vroom on 18 April 1728, and they had seven children, but only one survived, which survival was just as well for me. He was Jacob, my two children's atavism, born at Oostzaan on 6 February 1738.

Jacob van Heyningen was first a baker, then in 1762 he built the 'Snuff or Powder Mill De Heyning'. He became Alderman, and then Burgomaster of the juridical district of Oostzaan. At this stage the van Heyningen line again nearly came to an end. Jacob married three times. First in 1755 to Lijsje Jans de Jong, who bore him two children who died young; then in 1758 to Jouki Boekhout, who bore him five children, all of whom died young; then, and finally, in May 1780, to Maria van Weenen, who bore him four children, two of whom died young. It must have been dreadfully sad, those nine children dying so young, and those three unfortunate wives. The second of the surviving children was Hendrik van Heyningen, the atavism of my four grandchildren, born at Oostzaan on 22 October 1787, the year the Philadelphia Convention met under George Washington to frame the Constitution of the United States of America, and the MCC moved to Lord's.

Hendrik van Heyningen was the father of my grandfather. He was a distinguished man. He went to the Latin School and the Athenaeum in Amsterdam, and then to the University of Leiden. He became a predikant in the established Dutch Church, known as the *Nederduitse Hervormde Kerk,* first in Langerak just north of Amsterdam, then in Rijswijk, now a suburb of The Hague, and then Meppel in the province of Drenthe. He was also chaplain with the Dutch Army in Holland and Belgium. He served on the high councils of the church, and wrote many theological books and articles, not, I fear, of interest to me. In 1842 King Willem II appointed him Knight of the Order of the Netherlands Lion. Ruthie and I recently visited Meppel and were well received at his immense magnificent church, beautiful inside and outside, with a striking tall clock tower.

Now enter Wilhelmina Gerardina Kits. She was born in Maastricht on 2 May 1794, the daughter of George Philip Kits and Maria Schermbeek. According to Adrienne Kits van Heyningen van Beusekom (p.2), Wilhelmina Kits was a proud and aristocratic woman. Proud she certainly was, but I have not been able to confirm her aristocratic quality. All the *Centraal Bureau voor Genealogie* in The Hague could tell me was that her father was a *kapitein van kleeding* (captain of clothing) in the *Bataillon Infanterie* of Ligne. Adrienne told me that when Hendrik proposed marriage to Wilhelmina, she agreed to it on condition that their first-born son should assume the surname Kits van Heyningen, and that is what he did. As if to make up for the terrible losses suffered by his father, Hendrik and his (only) wife produced thirteen children between 1816 and 1833, who died at an average age of 65 years, the last of them being my grandfather. The first child was a girl, Maria. The second was a boy, born at Rijswijk on 4 April 1817, christened and officially registered as George Philips [*sic*] Kits with the surname van Heyningen. However, he has his own sub-heading in the *Patriciaat*, and in a Dutch ecclesiastical biography, under the surname Kits van Heyningen, and all his successors, including Adrienne, have that surname, so it must be that George Philips' surname was deliberately changed to Kits van Heyningen, and I shall produce some heraldic evidence of this.

George Philips Kits van Heyningen followed his father in a scholarly and distinguished career in the Church. In 1844 he married Johanna Abrahamina Trip, who came from a grand family to judge by the fact that there are three slightly varying armorials for Trip in J.-B.Rietstap's well-known *Planches de l'Armorial Géneral* [28]. My father's youngest sister, Caroline (Cara) Hill, remembers meeting George Philips and Johanna Abrahamina in 1902. She had sailed after the Boer War with her father and her sister Ada from South Africa to Holland, and they had arrived late one night to visit them in The Hague (where they spent the first night in a hotel near the station, which they learned the next day was in fact a brothel). She found them 'a real Darby-and-Joan couple', and very well-off, having been left a great deal of money by one of his parishioners.

After George Philips there were six more girls and five more boys, all plain van Heyningens. Philippina married a bookseller in Delft called Willem Beets, brother of the poet Nicolaas Beets. (Once in a coffee shop Nicolaas competed with another poet to produce the shortest poem. The other poet put his knife in the butter and smeared it on Nicolaas's coat, crying '*Vet smet*!' [fat dirties!]; Nicolaas instantly smashed his fist into his opponent's nose, roaring '*Ik tik*!' [I hit!]). Jacoba was a well-known literary figure; Willem Hendrik was Editor of the *Middelburgsche Courant*; Frederik Willem is said by my Aunt Cara to have eloped with an heiress, run through her money, fought a duel and killed his opponent, and fled to England, where he started a margarine factory and became very rich; the next one, Hendrik, was not such a black sheep — he was a Lieutenant-Colonel in the army, and like his father, a Knight of the Order of the Netherlands Lion; finally there was my grandfather, Petrus Arnoldus Conradus (whose first names were carried on by my younger brother), born in Meppel on 29 July 1833. In that year Johannes

Brahms, Edward Burne-Jones and Alfred Nobel were also born; and Britain proclaimed sovereignty over the Falkland Islands; and — two events that were later to affect my life — John Keble started the Oxford Movement (not the much later odious Oxford Group!), and the Second Cholera Pandemic was raging for the first time in Europe and North America. Twenty-five years later he went to South Africa.

None of George Philips Kits' siblings were given the name Kits, nor, as far as I know, were any of their offspring, but my elder brother has practically the same first names, George Philipus Kits, and the name has its place on two of the family escutcheons and on the crest of my coat of arms (fig.3e) The van Heyningen escutcheon is displayed in Rietstap's armorial and in Vosterman van Oyen's *Stam- en Wapenboek van Aanzienlijke Nederlandsche Familien*. It is divided horizontally with a rampant lion in chief and three lozenges in base, as shown in fig.3b. Since it displays a rampant lion, and since we have seen that Hendrik's forebears were not particularly distinguished, I now conclude that it was Hendrik's escutcheon, which he acquired on being appointed Knight of the Order of the Netherlands Lion in 1842. What had diverted me from this escutcheon previously was the fact I have a sketch, made I don't know when, and sent to me many years ago by my cousin Margaret Hoskyn, of a van Heyningen coat of arms, the impaled escutcheon of which is copied in fig. 3a. On the dexter side there is a tree of indeterminate character, and on the sinister three trefoils (in heraldry the sides of an escutcheon are reversed in the eye of the beholder because they are given from the eye of the holder behind it). Now this becomes interesting — to me at any rate — because of what I learned in the early 1970s, when I met Mr John Brooke-Little, then Richmond Herald of Arms, now Norroy and Ulster King of Arms, of the College of Arms in London. It was he who introduced me to Lewis Kirby, whom I mentioned in Chapter 9. Lewis Kirby has a really profound knowledge of heraldry, and in 1972 he urged me to apply to the College of Arms for a Grant of Armorial Bearings. I had no particular interest in having my own armorial bearings, but I thought it expedient, in order to retain his interest, to apply for them. These were granted to me in November 1972. In the Certificate of the Grant of Arms there is a statement based on enquiries made in The Netherlands by a Dutch correspondent of the College of Arms which reads in part as follows : 'he is descended from a family once seated in Oostzaan in The Netherlands and which later settled in South Africa ... his family had ... certain armorial bearings (videlicet: Per pale Argent and Or on the dexter side three Trefoils slipped Sable and on the sinister upon a Mount in base proper a Poplar Tree Vert)', see fig. 3c. Thus the arms described by the College of Arms differ from those in fig. 3a in that the sides of the tree (now a recognizable poplar) and the trefoils are reversed. Since the dexter side is the more important, it seems likely that the arms studied by the College of Arms are those of George Philips Kits van Heyningen, the first-born son of Hendrik van Heyningen and Wilhelmina Gerardina Kits. Indeed, it must certainly be so, since I had specifically asked Richmond Herald to inquire into the Kits van Heyningen family, thinking at that time that we were all Kits van Heyningens, and knowing that the name van Heyningen, though not common, was not particular to our family. When I recently studied the van Heyningen section in the *Nederlands Patriciaat* in The Hague, showing Hendrik van Heyningen's escutcheon, I found the section had a sub-heading 'Kits van Heyningen', and a note describing the Kits van Heyningen escutcheon in the same terms as those used by the Dutch correspondent of the College of Arms, and recently Adrienne Kits van Heyningen van Beusekom sent me a photocopy of the same escutcheon, maintaining that the three trefoils were Kits trefoils. This is also maintained in an article on the Kits van Heyningen arms by H. M. W. Kits Nieuwenkamp in *De Navorscher,* 1927, on the grounds that trefoils are a heraldic device of the North Dutch provinces of Friesland and Groningen, and that since George Philips Kits van Heyningen was a predikant in Akkrum in Friesland it was natural that he should adopt it. How does that make it a Kits symbol? And what about the tree, which the author does not mention? I think his idea of the origins of the trefoils is poppycock, and I suggest that after Hendrik van Heyningen and the imperious Wilhelmina Gerardina Kits moved to Meppel in 1830, and before he was made Knight of the Order of the Netherlands Lion in 1842, and so acquired the escutcheon at 3b, he made up the escutcheon shown at 3a. The tree, I suggest with not too much confidence, might have been the best representation he could think of for his own name, since a *heyning* is a hedge (cf the English surname Hedges), and a hedge is made up of trees. As to the acquisition of the trefoils, I think it pre-dates George Philips Kits' growing up and becoming a predikant in Akkrum. Three trefoils, I found recently in Meppel, have been connected with Hendrik's beautiful church since 1657 at the latest. I suggest that Hendrik gave them to his wife, put the tree on the more important dexter side of his escutcheon and impaled his wife's newly acquired trefoils to signify van Heyningen Kits; and his first-born son many years later reversed the order to signify Kits van Heyningen.

Fig. 3e is a sketch of the Achievement of Arms granted to me by the College of Arms. It is the outcome of discussions I had with Lewis Kirby. He suggested that my family connections, that is, the van Heyningen tree and the Kits trefoils, should be incorporated in the Crest, but instead of a poplar tree I chose the only tree I used to know in the South West African desert where I spent my boyhood, the camel thorn tree, officially known as *Acacia giraffae*, because in other parts of Africa it is much favoured by those animals. On the shield, Mr Kirby suggested I should display something of myself, something I was proud of. Naturally I thought immediately of the College in Oxford of which I was the founding Master, St Cross College. But a cross by itself would not be interesting or uncommon. What other interests did I have? The answer was easy to find — bacterial toxins, on which I had done research for most of my scientific life. The word 'toxin' is derived from the Greek for arrow poison, *pharmakon toxikon*; *pharmakon* meaning poison, and toxikon relating to bows and arrows (e.g. toxophily). In the course of time, as often happened, the key word was lost in the mists of time; for example, the words 'whisky' and 'vodka' both in fact mean 'water', and are all that remain of 'water of life'. In the same way, *pharmakon* was lost, and toxin came to stand for poison, and particularly for bacterial poisons. So I thought of two arrows crossed, but they looked thin. Then I thought of four arrows crossed parted and fretty two by two, because my modest reputation was based on my work on four bacterial toxins, those of gas gangrene, dysentery, tetanus and cholera. And then I entwined them with a serpent, because arrow poisons were often snake venoms, which are similar in chemical constitution to bacterial toxins, but not nearly so toxic. And the serpent-entwined arrows would remind one of the caduceus, and so the medical connotations of my work would be expressed. A coat of arms should have a motto. I believe that one should never despair. If you are faced by a disaster, you should recover you composure as soon as you can, walk around the ruins of the disaster, and find a way of turning it to your advantage. *Nil desperandum* would have done, but the best heraldic mottoes seemed always to be in incomprehensible mediaeval French, so

I asked my friend Jean Seznec, Marshal Foch Professor of French Literature, to find me such a motto. After several weeks he came up with one — *Fol qui se desconforte,* from the *Le Roman de la Rose* — he's a fool who despairs. (I decided to ignore the other half of this statement, that goes on to say that he is also a fool who rejoices when things go well, in other words, keep your cool.)

The Hutois

As related in the beginning, when my grandfather emigrated from Holland to South Africa, he is said to have garnished his name not only with the name Kits before but also with van Hoei Schildhouder after. He was newly married to Boudina Ketel, the fruit of the elopement of her mother with an inn-keeper called Ketel. I am proud to have Meneer Ketel as a great-grandfather (and we have seen that one of my maternal great-grandfathers was also an inn-keeper), but it was a social come-down for her, for she had been a van Hoei Schildhouder, whose two escutcheons are shown at Fig. 3d. My family have always been proud of this connection, both because of her mother's maiden surname, which was of Hutois origin, and perhaps even more because of her own first name, which is thought to be of high Flemish origin.

It is easy to see that Schildhouder means shield holder, arms bearer, armiger, *écuyer*. I wondered whether this referred to a bearer of arms of or from a place called Hoei in Holland, but I could find no such place. Eventually I found a town in Belgium that had been called Hoei in the days of Dutch rule, but was now called Huy, with the alternative name of Hoei. It is a sizeable town at the confluence of the River Hoyoux with the River Meuse, halfway between Namur and Liège. I wrote to the *Maire* of Huy to ask for a picture of the escutcheon of his town, but it bore no resemblance to either of those of the van Hoei Schildhouders, consisting as it did of a castle with three turrets. I also received a pleasant letter from the *Archives de l'Etat à Huy*, suggesting that the name meant '*de Huy, écuyer*', and continuing: '*. . . je vous signale que la famille en question a été très connu au moyen âge et qu'elle entretenait des rapports commerciaux avec l'Angleterre. Voir à ce sujet l'ouvrage suivant: A.Joris, La Ville de Huy au Moyen Age. 'Des origines à la fin du XIV siècle. 1959''* [17]. [' . . . the family in question was well known in the Middle Ages and maintained commercial relations with England, see Joris.] I looked this up in the Bodleian, as well as another it led me to, Berlière, *Monasticon* *belge* [3]. In the latter part of the Middle Ages the southern lowlands, the ancient territory of the Belgae, was divided, and ruled by different powers. On the west, Flanders was governed from 862 to 1369 by Counts subject to the King of France; in the middle, Brabant was a Duchy of Charlemagne's empire from 959 to 1429, when it descended to Philip II of Burgundy; in the east, Liège, including Huy, was a bishopric under the German empire until 1467, when it was taken by Charles the Bold, Duke of Burgundy. Belgium did not become a unified and independent state until 1831, when it separated from Holland and became a constitutional monarchy, two years before my grandfather was born. The de Huys were concerned with spiritual matters as well as temporal. The earliest mention I can find of them in *Monasticon Belge* concerns Jean de Huy, abbot of Leffe, who signed an agreement between the abbeys of Ninove and Hautmont in 1186; in 1246 the abbot Dolmitien de Huy caused altars to be built to the Holy Cross and to St Dolmitien, and he settled a difference between the abbots of Villers and Averbode; in 1391 Agnès de Huy was an abbot in the Abbey of Moulins. On the temporal side the de Huys were largely concerned with the cloth trade. They were trading cloth in Vienna in 1221, and three of them, Jacques, Nicolas and Colin, are mentioned as being citizens of Vienna at the turn of the 13th and 14th centuries, while their brother Lambert was the abbot of a convent in Scotland. Jacquemin de Huy and others of his ilk were also trading cloth in England, notably Winchelsea and Winchester, between 1327 and 1339. From the middle of the 13th century until the end of the 14th the 'grand' Hutois played an important political role, because the functions of magistrature and mayoralty were their uncontested domain. In this way they kept civil and penal justice, and financial jurisdiction, in their hands. They were important people, and perhaps my ancestors numbered among them.

After our visit to The Netherlands Ruthie and I went to Huy. It is a handsome town, with which I am glad to be connected, if only in a distant way. In Fodor's *Guide to Belgium* it is known as 'Romantic Huy'.

The Flemish?

Since my grandfather married Boudina Ketel, the name Boudina has been given to many of the girls in my family, including my Aunt Boudina Fivaz, who died of typhoid in the dreadful Bloemfontein concentration camp during the Boer War, my sister Boudina Cornelia, who looked after us when our mother died in 1918, and my cousin Boudine van Braam. Now I am a little sorry I did not keep up this tradition with my own dear daughter Joanna, but perhaps neither her mother nor she would have liked it. I wondered how far back the name went, and made enquiries about the van Hoei (or Hoey) Schildhouders (or Schildhouwer, Schilthouder, Schilthouwer; or reversed as variants of Schildhouder van Hoei) in the *Jaarboek 1972* at the Centraal Bureau voor Genealogie in The Hague. There are a number of Boudinas, Boudines, Boudewinas and Boudewijns (the masculine version) scattered about, and the earliest seems to have appeared in 1752, when Johan Schilthouwer van Hoei married Cornelia Boudina Mathia van Oostzee. All the subsequent Boudinas etc. seemed to be derived from this one, and are therefore irrelevant to my present concern, which goes much further back than 1752, indeed to Baldwin (i.e. Boudewijn) IX (1171-1206), Count of Hainault and of Flanders, who took part in the fourth crusade, and was elected First Latin Emperor of Constantinople in 1204. It is the tradition in the family that we are descended from him, but I think perhaps the family has been barking up the wrong family tree, since 1925.

The two escutcheons shown in Fig. 3d are engraved on Boudina Ketel's silver which she brought with her from Holland when she sailed with my grandfather to South Africa in 1858. At the beginning of the Boer War my Aunt Cara buried all the silver, and after the war it was dug up, with some loss, and shared among my father's sisters, not, I understand, without some quarrelling. In April 1984 I saw a piece of this silver when I visited my cousin Margarieta van Rooyen (daughter of Boudina Fivaz) in Johannesburg. I have among my papers a letter (or a copy) dated August 1925 and sent to a relation in South Africa by a genealogist in Ghent in the West Flanders province of Belgium. The letter I have is handwritten on ruled paper without a letter-head; Margarieta has the same letter, roughly typewritten, and also without a letterhead. One is a copy of the other, but we cannot tell which is which — all I will say is that the genealogist seems amateur to me, and I do not trust his information. He states that the escutcheon on the right (and I do not mean dexter) is that of the Belgian family Tulleken. Rietstap's Armorial confirms that it is the Tulleken family — on gold a black fess with two silver ram's heads with golden horns — but it is not a Belgian family. According to the *Nederlands Adelsboek* (Book of Nobles), it is a Dutch family from the province of Gelderland, of which

Arnhem is the main town, where the first sighting of one Wilhelmus Tolleken was made in 1267. The Ghentish genealogist states that the escutcheon on the left is that of the Velse family of Holland, and that of the four quarterings (1 — three fishes naiant the one above the other in the dexter chief position, 2 — an aesculapean staff, 3 — a *Fer-de-moline*, 4 — three bars), the last three belong respectively to the Dutch family Koeneman, the German family Stynen, and an unidentified Danish family. All this is confirmed by Rietstap, but what bothers me is that first quartering of three fishes. The Ghentish genealogist states that this is the escutcheon of 'Messire Robert Tencke, called Marishal, Marshal of the Count' (Louis de Nevers, Count of Flanders). Robert Tencke married one of Louis de Nevers' two natural daughters, Beatrix of Flanders. Louis de Nevers was the son of Robert Bethune, Count of Flanders, who was the son of Guy de Dampierre, Count of Flanders, who was the son of Guy de Dampierre, Duke of Flanders, who married Marguerite (Zwart Magriet, Black Margaret), Countess of Flanders and of Hainaut, second daughter of the aforementioned Baldwin IX, First Latin Emperor of Constantinople. Robert Tencke of the three fishes had three daughters, two of whom were married to members of the de Masmines family, and one or the other of these is said by the Ghentish genealogist to be connected (in a way he does not define) with the Velse family. My search for the escutcheon of Robert Tencke, and of de Masmines, in the well-provided Duke Humphrey's Library of the Bodleian Library was quite fruitless, so I am unable to confirm that Tencke's escutcheon has three fishes. And even if I could, it would not mean much. Heraldry is notorious for being a rotten guide to ancestry, and this is exemplified by the fact that three little fishes, the one above the other, naiant from east to west, are far from uncommon — they could belong to anybody. One of the handbooks on heraldry I looked up in Duke Humphrey's Library had about fifty pages devoted to fish alone, and amongst the thirty or so escutcheons containing three fishes naiant the one above the other, none was ascribed to Tencke or de Masmines.

I don't know whether the idea of our being derived from the Emperor of Constantinople goes back any further than 1925, when the Ghentish genealogist wrote his letter. In this letter he stated that the de Masmines family once occupied the Château of Laarne, about 8 miles east of Ghent, and that may be the reason why my Uncle Pieter and my Aunt Ada van Braam took my sister Christina to see that Château in 1933. Christina once told me she thought that the van Hoei Schildhouder arms were to be seen there. After our visit to Huy, Ruthie and I went to visit this Château of Laarne, and a very fine moated château it is. I wish I could claim it for my family, but I doubt if I can. It certainly was once occupied by the de Masmines, but we could see no van Hoei Schildhouder arms. There just may have been: over the entrance there is a large block of stone showing obvious evidence of something having been chopped off it, I should think almost certainly a coat of arms, but whose? I doubt if it was that of the van Hoei Schildhouders. I think it was all a lot of Hoei. (When I was editing this appendix, I happened to check my name in the new Oxford and district telephone directory. There, directly following my name was a new name — a Mr Van Hoey Smith. I telephoned him and asked: 'Are you descended from Baldwin IX, Emperor of Constantinople?' He said no, the Van Hoey's were descended from robber barons in Northern Island. That's when I gave up.)

The English

My maternal great-grandfather, Charles Higgs, was born in England, in Kent, in 1815. We know that he was in Cape Town in 1837, but we are not clear about when he arrived in the Cape. There are those of my Higgs relations who say he arrived as a young man of 22 in 1837, and this would not be inconsistent with the entries in the Births, Deaths and Marriages section in the middle of the huge Higgs family Bible that used to be kept by my beloved Uncle Willie Higgs at Boomplaats. In this register Charles' name is the first to be recorded, and he is also labelled as the 'founder of the Higgs family in South Africa' at the head of the Higgs family tree that was drawn up by my cousin Alan Higgs. This family Bible is now kept by Alan on his farm near Tweespruit in the Orange Free State, and on our visit there in 1984, I saw that Bible myself and could see no sign of an earlier Higgs. But my elder brother Kits was with us, and he swears that when the Bible was kept at Boomplaats, there were written on a blank front page (well away from the Births, Deaths and Marriages section in the middle) words to the effect that Charles *and two other Higgses* arrived in Cape Town in 1820 (nothing to do with the 1820 Settlers, who landed much further east in Algoa Bay). Unfortunately that page is now missing, but my brother Kits is never wrong, so I must conclude that Charles Higgs arrived in Cape Town in 1820, and since he was aged 5 at the time, he was presumably accompanied by the two relations referred to by Kits. Inez Heunis, daughter of my cousin Jack Higgs, and well-informed about the Higgs family, has told me we are descended from a farmer in Kent who died leaving three sons. The oldest inherited the farm, and the other two emigrated to South Africa, one of these possibly being a doctor, and perhaps the other was the father of Charles Higgs. But why was he only on the lost front page, and not in the formal Births, Deaths and Marriages section of the family Bible at Boomplaats? All my efforts to take this matter any further in South Africa failed. I have been in touch with the Kent Archives Office in Maidstone, but their reply was: 'It is virtually impossible to trace a person, except members of well-known families, unless you can narrow your search down to one, or at least a very small number of, parishes in Kent'. That I am unable to do, so I must give up the search, which grieves me.

REFERENCES

1. Abraham, E., *Ernst Boris Chain*. Biograph. Mem. Fell. Roy. Soc. 28, 43, 1983.
2. Belfield, E., *The Boer War*. London: Leo Cooper, 1975.
2a. Bell, E., *The Anatomy and Philosophy of Expression*, 2nd Edition, 1834.
3. Berlière, *Monasticon belge, tome I, Province de Namur et de Hainault; tome II, Province de Liège*. Liège: Centre National de Recherches d'Histoire Religeuse, 1890.
4. *Biographie Nationale publiée par l'Academie Royal des Sciences, des Lettres et des Beaux-Arts de Belgique*. 1–28. Bruxelles: Thiry-van Bruggenhout, 1866-1976.
5. *Biographie du Royaume des Pays-Bas, Ancienne et Moderne*. Liège, Desoer, 1828.
6. *Biographisch Woordenboek de Nederlanden*, 1867.
7. Caesar, Julius, *Gallic Wars*, Book V, Ch. XXIII.
8. Calvert, A.E., *South-West Africa* (1884-1914). London: T. Werner Laurie, 1915.
9. Conan Doyle, A., *The Great Boer War* (8th Impression), p. 356. London: Smith, Elder & Co., 1900.
10. Delvenne père, *Biographie du Royaume des Pays-Bas, Ancienne et Moderne*. Liège: Desoer, 1928.
11. de Renesse, *Dictionnaire des Figures Héraldiques*, p.199 Poissons. Bruxelles: Société Belge de Librarie, 1892.
12. *Dictionary of South African Biography*. Van Heyningen, Petrus (Pieter) Arnoldus (Adriaan) Conradus (Coenraad), I, 827. Cape Town: Nasionale Boekhandel, 1968.
13. Ellenberger, D.F. and MacGregor, J.C., *The History of the Basuto. Ancient and Modern*. London: Caxton Publishing Company, 1912.
14. Farwell, B. *The Great Boer War*. London: Allen Lane, 1977.
15. *Grand Armorial de France*. Société de Grand Armorial de France Editeurs, 1939.
16. Hobhouse, Christopher, *Oxford. As it was and as it is today*. London: Batsford, 1939.
17. Joris, A., *La Ville de Huy au Moyen Age. Des origines à la fin du XIVe siècle*. Paris: Société d'Edition 'Les Belles Lettres', 1959.
18. Marquard, Leo, *The Story of South Africa*. London: Faber and Faber: Ltd, 1955.
19. Maurois, André, *La Vie de Sir Alexander Fleming*. Paris: Librairie Hachette, 1959.

20. Michener, J.A., *The Covenant*. New York: Fawcett Crest Books, 1980.
21. Macfarlane, Gwyn, *Howard Florey. The Making of a Great Scientist*. Oxford: Oxford University Press, 1979.
22. Macfarlane, Gwyn, *Alexander Fleming. The Man and the Myth*. London: Chatto and Windus, The Hogarth Press, 1984.
23. *Nieuw Nederlandsch Biografisch Woordenboek*. Leiden: A.W.Sijthkoff's Uitgewersmaatschappy, 1914.
24. Pakenham, Thomas, *The Boer War*. London: Weidenfeld and Nicolson, 1979.
25. Papacostas, G. and Gaté, J., *Les Associations Microbiennes*. Paris: Doin et Cie, 1928.
26. Philip, I. *The Bodleian Library in the Seventeenth and Eighteenth Centuries*. Oxford: Clarendon Press, 1983.
27. Pirie, A. and van Heyningen, R.E., *The Biochemistry of the Eye*. Oxford: Blackwell Scientific Publications, 1956.
28. *Planches de l'Armorial Général* (de J.-B. Rietstap par V. Rolland). Paris: Institut Héraldique, 1909.
29. Sitwell, S., *The Netherlands*. London: Batsford, 1974.
30. Snow, C.P., *Corridors of Power*. London: Macmillan, 1964.
31. Snow, C.P., *Corridors of Power*. Harmondsworth: Penguin Books, 1966.
32. *Standard Encyclopaedia of Southern Africa*, 2, 516-324, 1970.
33. Steel, T., *The Life and Death of St Kilda*. London: Collins, 1975.
34. van Heyningen, Caroline (Mrs C. Hill), *Orange Days. Memoirs of Eighty Years Ago in the Old Orange Free State*. Pietermaritzburg: University of Natal Press, 1965.
35. van Heyningen, Ruth, *Sugar Alcohols — Galactose and Diabetic Cataracts in The Eye and Inborn Errors of Metabolism*, New York: Alan R. Liss Inc. 1976, pp. 295-303.
36. van Heyningen, W.E., *Stable Isotope as Indicators in Biology*. Biol. Rev. 14, 420, 1939.
37. van Heyningen, W.E., *Bacterial Toxins*. Oxford: Blackwell Scientific Publications, 1950.
38. van Heyningen, W.E. and Mellanby, J., 'Tetanus Toxin', in Microbial Toxins. New York: Academic Press, Vol. 2A, p.69.
39. van Heyningen, W.E. and Seal, J.R., *Cholera: The American Scientific Experience, 1947-1980*. Boulder: Colorado, The Westview Press.

INDEX